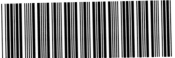

369 0246796

OXFORD MEDICAL PUBLICATIONS

Emergencies in Gastroenterology and Hepatology

KU-875-865

Published and forthcoming titles in the Emergencies in... series:

Emergencies in Adult Nursing
Edited by Philip Downing

Emergencies in Anaesthesia
Edited by Keith Allman, Andrew McIndoe, and Iain H. Wilson

Emergencies in Cardiology
Edited by Saul G. Myerson, Robin P. Choudhury, and Andrew Mitchell

Emergencies in Children's and Young People's Nursing
Edited by E.A. Glasper, Gill McEwing, and Jim Richardson

Emergencies in Clinical Surgery
Edited by Chris Callaghan, Chris Watson and Andrew Bradley

Emergencies in Critical Care, 2e
Edited by Martin Beed, Richard Sherman, and Ravi Mahajan

Emergencies in Gastroenterology and Hepatology
Marcus Harbord and Daniel Marks

Emergencies in Mental Health Nursing
Edited by Patrick Callaghan

Emergencies in Obstetrics and Gynaecology
Edited by S. Arulkumaran

Emergencies in Oncology
Edited by Martin Scott-Brown, Roy A.J. Spence, and Patrick G. Johnston

Emergencies in Paediatrics and Neonatology, 2e
Edited by Stuart Crisp and Jo Rainbow

Emergencies in Palliative and Supportive Care
Edited by David Currow and Katherine Clark

Emergencies in Primary Care
Chantal Simon, Karen O'Reilly, John Buckmaster, and Robin Proctor

Emergencies in Psychiatry, 2e
Basant Puri and Ian Treasaden

Emergencies in Radiology
Edited by Richard Graham and Ferdia Gallagher

Emergencies in Respiratory Medicine
Edited by Robert Parker, Catherine Thomas, and Lesley Bennett

Emergencies in Sports Medicine
Edited by Julian Redhead and Jonathan Gordon

Head, Neck and Dental Emergencies
Edited by Mike Perry

Medical Emergencies in Dentistry
Nigel Robb and Jason Leitch

Emergencies in Gastroenterology and Hepatology

Daniel Marks
BSc MB PhD MRCP
Wellcome Trust Postdoctoral Fellow
University College London Hospital

Marcus Harbord
BSc MB PhD FRCP
Consultant Gastroenterologist
Chelsea and Westminster Hospital, London

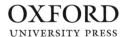

OXFORD
UNIVERSITY PRESS

OXFORD
UNIVERSITY PRESS

Great Clarendon Street, Oxford, OX2 6DP,
United Kingdom

Oxford University Press is a department of the University of Oxford.
It furthers the University's objective of excellence in research, scholarship,
and education by publishing worldwide. Oxford is a registered trade mark of
Oxford University Press in the UK and in certain other countries

© Oxford University Press 2013

The moral rights of the authors have been asserted

First edition published in 2013

Impression: 1

British Library Cataloguing in Publication Data

Data available

ISBN 978-0-19-923136-2

Special trade edition ISBN 978-0-19-968773-2

Printed in China by
C&C Offset Printing Co. Ltd.

Foreword

I am delighted to write a Foreword for this excellent practical book written by two young gastroenterologists. Each chapter is headed by a symptom or condition, and the reader is then led quickly into clear and up-to-date advice on managing them, without expanding into aetiology. I was particularly pleased to see useful advice on difficult-to-manage symptoms, such as nausea and vomiting and thoracic pain, and the inclusion of nutritional treatment. The chapter on HIV disease will be especially useful to the average gastroenterologist or general physician faced with the myriad of potential complications of this disease and side effects of treatment.

The authors are to be congratulated. I predict this will be a handy reference book (in the hand or on a screen), for all grades of doctors faced with these common problems.

Sir Richard Thompson
President
Royal College of Physicians
London, UK
January 2013

Foreword

Preface

This book focuses on managing the sick gastroenterology and hepatology patient, providing a point of rapid reference for use at the bedside. We make no apologies for covering a wide range of problems, as what may seem mundane to the visiting physician can be an emergency for the patient. Throughout, we have focused on giving practical advice, trying to answer the sorts of questions we have both faced over the years, as well as addressing emergency topics that are minimally covered or absent in other texts. This book provides contemporary guidance for doctors training in gastroenterology and hepatology, their seniors, and other team members responsible for the assessment and care of the acute medical patient. It complements the *Oxford Handbook of Gastroenterology and Hepatology* that one of us co-authored. We are grateful to its other co-authors Stuart Bloom and George Webster for their advice and friendship over many years.

On a personal note, we would also like to thank the following experts, who have peer-reviewed many of the chapters or provided some of the images: Mike Anderson, Martyn Caplin, Tom Doherty, Matthew Foxton, Brian Gazzard CBE, John Karani, Aamir Khan, Nas Khan, Rob Miller, Iain Murray–Lyon, David Nott OBE, James O'Beirne, Alastair O'Brien, David Patch, and Stephen Wright. We are particularly grateful to Kevin Moore, editor of the *Oxford Handbook of Acute Medicine*, who was instrumental in this book's early stages and who has contributed some new content. We also thank our families for their support, and OUP for its patience. Finally, we thank you, the reader, without whom the written word has no purpose. We invite you to contact us with any suggestions to improve the text.

Daniel Marks, BSc MB PhD MRCP
University College London Hospital
d.marks@ucl.ac.uk

Marcus Harbord, BSc MB PhD FRCP
Chelsea and Westminster Hospital
marcus.harbord@chelwest.nhs.uk

Contents

Contents

Symbols and abbreviations

~	approximately
≈	approximately equal to
+	plus
%	percentage
&	and
>	more than
<	less than
°C	degrees Celsius
📖	cross-reference
↑	increasing
↓	decreasing
®	registered trademark
α	alpha
β	beta
δ	delta
γ	gamma
μ	mu
A1AT	alpha1-antitrypsin
Ab	antibody
ABG	arterial blood gases
ACD	anaemia of chronic disease
ACE	angiotensin-converting enzyme
ACTH	adrenocorticotropic hormone
ADH	anti-diuretic hormone
A & E	Accident and Emergency department
AF	atrial fibrillation
α-FP	alpha-fetoprotein
AIDS	acquired immunodeficiency syndrome
ALD	alcoholic liver disease
ALF	acute liver failure
ALP	alkaline phosphatase
ALT	alanine aminotransferase
AMA	anti-mitochondrial antibodies
ANA	anti-nuclear antibodies

APC	argon plasma coagulation
APTT	activated partial thromboplastin time
ARDS	acute respiratory distress syndrome
ASA	aminosalicylic acid; American Society of Anesthesiologists
AST	aspartate aminotransferase
ATLS	Advanced Trauma and Life Support
AXR	abdominal X-ray
bd	*bis die* (twice daily)
BHIVA	British HIV Association
BMI	body mass index
BNF	British National Formulary
cal	calorie
cAMP	cyclic adenosine monophosphate
CAP	cellulose acetate precipitation
CBD	common bile duct
CCF	congestive cardiac failure
CD	Crohn's disease
CDAD	*Clostridium difficile*-associated diarrhoea
CDAI	Crohn's disease activity index
CDT	*Clostridium difficile* toxin
CEA	carcinoembryonic antigen
cfu	colony-forming unit
CK	creatine kinase
Cl$^-$	chloride ion
cm	centimetre
cmH$_2$O	centimetre water
CMV	cytomegalovirus
CNS	central nervous system
CO$_2$	carbon dioxide
COPD	chronic obstructive pulmonary disease
COX	cyclo-oxygenase
CRP	C-reactive protein
CSM	Committee on the Safety of Medicines
CT	computed tomography
CVP	central venous pressure
CVVHF	continuous veno-venous haemofiltration
d	day
DAT	direct antiglobulin test
DI	discriminant index
DIC	disseminated intravascular coagulation

DILI	drug-induced liver injury
dL	decilitre
DNA	deoxyribonucleic acid
DPA	diagnostic peritoneal aspiration
DVT	deep vein thrombosis
EASL	European Association for the Study of the Liver
EBV	Epstein–Barr virus
ECG	electrocardiogram
EDNOS	eating disorder not otherwise specified
EDTA	ethylenediaminetetraacetic acid
EEG	electroencephalography
e.g.	*exempli gratia* (for example)
eGFR	estimated glomerular filtration rate
EHEC	enterohaemorrhagic *E. coli*
EIEC	enteroinvasive *E. coli*
ELISA	enzyme-linked immunosorbent assay
EMG	electromyography
EPEC	enteropathogenic
ERCP	endoscopic retrograde cholangiopancreatography
ESR	erythrocyte sedimentation rate
ET	endotracheal tube
ETEC	enterotoxigenic *E. coli*
ETT	exercise tolerance test; endotracheal tube
EUA	examination under anaesthesia
EUS	endoscopic ultrasound
FAST	focused assessment with sonography for trauma (scan)
FBC	full blood count
FDG	^{18}F-fluorodeoxyglucose
FFP	fresh frozen plasma
FiO$_2$	fraction of inspired oxygen
fL	femtolitre
FNA	fine needle aspiration
FSH	follicle-stimulating hormone
g	gram
G	Gauge
GAHS	Glasgow alcoholic hepatitis score
GCS	Glasgow coma score
G-CSF	granulocyte colony-stimulating factor
GFR	glomerular filtration rate
γGT	gamma-glutamyl transpeptidase

GI	gastrointestinal
GIST	gastrointestinal stromal tumour
G & S	group and save
GTN	glyceryl trinitrate
Gy	gray
h	hour
HAART	highly active anti-retroviral treatment
HAS	human albumin solution
HAV	hepatitis A virus
Hb	haemoglobin
HBIg	hepatitis B immunoglobulin
HBV	hepatitis B virus
HCC	hepatocellular carcinoma
HCG	human chorionic gonadotrophin
HCl	hydrochloric acid
HCO_3	bicarbonate
Hct	haematocrit
HCV	hepatitis C virus
HDL	high-density lipoprotein
HDU	high dependency unit
HDV	hepatitis D virus
HELLP	haemolysis, elevated liver enzymes, and low platelets
HEV	hepatitis E virus
HHV-8	human herpesvirus-8
HIAA	hydroxyindoleacetic acid
HIDA	hepatobiliary iminodiacetic acid
HIV	human immunodeficiency virus
HLA	human leukocyte antigen
HMG-CoA	3-hydroxy-3-methylglutaryl-coenzyme A
HPS	hepatopulmonary syndrome
HPV	human papilloma virus
HR	heart rate
HRS	hepatorenal syndrome
HRT	hormone replacement therapy
HSV	herpes simplex virus
5-HT	5-hydroxytryptamine
HTLV	human T-lymphotropic virus
HTN	hypertension
HUS	haemolytic uraemic syndrome
HVA	homovanillic acid

Hx	history
IBD	inflammatory bowel disease
ICP	intracranial pressure
IDA	iron deficiency anaemia
i.e.	*id est* (that is)
IFAT	immunofluorescence antibody testing
IFN	interferon
Ig	immunoglobulin
IGF	insulin-like growth factor
IM	intramuscular
IMA	inferior mesenteric artery
INR	international normalized ratio
IPAA	ileal pouch anal anastomosis
IRIS	immune reconstitution inflammatory syndrome
ITU	intensive therapy unit
IU	international unit
IV	intravenous
IVC	inferior vena cava
IVDU	intravenous drug user
Ix	investigation
J	Joule
JET	jejunal extension tube
JVP	jugular venous pressure
K^+	potassium ion
kcal	kilocalorie
KCl	potassium chloride
kg	kilogram
$KHCO_3$	potassium bicarbonate
kPa	kilopascal
KUB	kidneys, ureters, bladder
L	litre
LBO	large bowel obstruction
LCHAD	long-chain 3-hydroxyacyl-CoA dehydrogenase
LDH	lactate dehydrogenase
LFT	liver function tests
LH	luteinizing hormone
LMWH	low molecular weight heparin
LUQ	left upper quadrant
m	metre
MAHA	microangiopathic haemolytic anaemia

MAP	mean arterial pressure
MARSIPAN	management of really sick patients with anorexia nervosa
M, C, & S	microscopy, culture, and sensitivities
MCV	mean corpuscular volume
MELD	model for end-stage liver disease
MEN	multiple endocrine neoplasia
mEq	milliequivalent
µg	microgram
mg	milligram
Mg^{++}	magnesium ion
$MgSO_4$	magnesium sulphate
MI	myocardial infarction
MIBG	metaiodobenzylguanidine
min	minute
mL	millilitre
mm	millimetre
mmHg	millimetre mercury
mmol	millimole
µmol	micromole
mo	month
mOsm	milliosmole
MR	magnetic resonance
MRA	magnetic resonance angiography
MRCP	magnetic resonance cholangiopancreatography
MRI	magnetic resonance imaging
MRSA	meticillin-resistant *Staphylococcus aureus*
MRV	magnetic resonance venography
MSM	men who have sex with men
mSv	millisievert
mTOR	mammalian target of rapamycin
MU	million units
MUST	malnutrition universal screening tool
Na^+	sodium ion
NAC	*N*-acetylcysteine
NaCl	sodium chloride
NAFLD	non-alcoholic fatty liver disease
$NaHCO_3$	sodium bicarbonate
NAPQI	*N*-acetyl-*p*-benzoquinoneimine
NASH	non-alcoholic steatohepatitis

NASPGHAN	North American Society for Pediatric Gastroenterology, Hepatology and Nutrition
NBM	nil by mouth
NEB	via nebulizer
NET	neuroendocrine tumour
ng	nanogram
NG	nasogastric
NGT	nasogastric tube
NH_3	ammonia
NH_4^+	ammonium ion
NICE	National Institute for Health and Clinical Excellence
NJ	nasojejunal
NOMI	non-occlusive mesenteric ischaemia
NSAID	non-steroidal anti-inflammatory drug
O_2	oxygen
OCP	oral contraceptive pill
od	*omni die* (once daily)
OGD	oesophagogastroduodenoscopy
OP	outpatient
ORS	oral rehydration solution
PAIR	percutaneous aspiration, injection, and re-aspiration
PAN	polyarteritis nodosa
$PaCO_2$	partial pressure of carbon dioxide
PaO_2	partial pressure of oxygen
PCP	*Pneumocystis jirovecii* pneumonia
PCR	polymerase chain reaction
PCV	packed cell volume
PE	pulmonary embolism
PEG	percutaneous endoscopic gastrotomy
PEJ	percutaneous endoscopic jejunostomy
PEP	post-exposure prophylaxis
PET	positron emission tomography; pre-eclampsia toxaemia
pg	picogram
PMN	polymorphonuclear cells
PN	parenteral nutrition
PO	*per os* (by mouth)
PO_4^{3-}	phosphate ion
PPI	proton pump inhibitor
PR	per rectum
PRN	*pro re nata* (as needed)

PSA	prostate-specific antigen
PSC	primary sclerosing cholangitis
PTC	percutaneous transhepatic cholangiography
PTLD	post-transplant lymphoproliferative disease
PTT	prothrombin time
PUO	pyrexia of unknown origin
qds	*quater die sumendus* (four times daily)
RBC	red blood cell
RDW	red cell distribution width
RFA	radiofrequency ablation
RIF	right iliac fossa
RPF	retroperitoneal fibrosis
RNA	ribonucleic acid
RR	respiratory rate
RUQ	right upper quadrant
Rx	treatment
s	second
SAAG	serum-ascitic albumin gradient
SaO_2	oxygen saturation
SBP	spontaneous bacterial peritonitis
SBO	small bowel obstruction
SC	subcutaneous
SCC	squamous cell carcinoma
SIRS	systemic inflammatory response syndrome
SLE	systemic lupus erythematosus
SMA	superior mesenteric artery
SMV	superior mesenteric vein
SNRI	serotonin-noradrenaline reuptake inhibitor
SRUS	solitary rectal ulcer syndrome
SSRI	selective serotonin reuptake inhibitor
SVC	superior vena cava
T3	triiodothyronine
TACE	trans-arterial chemoembolization
TB	tuberculosis
tds	*ter die sumendum* (three times daily)
TFT	thyroid function tests
TIBC	total iron binding capacity
TIPS	transjugular intrahepatic portosystemic shunting
TNF	tumour necrosis factor
tPA	tissue plasminogen activator

TPMT	thiopurine methyltransferase
TPN	total parenteral nutrition
TTG	tissue transglutaminase
TTP	thrombotic thrombocytopaenic purpura
U	unit
UC	ulcerative colitis
UDCA	ursodeoxycholic acid
U & E	urea and electrolytes
UK	United Kingdom
ULN	upper limit of normal
USA	United States of America
US	ultrasound
UTI	urinary tract infection
VBG	venous blood gases
VIP	vasointestinal peptide
VMA	vanillylmandelic acid
V/Q	ventilation/perfusion
vs	versus
VZV	varicella zoster virus
W	Watt
WCC	white cell count
WDP	Wilson's disease protein
WHO	World Health Organization
wk	week

Acute upper gastrointestinal bleeding

☼ / ☼ Presentation

- *Haematemesis*. Vomiting fresh blood or 'coffee grounds'; 29% of patients with coffee grounds in nasogastric aspirate have a significant high-risk lesion at endoscopy.
- *Melaena*. Black, sticky, smelly stool. This occurs following bleeding proximal to the transverse colon. Blood is cathartic, with melaena usually appearing 4–6h following a GI bleed, continuing for up to 2d after its cessation. Other causes of dark stool include iron therapy, bismuth (present in De-Noltab®), liquorice, or drinks such as Guinness and red wine.
- *Fresh rectal bleeding*. 11% of massive upper GI bleeds present in this way (Jensen and Machicado, 1988).
- *Shock*. Weakness, sweating, palpitations, postural dizziness, syncope.

Causes

- Peptic ulcer (35–50%).
- Mallory–Weiss tear (5–15%).
- Gastroduodenal erosions (8–15%).
- Oesophagitis (5–15%).
- Gastro-oesophageal varices (7–10%).
- Vascular malformations (5%):
  - Hereditary haemorrhagic telangiectasia.
  - Gastric antral vascular ectasia (GAVE).
  - Portal hypertensive gastropathy.
  - Angiodysplasia.
  - Dieulafoy lesion.
- Rare miscellaneous causes (5%):
  - Hiatus hernia.
  - Crohn's disease.
  - Aorto-enteric fistula.
  - TB.
  - Herpesviridae (HSV, CMV).
- Upper GI malignancy (1%).

Initial management

Upper GI bleeding has an overall mortality of 11–14%. Priorities are to:
- Stabilize the patient: protect the airway, restore circulating volume.
- Assess severity.
- Identify source of bleeding.
- Stop the bleeding.

Stabilize the patient

- *Protect the airway.* Position patient on left side if actively vomiting.
- *Rapidly assess circulatory status.* Feel temperature of hands and feet. Does the patient look unwell? Is there pallor or sweating? Measure BP (including postural drop: significant if >20mmHg drop in systolic pressure on standing) and HR.
- *IV access.* Insert two large IV cannulae (e.g. 14–16G). Jugular, subclavian, or femoral vein cannulation may be necessary to assess CVP or if peripheral access limited. If the patient is shocked (systolic BP <100mmHg, HR >100/min) or has other signs of hypovolaemia (such as pallor, sweating, cold peripheries, weak pulse, or postural hypotension), infuse 1L of 0.9% saline or 500mL colloid (e.g. Gelofusine®) 'stat'.

Blood tests

Request FBC, U & E, LFT, calcium and PO_4^{3-}, Mg^{++}, glucose, and clotting. Cross-match 4–8U if patient shocked on admission. 'G & S' serum only if patient is stable and history suggests only 'coffee ground' vomiting. Measure ABG in severely ill patients.
- Hb and PCV do not fall till the plasma volume has been restored, but if low at presentation suggest massive blood loss or acute-on-chronic bleeding.
- WCC may be elevated but usually is $<15 \times 10^9$/L. If elevated, look for evidence of sepsis, which can predispose to haemorrhage.
- Low platelet count may suggest hypersplenism and chronic liver disease. Other causes of thrombocytopaenia may predispose to GI bleeding.
- An elevated plasma urea out of proportion to plasma creatinine indicates renal hypoperfusion or the absorption of blood proteins from the gut. It signifies a significant GI bleed or dehydration. A ratio of (urea (mmol/L) x 100) divided by creatinine (μmol/L) of >7.0 indicates that the urea is disproportionately high.
- If there is massive haemorrhage, ask for 'O'-negative blood, which may be given without cross-matching. Avoid doing this unless absolutely necessary, and remember to save serum for retrospective cross-matching. 'O'-positive blood can also be used if necessary in men or post-menopausal women. Activate 'major haemorrhage protocol' (see Appendix, 📖 pp. 360–1).

History and examination

A brief history will probably already be available, but ask specifically about: use of NSAIDs anti-platelet drugs and anticoagulants; symptoms suggestive of peptic ulcer disease; a history of alcohol abuse or liver disease; previous GI bleeds, ulcers or surgery; and whether bleeding was spontaneous or followed retching and vomiting (occurs in 40% of Mallory–Weiss tears or variceal bleeds). Examine for stigmata of chronic liver disease (such as jaundice, spider naevi, hepatosplenomegaly, or ascites), which may suggest the bleed is variceal. Rectal examination may reveal melaena or semi-fresh blood.

Restore circulating volume

Tachycardia, hypotension, or postural hypotension suggest low intravascular volume. Initially, give 1–2L of crystalloid (0.9% saline or Hartmann's solution) or 500mL–1L of colloid (e.g. Haemaccel® or Gelofusine®) 'stat'. If there are no signs of hypovolaemia, use a slower rate of infusion. Continue infusing crystalloid/colloid to normalize the BP until blood is available (as of yet there are no definitive trials proving superiority of one fluid type over another). Try to maintain the systolic BP >100mmHg. There are no hard rules about the rate of IV infusion. In general, if the patient is >70–75y or has a history of heart failure, use a slower rate of infusion so as to avoid precipitating pulmonary oedema, but this has to be gauged against the degree of hypotension. Assess, infuse, and reassess again until you have a stable patient.

CVP monitoring is primarily used to prevent overfilling. It should be considered in the elderly, those with chronic liver disease or a history of heart failure, following resuscitation after a large bleed. Do not waste time doing this initially since it is easier to place a central line once the patient has been resuscitated. A rapid drop in CVP (fall >5cmH$_2$O) may indicate re-bleeding, although this may also occur in patients with chronic liver disease due to abnormal venous compliance.

Blood transfusion

Blood transfusion is indicated in moderate or massive, but not minor, haemorrhage (e.g. Hb >10g/dL after fluid resuscitation). Give blood at 1 unit/h until the circulating volume is restored or the CVP is between 5–10cm as measured from the mid-axilla with the patient supine. O-negative blood can be transfused immediately in massive bleeds. Serum calcium may fall after several units of citrate-containing blood. Give 10mL (4.5mEq) of 10% calcium gluconate for every 3–4U transfused. Supplement magnesium and phosphate as necessary (often low in alcoholics).

Monitor vital signs

Measure BP (aim systolic >100mmHg) and HR (aim <100/min) every 15min initially and then less frequently as the patient is stabilized. Although it is often not necessary to catheterize patients, monitor urine output (aim for >30mL/h), and insert a urinary catheter if low. Oliguria may indicate inadequate fluid resuscitation. Watch for fluid overload (raised JVP or CVP, pulmonary oedema). Rapid transfusion may precipitate pulmonary oedema, even before the total lost volume has been replaced. Consider elective intubation in obtunded patients who cannot protect their airway.

Keep patient nil-by-mouth

Inform the nursing staff to keep the patient nil-by-mouth for endoscopy. Inform the surgical team about the patient, especially if they remain unstable following endoscopy. If the patient is suffering a life-threatening bleed, make sure they are admitted to ITU/HDU or a Level 1 ward. Often, such patients are best managed by both medical and surgical teams. If in doubt, seek advice from the senior gastroenterologist/GI surgeon on-call.

Commence intravenous PPI

Patients with a significant GI bleed should be treated with high-dose IV PPI. Generally, 80mg IV omeprazole or pantoprazole is advocated, followed by an infusion at 8mg/h for 72h. This regimen has been shown to reduce re-bleed rates in patients with high-risk lesions (active bleeding, visible vessel, adherent blood clot) (Lau *et al.*, 2000). Alternatively, 20mg IV omeprazole od for 3d has been suggested to be as effective as high-dose omeprazole infusion (Udd *et al.*, 2001).

It is sensible to start PPI therapy at presentation in those with major bleeding, which has been shown to down-stage bleeding lesions, reducing the need for endoscopic therapy (Lau *et al.*, 2007). In the UK, pantoprazole 40mg bd IV is often given for less critical bleeds. This can be converted to an oral PPI (e.g. omeprazole 20mg bd) after 24–48h.

Imaging

CT scan (Mark *et al.*, 1985) should be carried out in all patients with a Dacron aortic graft unless immediate surgical intervention is required. Patients with confirmed aortoenteric fistulae require immediate stabilization followed by surgery, with about a 50% chance of long-term survival.

Suspected variceal bleeding

Until a patient has an endoscopy, you do not know whether bleeding is variceal. However, you should assume that bleeding is variceal in any patient with signs or a history of portal hypertension. Oesophageal (see Colour plate 1) and gastric varices develop in patients with portal hypertension, regardless of its aetiology. Bleeding from varices is typically vigorous and difficult to control. It often occurs in the context of abnormal clotting, thrombocytopaenia, and bacterial infections. A history, or clinical stigmata of chronic liver disease or portal vein thrombosis on examination, makes it more likely that there is a variceal source of bleeding.

☼ If the patient is stable and not actively bleeding

- Upper GI endoscopy should be arranged as soon as possible. It is inadvisable to delay endoscopy too long since variceal bleeding can be high-volume and a stable patient can rapidly become unstable. The incidence of re-bleeding is high.
- Provide metoclopramide 10mg IV or erythromycin 250mg IV, between 20min and 2h before endoscopy, to help clear the stomach of blood.
- When undertaking resuscitation with blood products and fluids, avoid over-transfusion, as this may increase portal pressure and risk of re-bleeding (aim for CVP of $5cmH_2O$ and Hb ~10g/dL).

- Give vitamin K 10mg IV once only since many patients will have a prolonged PTT, and it is important to correct any underlying vitamin K deficiency.
- Studies have shown that variceal bleeding is associated with bacterial infections (Bernard *et al.*, 1999). Take blood, urine, and (if present) ascitic fluid for culture (transport in blood culture bottles) and microscopy.
- Start broad-spectrum IV antibiotics: a third generation cephalosporin (e.g. ceftriaxone 1g IV od) or ciprofloxacin 400mg IV stat followed by 500mg bd PO plus amoxicillin 500mg tds PO. Treat for 5d.
- If the patient has bled within the last 24h, start terlipressin (glypressin) (2mg IV initially, and then 1mg IV every 4h for up to 72h). This causes splanchnic vasoconstriction, diverting blood from the bleeding lesion, and reduces relative mortality by ~34%. Serious side effects occur in 4%, including cardiac ischaemia and peripheral vasoconstriction, which may produce significant hypertension, and skin and splanchnic ischaemia. If the history suggests that their last episode of bleeding was >24h ago and they remain stable, it is probably safe to delay giving terlipressin until endoscopy has been performed, provided it will be carried out within the next 12h.
- Use of somatostatin or octreotide? Somatostatin (250µg bolus followed by 250µg/h IV for 5d) reduces bleeding compared to placebo. A Cochrane review (Gøtzsche and Hróbjartsson, 2005) found that octreotide had no effect on mortality and a minimal effect on transfusion requirements. Many liver centres do not use octreotide since terlipressin is associated with a reduction in mortality compared to placebo.
- Give lactulose 10–15mL PO tds to prevent encephalopathy. Use magnesium or phosphate enemas for patients with severe encephalopathy.
- If the patient is alcoholic or malnourished, start Pabrinex® 1 & 2 IV tds for 3–5d and supplement with oral thiamine 200mg PO od.

If the patient is unstable or appears to be actively bleeding

The most important part of management of these patients is *airway protection, airway protection, and airway protection*. Emergency endoscopy must occur as soon as the patient is stabilized, with anaesthetic assistance. Some gastroenterologists recommend bolus injection of metoclopramide 20mg IV, which transiently increases lower oesophageal pressure and decreases azygous blood flow, although many do not use this simple approach. The remainder of the care, detailed in 'If the patient is stable and not actively bleeding' (see p. 5), should also be provided.

Correcting coagulopathy

Risk of reversing anticoagulation should always be weighed against the risk of continued bleeding without reversal. In general, active bleeding is more life-threatening than any of the conditions whose risk is enhanced by reversal of anticoagulation.

- Annual risk of embolization in non-anticoagulated patients with prosthetic heart valves is 4% for aortic and 8% for mitral valves overall (Cannegieter *et al.*, 1994). The risk is greater with caged-ball valves, especially of the Starr–Edwards type. Routine use of antibiotics in patients with prosthetic valves undergoing endoscopy is no longer recommended unless there is a previous history of endocarditis.
- Overall annual risk of stroke in non-anticoagulated patients with AF is 3–5% (relative risk 2.5–3) but much lower in those <75y old without co-morbidity.

Thrombocytopaenia

Patients with active or severe GI bleeding with a platelet count <50 x 10^9/L should receive platelet support (5–10U ≈ 1–2 pools).

Warfarin reversal

Immediate reversal in actively bleeding patients requires replacement of vitamin K-dependent clotting factors (II, VII, IX, X). Although these are present in FFP, consider requesting Octaplex® or Beriplex® (concentrated vitamin K-dependent clotting factors) as well as with vitamin K for major bleeding (see 'What should I do if the patient continues to bleed despite these measures?', 🕮 p. 8), as this is the quickest and most effective means of normalizing the INR. Discuss with the haematology team (treatment is expensive, so there may be reluctance to use it, but don't let that put you off requesting it if required). In the stable patient, give low-dose vitamin K 0.5–1mg IV; INR corrects within a few hours.

Avoid large doses of vitamin K if re-anticoagulation is required once bleeding is controlled, particularly in patients with prosthetic heart valves. For conditions in which the need for anticoagulation is less definitive (e.g. AF) and a decision is taken to discontinue warfarin indefinitely, give high-dose vitamin K 10mg IV. If in doubt, consult haematology.

Heparin reversal

Unfractionated heparin can be reversed with protamine sulphate (1mg IV neutralizes 100U; bolus doses >25–50mg seldom required, as half-life of heparin is 30–60min). Use protamine (1mg/100 anti-Xa units) to neutralize LMWH, but halve the dose if LMWH administered >8h beforehand.

Other coagulopathies

If INR is elevated for reasons other than warfarin administration, correct clotting with FFP 10–15mL/kg IV. This contains all clotting factors, except substantial concentrations of fibrinogen. In patients in whom fibrinogen is also depleted due to widespread consumption (e.g. DIC), replace with cryoprecipitate. Be aware that transfusion of large volumes of blood leads to deficiency of various clotting factors.

ⓘ **What should I do if the patient continues to bleed despite these measures?**

There are no hard rules on what to do when patients continue to bleed despite attempts to correct the above. Clearly, the sooner they undergo urgent therapeutic endoscopy the better, and you can only use the resources available to you. The following manoeuvres may help, although there are no right answers or clear guidelines.

- Recombinant factor VIIa 90µg/kg every 2h until haemostasis achieved. May have a role in stabilizing INR in massive variceal bleeding in patients with Child–Pugh B and C cirrhosis (a very expensive treatment).
- Aprotinin for massive, life-threatening bleeds following thrombolysis (50–100mL ≈ 0.5–1MU) as slow IV bolus, followed by 20mL/h until bleeding stops.
- Tranexamic acid, 0.5–1.5g tds IV or 1–1.5g tds PO, increases levels of fibrinogen and can be given when bleeding is difficult to control. Likewise, desmopressin (DDAVP®) (0.3µg/kg in 50mL 0.9% saline over 30min) increases release of von Willebrand factor multimers from endothelium. These are particularly effective in renal failure. Effects last 4–24h.

Assessment of severity

It is essential to categorize patients on admission into high or low risk of death. Most deaths occur in elderly patients with co-morbid disease. In general, high-risk factors include:
- Age >60y (30% risk of death if >90y).
- Chronic liver disease.
- Other chronic disease (cardiac, respiratory, renal).
- Bleeding diathesis.
- Re-bleed or bleeding whilst an inpatient for another reason (3-fold mortality).
- Decreased conscious level.
- Shock (systolic BP <100mmHg in patients <60y or <120mmHg in patients >60y, or HR >100/min).

Risk prediction scores

The Glasgow–Blatchford score predicts need for medical intervention (see Table 1.1). The Rockall score and Forrest classification can be used post-endoscopy to determine re-bleeding and mortality risk (see Tables 1.2 and 1.3; Fig. 1.1). Whilst there is much enthusiasm for scoring systems, in practice, they are not used very much. Most clinicians recognize that a large bleed with high urea, shock, and melaena is high-risk and requires urgent active treatment.

The UK and USA guidelines for triaging patients with upper GI bleeds are available at: see 🐾 http://www.bsg.org.uk and see 🐾 http://www.asge.org/

Table 1.1 Glasgow–Blatchford score

Marker	Range	Score
Urea (mmol/L)	<6.5	0
	6.5–8	2
	8–10	3
	10–25	4
	>25	6
Hb (men, g/dL)	>13	0
	12–13	1
	10–12	3
	<10	6
Hb (women, g/dL)	>12	0
	10–12	1
	<10	6
Systolic BP (mmHg)	>109	0
	100–109	1
	90–99	2
	<90	3
Other	HR >100	1
	Melaena	1
	Syncope	2
	Liver disease	2
	Heart failure	2

Glasgow–Blatchford predicts need for inpatient admission and endoscopic therapy. Patients with scores <1 can be investigated as outpatients. A score <4 predicts low probability of requiring endoscopic therapy. Reprinted from *The Lancet*, 373, AJ Stanley *et al.*, 'Outpatient management of patients with low-risk upper-gastrointestinal haemorrhage: multicentre validation and prospective evaluation', pp. 42–47. Copyright 2009, with permission from Elsevier.

Table 1.2 Rockall score

Variable	0	1	2	3
Age		60–79	>80	
Shock		HR >100/ min	Systolic BP <100mmHg	
Co-morbidity			Cardiovascular, GI cancer	Renal or liver failure, metastases
Endoscopic diagnosis	Mallory–Weiss tear	Other	Malignancy	
Endoscopic stigmata of recent haemorrhage			Clot, bleeding, or visible vessel	

Rockall score predicts patient outcome (see Fig. 1.1). For example, patients with score ≤2 have a re-bleed and mortality rate of 4.3% and 0.1%, respectively. Usually, they can safely be discharged from hospital the same day as the endoscopy. Reproduced from Gut, TF Rockall et al., 'Risk assessment after acute upper gastrointestinal haemorrhage', 38, 3, pp. 316–321, copyright 1996, with permission from BMJ Publishing Group Ltd.

Table 1.3 Forrest classification of re-bleeding risk

Class	Endoscopic finding	Re-bleeding rate (%)
Ia	Spurting artery	80–90
Ib	Oozing	55–80
IIa	Non-bleeding visible vessel	50–60
IIb	Adherent clot	25–35
IIc	Black spot in ulcer base	0–8
III	Clean ulcer base	0–12

Reproduced from W. Heldwein et al., 'Is the Forrest classification a useful tool for planning endoscopic therapy of bleeding peptic ulcers?', Endoscopy, 21, 6, pp. 258–262, 1989, with permission from Thieme Publishing Group. DOI:10.1055/s-2007-1010729.

Endoscopy

It is important to identify patients with portal hypertension since these individuals have much higher mortality.

Diagnostic endoscopy

- *Consider 250mg IV erythromycin.* Although not yet standard practice, two controlled studies have shown injection of 250mg erythromycin IV 30–60min before endoscopy provides better views in patients with haematemesis. A clear stomach was observed in 80% of patients given erythromycin compared to 35% of controls (Frossart et al., 2002).
- *Timing of endoscopy.* Endoscopy should be performed as soon as possible in patients who need major resuscitation, those who remain shocked after 4L of fluid resuscitation, or when variceal bleeding is suspected. In all other patients, endoscopy should be done within 12h of the bleed (especially in elderly patients or those with co-morbidity)

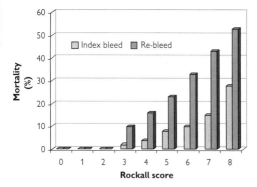

Fig. 1.1 Mortality from index and recurrent upper gastrointestinal bleed according to Rockall score. Data from Gut, TF Rockall et al., 'Risk assessment after acute upper gastrointestinal haemorrhage', 38, 3, pp. 316–321, copyright 1996, BMJ Publishing Group Ltd.

and certainly within 24h. Patients must be adequately resuscitated before endoscopy.

- *Call the senior endoscopist on-call.* Within working hours, liaise with the endoscopy unit and tell them you have a patient with a GI bleed who needs urgent endoscopy. Pregnancy or recent MI are not necessarily contraindications (see Box 1.1). Young patients with an insignificant bleed and a normal BP and Hb can often safely be discharged from A & E but should be endoscoped within 1wk (Rockall et al., 1996).
- *Consent.* Patients with capacity must provide, at least, verbal consent. If the bleed is life-threatening and the patient cannot provide consent, endoscopy may proceed if in best interests in the absence of express consent, so long as the patient has not expressed a prior wish not to have the procedure. A senior doctor should provide consent in patients who lack capacity (in the UK, this is the Consent Form IV).
- *Sedation.* Usually patients are sedated using a short-acting benzodiazepine such as midazolam 1–5mg IV. Oxygen, oxygen saturation and pulse rate monitoring are mandatory. At least three trained individuals should be present when endoscopy is performed. General anaesthesia should be considered for agitated patients, especially if there is a large haemorrhage or suspected variceal bleed.

Therapeutic endoscopy

It is important to perform quick, but thorough, endoscopy and therefore someone experienced should undertake the procedure. Therapy can be applied once the bleeding lesion has been discovered (see Box 1.2). The absence of bleeding suggests mid- or hind-gut haemorrhage, which has lower mortality risk. Further investigations may be warranted in such situations (see Chapters 2 and 3). If too much blood is present to determine the bleeding site, repeat endoscopy after 6–12h should be performed, following IV erythromycin or metoclopramide administration.

Box 1.1 Risks of endoscopy during pregnancy and post-MI

Risks of endoscopy during pregnancy

Guidelines have been published (Qureshi et al., 2005). Endoscopy is safe in pregnancy, but deep sedation should be avoided. Have a low threshold for anaesthetic involvement. Be aware of effects of drugs on the foetus.

Risks of endoscopy post-MI

The overall risk of cardiovascular complications in upper GI endoscopy is ~0.3% (Gangi et al., 2004). In 200 patients undergoing upper GI endoscopy within 30d of MI, the risk of a significant cardiovascular complication was 7.5%, exclusively in unwell patients or those with ongoing hypotension (Cappell and Iacovone, 1999). There are no clear guidelines for endoscopy in patients within 7d of an MI. The risks have to be balanced against those of no intervention in patients in whom therapeutic endoscopy may be life-saving. There are data to show that even PEG placement is relatively safe in patients following a recent MI (Cappell and Iacovone, 1996).

Box 1.2 Endoscopic therapies

- *Injection therapy* involves injection with adrenaline (1:10,000). While adrenaline is good at achieving initial haemostasis, re-bleeding rate is 18% in the short term. Therefore, endoscopists follow this with either thermal coagulation or placement of haemoclips (endoclips).
- *Thermal coagulation* involves application of a contact heater probe to the bleeding ulcer base. Bipolar devices are preferred, as desiccated tissue limits the penetration of alternating current (e.g. 'gold' probe 15W applied for 6s, re-positioned as necessary). Use 30J for four pulses before re-positioning if using the 'heater' probe (direct current).
- *Endoclips* are effective in Dieulafoy lesions and small visible vessels but are of limited value for large ulcers.
- *Argon plasma coagulation (APC)* is a thermoablative technique with limited penetration of the mucosa. The non-contact nature of application allows large areas to be treated rapidly, in contrast to contact thermal techniques such as the heater probe. APC also allows treatment of lesions that are not directly 'en face' or behind folds. It is mainly used to treat GAVE (use 40W).
- *Fibrin sealant* can be injected into a bleeding ulcer. In one trial (Rutgeerts et al., 1997), this resulted in less re-bleeding than injection of a sclerosant (policanol) and fewer treatment failures, although differences were not large. It is not widely used. Histoacryl glue injection is used for bleeding gastric varices but requires expertise.

Endoscopic therapy for bleeding peptic ulcers

Bleeding peptic ulcers are the commonest cause of upper GI bleeding, accounting for 35–50% of all cases (see Colour plate 2). The majority are caused by *Helicobacter (H.) pylori,* while NSAIDs are responsible for ~30%. It is said that upper GI bleeding in cirrhotic patients has a non-variceal origin in ~30% of cases. Without endoscopic therapy, there is high risk of peptic ulcer re-bleeding in the case of:

- Active bleeding (90%).
- A visible vessel (50%).
- Adherent clot (25–30%).

The endoscopist should inject these lesions quadrantically and centrally with 0.5–1mL 1:10,000 adrenaline *AND* apply a second therapeutic modality (e.g. bipolar coagulation or endoscopic clips), which reduces re-bleed and mortality rates from 18.4% to 10.6% and 5.1% to 2.6%, respectively (Calvet *et al.,* 2004). If an adherent clot obscures the bleeding lesion, experienced endoscopists should inject the clot as above before removing it using a 'cold' snare, and then apply a second therapy (Jensen *et al.,* 2002). Low-risk lesions (clean ulcer base ± a red spot) do not require any endoscopic therapy since their risk of re-bleeding is low (<10%).

Endoscopic therapy for varices

Band ligation is the preferred method for variceal obliteration (see Colour plate 3) and has largely replaced intra-variceal injection of sclerosant (e.g. 1mL ethanolamine, thrombin, or cyanoacrylate glue). However, initial treatment with sclerosant is indicated for gastric varices, which are often harder to obliterate. Serious side effects occur in 7%, mainly retrosternal pain and fever immediately post-injection with subsequent mucosal ulceration.

Endoscopic therapy for other conditions

Mallory–Weiss tears are longitudinal mucosal tears at the gastro-oesophageal junction following severe retching, and are particularly common following alcohol binges. They can be precipitated by increased intra-abdominal pressure due to vomiting, straining at stool, coughing, lifting, or convulsions; >40% patients have hiatus hernias. The first vomit is usually normal, then it becomes bright red. There may be associated back or abdominal pain. Most stop bleeding spontaneously. Endoscopic therapy can be applied as for peptic ulcers if bleeding is ongoing; clips may be particularly effective (see Colour plate 4). Tamponade with a Sengstaken–Blakemore tube has been used with very severe bleeding.

Erosive gastritis/oesophagitis (see Colour plate 5) generally presents as relatively minor bleeds but may be significant in patients with a bleeding diathesis. They may occur due to 'stress' in the critically ill patient. At endoscopy, there is commonly a generalized ooze of blood from the inflamed mucosa. Endoscopic therapy is not beneficial. If the bleeding continues, partial gastric resection may be necessary, but this is very rare. Overall mortality rate is very low.

Uncommon causes of upper GI bleeding

- A *Dieulafoy lesion* is a dilated, aberrant blood vessel, which erodes through the gastric lining in the absence of an ulcer. They are usually located in the upper stomach along the lesser curvature near the oesophago-gastric junction and can be hard to locate endoscopically. They are thought to be congenital, although bleeding tends to occur in men with cardiovascular or renal disease, or alcohol abuse. Re-bleeding is common (10–35%). Haemoclips are said to reduce risk of re-bleeding (Park *et al.*, 2003), best applied in conjunction with endoscopic injection (Cui *et al.*, 2011).

- *Gastric antral vascular ectasia (GAVE)*, or 'watermelon stomach', is a rare cause of GI bleeding. There are longitudinal rows of reddish stripes radiating from the pylorus to the antrum due to the presence of ectatic mucosal vessels. The cause is unknown, but it is more common in cirrhosis and systemic sclerosis. Bleeding is rarely massive. Therapy is by thermal or argon plasma coagulation. It does not respond to TIPS.

- Bleeding from *portal hypertensive gastropathy* (see Colour plate 6) is rare and generally due to oozing rather than haemorrhage from a specific point. The risk seems to increase post-sclerotherapy. Bleeding can be prevented by TIPS or thermal coagulation.

- *Haemobilia*. Bleeding from the hepatobiliary tract is very rare and suggests hepatic or biliary tract injury, often caused by liver biopsy. Bleeding can occur up to 2wk following a procedure, with associated pain and jaundice. Treatment may require surgical resection or angiography with embolization. Rarely, one may also get bleeding from the pancreatic duct due to chronic pancreatitis or tumours.

- *Aorto-enteric fistulae*. These rare lesions tend to occur in the third or fourth portion of the duodenum. They cause massive GI bleeding and carry high mortality. The most common cause is secondary to an atherosclerotic aortic aneurysm, usually following repair with a prosthetic graft which has become infected, but they can occur due to syphilis or TB. A small 'herald' bleed can occur, therefore, have a low threshold for organizing a contrast CT in such patients; ask the vascular team to review the scan, as the changes can be subtle.

- *Post-ERCP bleeding*. This is relatively rare (1–2%) and usually occurs post-sphincterotomy. Risk increased by thrombocytopaenia, high INR, and renal failure. It is rarely life-threatening. Patients should undergo endoscopic therapy with injection of adrenaline or fibrin sealant, or application of a haemoclip. Other therapeutic modalities can be used but, as a last resort, patients may need angiography or surgery.

After the endoscopy

Patients with high-risk lesions or varices should be kept nil-by-mouth until reviewed the next morning, in case repeat endoscopy is needed. If stable (no Hb drop and observations stable), they should be fed and possibly discharged after another 24h. If endoscopy demonstrates a low-risk lesion, the patient can probably be safely discharged the same day as the endoscopy, with anti-ulcer therapy (for Rockall score, see Table 1.2).

What should I do if endoscopic therapy fails?

There is no clear definition of endoscopic failure for non-variceal bleeding but, in general, it is regarded as failure to control bleeding after two attempted therapeutic endoscopies by an experienced endoscopist. Re-bleeding usually occurs in the first 24h (defined as reduction in Hb >2g/dL after allowing for haemodilution, re-development of shock, or fall in CVP >5cmH$_2$O). It increases mortality 3-fold (for Rockall score, see Table 1.2), so consider admitting the patient to HDU or a Level 1 ward. It is more common with ulcers on the incisura or posterior duodenal bulb. Repeat therapeutic endoscopy should be performed if the bleeding has been partially controlled following initial endoscopy (Lau et al., 1999). Relative indications for surgery or angiography include:

- Exsanguinating haemorrhage (too fast to replace).
- Profuse bleeding:
  - Initial resuscitation with >6U blood.
  - Continued bleeding at >1 unit/8h.
  - Persistent hypotension.
- Re-bleed in hospital, uncontrolled by a second therapeutic endoscopy.
- Lower thresholds in elderly or with lesions at high risk of re-bleeding (e.g. posterior duodenal ulcer with visible vessel or large gastric ulcer).
- Complex patients (such as those with a rare blood group, multiple anti-red cell antibodies, or those refusing blood transfusion) in whom bleeding is not readily controlled.

It is useful to invite a senior member of the surgical team to attend the endoscopy of patients who may require operative intervention. If endoscopy fails to identify the bleeding lesion in a patient with haematemesis and haemodynamic compromise, consider proceeding to CT angiography ± interventional angiography to help define ± control the point of haemorrhage.

If surgery is declined, ask the interventional radiologists to undertake transvenous arteriography of the coeliac axis and superior mesenteric artery to enable selective embolization of the bleeding vessel. Intra-arterial vasopressin can temporarily control haemorrhagic gastritis and is used if the collateral blood supply is poor following previous surgery. Embolization with a biodegradable long-acting gelatin sponge is used for other causes of upper GI bleeding as long as the bleeding is brisk (0.5–1mL/min). Both are effective in ~70%.

Continued bleeding from varices should be treated with placement of a Sengstaken–Blakemore tube, and patients should be referred to a liver unit for emergency TIPS (see Box 1.3). Emergency TIPS is successful in 90% of cases, with 6wk survival of 60–90% (Sanyal et al., 1996). Elective TIPS within 72h of successful endoscopic treatment has been shown to reduce both re-bleeding and mortality (Garcia–Pagán et al., 2010). TIPS is often the preferred treatment for gastric varices (see Colour plate 7).

⚙ Box 1.3 **Management of continued variceal bleeding**

Balloon tamponade

A Sengstaken–Blakemore, or Minnesota or Linton, tube should be inserted if the patient continues to bleed despite therapeutic endoscopy (see Colour plate 8). The tube should be removed from the fridge at the last possible moment to maintain stiffness. The airway must be protected prior to insertion, which usually requires a general anaesthetic. After insertion, inflate the gastric balloon with 250mL water and apply traction, fixing the tube at the mouth by anchoring it between two tongue depressors taped together. The oesophageal balloon should not be inflated unless the patient is known to be bleeding from a mid-oesophageal ulcer or varix (usually as a result of previous injection sclerotherapy). Arrange a repeat therapeutic endoscopy within 12h, otherwise ischaemic ulceration may occur (a risk that may be increased by co-administration of terlipressin). Major complications occur in 15%, of which the most lethal is oesophageal rupture.

Transvenous intrahepatic portosystemic shunting (TIPS)

TIPS is available in specialized units to provide definitive treatment for uncontrolled variceal bleeding (see Fig. 1.2). The hepatic veins are cannulated using a jugular or femoral approach, and an expandable stent is placed between the hepatic veins (low pressure) and portal venous system (high pressure). The portal pressure should be decompressed to <12mmHg. This has largely superseded surgical management (emergency portocaval shunting or oesophageal transection).

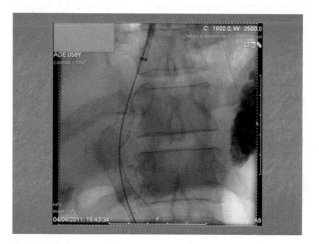

Fig. 1.2 TIPS following deployment. Reproduced with kind permission from John Karani.

Post-discharge management

Non-variceal haemorrhage

- Treat all patients with a PPI (e.g. omeprazole 20mg od for 6–8 wk). This may need to be continued in patients who had life-threatening bleeding (especially the elderly) and those requiring ongoing treatment with steroids, NSAIDs, aspirin, or clopidogrel.
- Patients with peptic ulceration not associated with NSAID use should receive empirical *H. pylori* eradication (Garcia–Altés *et al.*, 2000). Alternatively, in patients taking steroids, NSAIDs, and probably antiplatelet drugs, biopsy should be taken at the original endoscopy for the *H. pylori* urease test. As patients are usually on PPI therapy by this time, also check for *H. pylori* using another method (e.g. faecal antigen testing). Eradicate *H. pylori* (e.g. with amoxicillin 500mg bd PO plus clarithromycin 500mg bd PO for 1 wk) in individuals found to be colonized, and re-check 2mo following cessation of acid-lowering therapy.
- Repeat endoscopy for gastric ulcers at 6–8wk to ensure the ulcer was not malignant (see Colour plate 9). Duodenal ulcers do not usually need to be reviewed endoscopically. Endoscopic surveillance should be considered in those requiring ongoing treatment with steroids, NSAIDs, or antiplatelet drugs, although if possible such treatments should be discontinued. Of the NSAIDs, ibuprofen and naproxen have lower risks of causing bleeding.

Post-discharge management of variceal haemorrhage

- Treat all patients with a PPI (e.g. omeprazole 20mg od for 6–8wk). This reduces risk of early loosening of variceal bands.
- Band ligation is normally carried out at weekly intervals until variceal obliteration and then considered at 3-monthly intervals or longer. It is more effective and rapid than injection sclerotherapy (39d vs 72d) and has fewer complications (2% vs 22%) (Stiegmann *et al.*, 1992). Following a banding programme, some centres obliterate any remaining varices with injection sclerotherapy.
- Propranolol (20–40mg tds) reduces rate of bleeding and re-bleeding from varices and portal hypertensive gastropathy. Aim for a 25% reduction in resting HR or a rate of 50–60/min. Ideally, a reduction of portal pressure should be confirmed by measurement of wedged hepatic venous pressure gradient in specialist centres.
- TIPS provides more definite cure, and bleeding tends to recur only when the shunt blocks, but there is increased incidence of chronic hepatic encephalopathy (~20%). Its use is increasing.

Prognosis

Overall mortality of non-variceal bleeding is <10% and can be estimated by the Rockall score. Mortality is reduced by early surgery in high-risk patients. Overall mortality following variceal haemorrhage is 30%. This is highest in those with severe liver disease (Child–Pugh grade C, see 📖 p. 256). Terlipressin controls bleeding in ~70%, which is increased to 80–85% if combined with band ligation or injection sclerotherapy. Balloon tamponade has similar efficacy, although it is only a temporizing measure.

Acute upper gastrointestinal bleeding

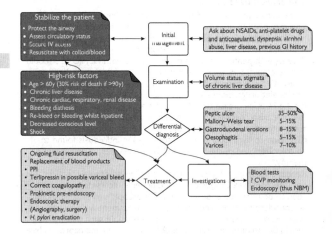

Stabilize the patient
- Protect the airway
- Assess circulatory status
- Secure IV access
- Resuscitate with colloid/blood

Initial management

Ask about NSAIDs, anti-platelet drugs and anticoagulants, dyspepsia, alcohol abuse, liver disease, previous GI history

High-risk factors
- Age > 60y (30% risk of death if >90y)
- Chronic liver disease
- Chronic cardiac, respiratory, renal disease
- Bleeding diathesis
- Re-bleed or bleeding whilst inpatient
- Decreased conscious level
- Shock

Examination

Volume status, stigmata of chronic liver disease

Differential diagnosis

Peptic ulcer	35–50%
Mallory–Weiss tear	5–15%
Gastroduodenal erosions	8–15%
Oesophagitis	5–15%
Varices	7–10%

- Ongoing fluid resuscitation
- Replacement of blood products
- PPI
- Terlipressin in possible variceal bleed
- Correct coagulopathy
- Prokinetic pre-endoscopy
- Endoscopic therapy
- (Angiography, surgery)
- *H. pylori* eradication

Treatment

Investigations

Blood tests
? CVP monitoring
Endoscopy (thus NBM)

Further reading

Bernard B, Grangé JD, Khac EN, et al. (1999) Antibiotic prophylaxis for the prevention of bacterial infections in cirrhotic patients with gastrointestinal bleeding: a meta-analysis. *Hepatology* 29: 1655–61.

Calvet X, Vergara M, Brullet E, et al. (2004) Addition of a second endoscopic treatment following epinephrine injection improves outcome in high-risk bleeding ulcers. *Gastroenterology* 126: 441–50.

Cannegieter SC, Rosendaal FR, Briët E (1994) Thromboembolic and bleeding complications in patients with mechanical heart valve prostheses. *Circulation* 89: 635–41.

Cappell MS, Lacovone FM Jr (1996) The safety and efficacy of percutaneous endoscopic gastrostomy after recent myocardial infarction: a study of 28 patients and 40 controls at four university teaching hospitals. *Am J Gastroenterol* 91: 1599–603.

Cappell MS, Lacovone FM Jr (1999) Safety and efficacy of esophagogastroduodenoscopy after myocardial infarction. *Am J Med* 106: 29–35.

Cui J, Huang LY, Liu YX, et al. (2011) Efficacy of endoscopic therapy for gastrointestinal bleeding from Dieulafoy's lesion. *World J Gastroenterol* 17: 1368–72.

Frossard JL, Spahr L, Queneau PE, et al. (2002) Erythromycin intravenous bolus infusion in acute upper gastrointestinal bleeding: a randomized, controlled, double-blind trial. *Gastroenterology* 123: 17–23.

Gangi S, Saidi F, Patel K, et al. (2004) Cardiovascular complications after GI endoscopy: occurrence and risks in a large hospital system. *Gastrointest Endosc* 60: 679–85.

García–Altés A, Jovell AJ, Serra–Prat M, et al. (2000) Management of Helicobacter pylori in duodenal ulcer: a cost-effectiveness analysis. *Aliment Pharmacol Ther* 14: 1631–8.

García–Pagán JC, Caca K, Bureau C, et al. (2010) Early use of TIPS in patients with cirrhosis and variceal bleeding. *N Engl J Med* 362: 2370–9.

Gøtzsche PC, Hróbjartsson A (2005) Somatostatin analogues for acute bleeding oesophageal varices. *Cochrane Database Syst Rev* 1: CD000193.

Jensen DM, Kovacs TO, Jutabha R, et al. (2002) Randomized trial of medical or endoscopic therapy to prevent recurrent ulcer hemorrhage in patients with adherent clots. *Gastroenterology* 123: 407–13.

Jensen DM, Machicado GA (1988) Diagnosis and treatment of severe hematochezia. The role of urgent colonoscopy after purge. *Gastroenterology* 95: 1569–74.

Lau JY, Sung JJ, Lam YH, et al. (1999) Endoscopic retreatment compared with surgery in patients with recurrent bleeding after initial endoscopic control of bleeding ulcers. *N Engl J Med* 340: 751–6.

Lau JY, Sung JJ, Lee KK, et al. (2000) Effect of intravenous omeprazole on recurrent bleeding after endoscopic treatment of bleeding peptic ulcers. *N Engl J Med* 343: 310–16.

Lau JY, Leung WK, Wu JC, et al. (2007) Omeprazole before endoscopy in patients with gastrointestinal bleeding. *N Engl J Med* 356: 1631–40.

Mark AS, Moss AA, McCarthy S, et al. (1985) CT of aortoenteric fistulas. *Invest Radiol* 20: 272–5.

Park CH, Sohn JH, Lee WS, et al. (2003) The usefulness of endoscopic hemoclipping for bleeding Dieulafoy lesions. *Endoscopy* 35: 388–92.

Qureshi WA, Rajan E, Adler DG, et al. (2005) ASGE Guideline: Guidelines for endoscopy in pregnant and lactating women. *Gastrointest Endosc* 61: 357–62.

Rockall TA, Logan RF, Devlin HB, et al. (1996) Selection of patients for early discharge or outpatient care after acute upper gastrointestinal haemorrhage. National Audit of Acute Upper Gastrointestinal Haemorrhage. *Lancet* 347: 1138–40.

Rutgeerts P, Rauws E, Wara P, et al. (1997) Randomised trial of single and repeated fibrin glue compared with injection of polidocanol in treatment of bleeding peptic ulcer. *Lancet* 350: 692–6.

Sanyal AJ, Freedman AM, Luketic VA, et al. (1996) Transjugular intrahepatic portosystemic shunts for patients with active variceal hemorrhage unresponsive to sclerotherapy. *Gastroenterology* 111: 138–46.

Stanley AJ, Ashley D, Dalton HR, et al. (2009) Outpatient management of patients with low-risk upper gastrointestinal haemorrhage: multicentre validation and prospective evaluation. *Lancet* 373: 42–7.

Stiegmann GV, Goff JS, Michaletz–Onody PA, et al. (1992) Endoscopic sclerotherapy as compared with endoscopic ligation for bleeding esophageal varices. *N Engl J Med* 326: 1527–32.

Udd M, Miettinen P, Palmu A, et al. (2001) Regular-dose versus high-dose omeprazole in peptic ulcer bleeding: a prospective randomized double-blind study. *Scand J Gastroenterol* 36: 1332–8.

Acute lower gastrointestinal bleeding

:✪: Lower gastrointestinal bleeding

Lower GI bleeding is common but usually of only modest severity. Most can be managed on an outpatient basis, although unwell patients need admission (have a lower threshold for patients with severe co-morbidity). In total, ~35% of significant bleeds require transfusion and 5% urgent surgery (see the *Oxford Handbook of Gastroenterology and Hepatology*, p. 579). Nonetheless, ~80% of bleeds will stop spontaneously without specific treatment.

Initial management

Resuscitation and initial assessment

- IV access: two wide-bore cannulae (at least 16G).
- Consider catheter and CVP line.
- IV fluids if shocked or bleeding >500mL. Initially, use colloid (e.g. Gelofusine®), alternating with crystalloid (e.g. Hartmann's), at a rate to maintain systolic BP >100mmHg. A total of 2L in the first hour is often required.
- Estimate volume of blood loss and consider transfusion.
- Contact the surgical team if haemodynamic instability (i.e. absent or only transient response despite initial resuscitation with 2L), or immediately if the bleed is large.
- Consider need to activate 'major haemorrhage protocol' (see Appendix, 📖 pp. 360–1).

Observations of concern

- HR >100.
- Systolic BP <100mmHg, especially with narrowed pulse pressure.
- RR >30/min.
- Urine output <0.5mL/kg/h.
- Blood loss >500mL.
- Confusion.
- Haemodynamic instability despite initial resuscitation.

History

- Are aspirin, clopidogrel, NSAIDs, or warfarin taken? All increase the rate of bleeding. For guidelines on reversal of anticoagulation, see 📖 p. 7.
- Is there a history of bleeding (suggestive of a bleeding disorder, the commonest being von Willebrand's disease)?
- Is chronic liver disease likely (causes prolonged PTT and increases likelihood of variceal bleeding)? Prolonged PTT also occurs in malnutrition. Renal disease, causing significant uraemia, impairs platelet function.
- Are there alarm features (see Box 2.1), in which case neoplasia is more likely?
- Is there a past history of colonic pathology?
- Is the blood mixed with the stool or separate? Bright red blood on toilet paper suggests anorectal aetiology.

Examination

- Assess degree of dehydration.
- Guarding/rebound occurs with colonic dilatation/intestinal perforation.
- Rectal exam. It's been said, 'If you don't put your finger in, you put your foot in it.' Helps define nature and magnitude of bleeding, and presence of rectal mass.
- Mouth ulcers and peri-anal disease suggest IBD. Erythema nodosum, uveitis, or arthralgia occur in IBD but occasionally also with infective diarrhoea.

---

① Box 2.1 Alarm features in patients presenting with lower GI bleeding

- Unexplained weight loss >5–10% normal body weight.
- Age >60y.
- Looser stools or increased frequency defaecation >6wk.
- Right-sided abdominal mass.
- Rectal mass.
- Iron-deficiency anaemia without obvious cause.
- Strong family history of colorectal carcinoma.*
- High-volume bleeding.*
- Passage of altered blood.*

* Although not part of NICE guidance, evidence shows these are logical 'alarm' criteria.

Investigations to be performed in Accident & Emergency

- Blood tests:
  - FBC. Is the patient anaemic? Remember Hb may be deceptively normal or high due to haemoconcentration.
  - U & E. Indicates extent of volume depletion, and urea is often disproportionately raised compared to creatinine if upper GI source. Bleeding often more severe if renal failure present.
  - LFT. Low albumin occurs in decompensated liver disease (look for coagulopathy), IBD, or malignancy.
  - Clotting. Correct coagulopathy if bleeding severe (see 📖 p. 7).
  - G & S. In all patients.
  - Cross-match. Total of 4U in severe bleeding.
  - ESR and CRP. If raised, consider colitis.
- AXR. To exclude toxic megacolon. Present if the transverse colon diameter is greater than vertebral body or >6cm, and the patient is toxic (fever, leukocytosis, anaemia, tachycardia). Thumb-printing suggests infectious or inflammatory disease.
- If haemodynamic compromise or significantly rise in urea, insert NGT and lavage stomach with 250mL water. Arrange emergency upper GI endoscopy if aspirate is bloody or bilious fluid absent. (11% of massive upper GI bleeds present as apparent lower GI bleeding).
- Stool analysis. Relevant if dysentery possible (see Chapter 6). *Clostridium (C.) difficile* does not cause rectal bleeding but is found in up to 5% of IBD relapses, in whom it should be tested.

Causes of severe rectal bleeding

Aetiologies and their frequencies are shown in Table 2.1.

Table 2.1 Causes of acute lower GI bleeding

Cause	Frequency (%)
Diverticular disease	5–42
Other colitis (infectious, antibiotic-associated)	3–29
Unknown aetiology	6–23
Ischaemic colitis	6–18
Anorectal (haemorrhoids, fissures, rectal ulcers)	6–16*
Upper GI/small bowel bleed	3–13
Post-polypectomy	0–13
Cancers/polyps	3–11
Other (anastomotic bleeding, aorto-enteric fistula)	1–9
Inflammatory bowel disease	2–4
Radiation colitis	1–3
Angiodysplasia	0–3

* Note, however, that haemorrhoidal bleeding is the most common cause of small-volume, fresh bleeding in those aged <50y. Reprinted from Gastroenterology Clinics of North America, 34, 4, Lisa L. Strate, 'Lower GI bleeding: epidemiology and diagnosis', pp. 643–664, Copyright 2005, with permission from Elsevier.

Admission

Recommended when haemodynamic compromise or severe disease:
- Pulse rate >100/min.
- Systolic BP >20mmHg less than normal.
- Postural BP drop >20/10mmHg.
- >10 bloody stools/day.
- Severe co-morbidity (significant heart, renal, or liver failure).

Most patients are admitted under the surgical team. However, patients likely to have IBD or dysentery should be looked after by physicians, with surgical review if fulminant colitis is suspected (see [] pp. 69, 98). Patients with haemodynamic instability or cardiopulmonary disease may require invasive monitoring (CVP line ± arterial line) and should be admitted to a high dependency bed. Patients that remain shocked despite resuscitation should be managed in ITU.

Following admission, basic resuscitation should be continued. Further investigation can be delayed to the following morning in stable patients (no ongoing haemodynamic compromise). Those that remain unstable should undergo angiographic localization of the bleeding site followed by embolization or surgery.

Definitive investigations

Stable patients should be investigated by colonoscopy, which reveals a bleeding site in ~75% (Angtuaco et al., 2001). There is limited evidence supporting urgent inpatient colonoscopy, which can provide therapeutic intervention to prevent further bleeding. If performed within 24–48h, it is more likely to:
• Reveal a source of bleeding.
• Result in cessation of diverticular bleeding.

In general, early outpatient colonoscopy probably does not increase mortality, transfusion requirements, or need for surgery. However, patients with continued bleeding need urgent inpatient investigation.

Colonoscopy

Excellent at diagnosing the principal causes of bleeding, namely cancer, diverticular disease, and angiodysplasia. It is very unusual to have to perform out-of-hours colonoscopy, but try and perform on the next list in severe bleeding (as you would for upper GI bleeding).
• Patients should receive bowel preparation (e.g. Klean-Prep®, Moviprep®): give 1L each 30min until effluent clear (usually 3–4L required) via NGT if in place. Blood is cathartic, so 'unprepared' colonoscopy can be attempted if absolutely necessary. There is no evidence that bowel preparation increases bleeding.
• Cover purge with diuretics if heart failure. Perform therapeutic paracentesis (see 📖 p. 262) prior to purge if tense ascites. If patient on dialysis, discuss with renal team.
• Give metoclopramide 10mg IV just prior to purge to reduce nausea and facilitate intestinal transit.
• Provide IV rehydration with bowel preparation (e.g. 1L 0.9% saline with 20mmol KCl over 12h).
• The diagnostic yield of colonoscopy is higher than arteriography, making it the first-line investigation for most patients.
• Therapy can be applied to control bleeding from arteriovenous malformations, diverticular disease, radiation proctitis/colitis, or polyps/ polypectomy sites. Argon plasma or bipolar coagulation are relatively safe despite the thin colonic wall.
• Colonoscopy should not be performed if toxic megacolon (although limited colonoscopy with minimal air insufflation has been shown to be safe in severe colitis; insufflation with CO_2 preferable).

Flexible sigmoidoscopy

May usefully identify haemorrhage in those suspected of having a distal colonic bleeding source.

Angiography

Interventional or CT angiography reveal bleeding source in ~50% cases. Useful for patients in whom colonoscopy is not feasible or diagnostic.

- Requires bleeding >0.5mL/min (~Hb drop >2g/dL/24h).
- Sensitivity 30–50% but specificity 100%.
- While CT angiography does not allow therapeutic intervention, it may guide subsequent direct selective catheter angiography or surgery, resulting in a lower overall complication rate.
- In primary direct selective angiography, superior mesenteric cannulation is most useful.
- Therapy comprises selective intra-arterial vasopressin injection to temporarily stop bleeding (rarely used), or embolization with metal coils. There is <10% risk of bowel infarction, which requires emergency laparotomy.

Labelled red cell scintigraphy

More sensitive than angiography (can detect bleeding >0.1mL/min) but requires active bleeding for a positive test. Provides poor localization of bleeding site and is non-therapeutic and time-consuming, so not widely used.

Surgery

Occasionally required to identify or treat bleeding site; preferably if endoscopy or angiography have already localized area of bleeding. Performed as an emergency if patient haemodynamically unstable despite attempted resuscitation (mortality 5–10%). If obscure bleeding continues (sometimes including patients with anaemia despite ongoing iron replacement), right hemicolectomy is sometimes performed (as bleeding often due to proximal colonic angiodysplasia).

Complications of endoscopy

Colonoscopy

- Some patients experience abdominal discomfort or pain.
- It is impossible to complete the procedure in 1 in 20 patients, who may then require a CT pneumocolon. Try and arrange same day, as the patient has already received bowel preparation (unless polypectomy has been performed, in which case delay for at least 2wk).
- Perforation occurs in ~1:800 examinations, although with modern equipment and training programmes it is likely this risk is lower. Perforations usually require surgical repair ± temporary stoma. Risk of perforation increases to ~1 in 600 post-polypectomy.
- Bleeding occurs in 1:1,500 cases although, if a polyp is removed, it occurs in 1:50–100 cases. It usually stops without any treatment but occasionally necessitates blood transfusion.
- Using sedation causes breathing complications in 1:200 procedures, which usually are not serious. To reduce this risk, pulse and oxygen levels are monitored throughout the test.

Flexible sigmoidoscopy

This is very safe and usually performed without sedation. Perforation occurs in 1:15,000 procedures, but otherwise there are no significant risks.

Gastroscopy

- Perforation occurs in about 1:10,000 procedures.
- Other rare complications include aspiration pneumonia, damage to loose teeth or to dental bridgework.
- Sedation risks are similar to colonoscopy.

Investigations if cause not identified

If the patient remains unstable (ongoing haemodynamic instability or transfusion requirement ≥3U/d after 3d), then surgery is indicated. Right hemicolectomy is usually performed if intraoperative endoscopy does not locate a bleeding site; results in cessation of bleeding in ~75%.

Stable patients with *ongoing* bleeding should be investigated further to try and locate the site of bleeding:

- Check colonoscopy was complete to caecum and that good views were obtained. If not, repeat.
- Check gastroscopy has been performed in patients with severe bleeding (Hb fall >3g/dL over 24h) or those who passed dark/altered blood.
- Request repeat colonoscopy in patients likely to have had colonic bleeding (i.e. fresh bleeding without haemodynamic compromise).
- Request urgent (within 24h) small bowel capsule endoscopy in patients who continue to bleed despite the above. This provides a diagnosis in >90% patients with ongoing bleeding, compared to <15% in those no longer bleeding. Prior small bowel follow-through, MRI follow-through (avoids radiation exposure), or patency capsule required if obstructive symptoms, history of adhesions, or (suspected) Crohn's disease.
- Double or single balloon enteroscopy are specialized techniques that can be used to provide endoscopic therapy to all parts of the small bowel if ongoing bleeding.
- Despite extensive investigations, no bleeding site is identified in ~5% patients. Consider Meckel's nuclear medicine scan in those <40y of age.

It is appropriate to perform no further investigation in stable patients who stop bleeding (as long as complete colonoscopy has been performed). Discharge the patient if they have remained stable for 48h with no fall in Hb. Re-investigate if they re-bleed.

⚙: Treatment of specific conditions

Diverticular disease

Patients with diverticulosis have a 15% lifetime risk of bleeding (see Colour plate 10), usually arising from right-sided diverticula. It is more common in elderly patients. Diverticulitis is rarely present at time of bleeding, which can be massive as diverticula often form where arteries penetrate the bowel wall. Bleeding stops spontaneously in 80%, but 25% will re-bleed. It can be successfully treated with endoscopic therapy (adrenaline injection and thermal coagulation), which has been shown to reduce inpatient stay from 5 to 2d and greatly reduce rate of re-bleeding. Arteriography is used mainly to locate bleeding site in patients requiring surgery: necessary in ~20% requiring transfusion, with 10% mortality (usually due to patient co-morbidities). Segmental colectomy performed in those with identified bleeding site, and subtotal colectomy in the remainder. Note that non-diverticular bleeding is the source in 50% of patients with severe rectal bleeding *and* diverticulosis.

① Colon cancer

Fresh rectal bleeding usually arises from tumours distal to the splenic flexure; more proximal tumours present with maroon blood, melaena, or iron-deficient anaemia (see Colour plate 11). Bleeding is often sporadic and small-volume. Endoscopically acquired biopsies establish the diagnosis. Request chest-abdomino-pelvic CT (and pelvic MRI if rectal cancer), and refer to the colorectal multidisciplinary team. Definitive treatment is surgery; endoscopic methods to curtail bleeding should only be employed in those unfit for operation.

⚙: Colon polyps and post-polypectomy bleeding

Spontaneous bleeding from polyps is usually sporadic and low-volume, and arises from left-sided polyps. Bleeding stops after snare resection (see Colour plate 12).

Delayed post-polypectomy bleeding occurs within 2wk in 1:50–100 cases. Request a colonoscopy, as it can usually be controlled endoscopically (although blood transfusion may be required).

⚙: Inflammatory bowel disease

See 'Inflammatory bowel disease' (📖 p. 31) and Chapter 7.

① Dysentery

See Chapter 6.

⚙: Colonic ischaemia and infarction

This is under-diagnosed. It is common in the elderly, especially those with atrial fibrillation (AF) or relative hypotension. Presentation is with mild abdominal pain and low-volume rectal bleeding. Increasing tenderness, distension, and diminished bowel sounds suggest pending infarction, which occurs in 15% and can be fatal. Suspect if blood gas demonstrates lactic acidosis. Colonoscopy should be performed with minimal instillation of air, or preferably CO_2, and shows segmental left-sided inflammation with rectal sparing. The mucosa appears pale with petechial haemorrhage; ulceration occurs with more severe ischaemia. Avoid colonoscopy if peritonitis or perforation likely. Histological appearances are not always specific. Further investigations, such as Doppler US of the mesenteric vessels and/or MRA/MRV, are rarely helpful as colonic ischaemic vessels are mostly arteriolar.

Treatment is directed at improving colonic blood flow and oxygenation with IV fluids, oxygen, antibiotics in moderate/severe cases, and avoiding hypotensive medication. Optimizing cardiovascular risk factors is important in the long term (diabetes mellitus, hypertension, hyperlipidaemia). Most patients completely recover within 1–2wk. Request urgent surgical opinion if peritonism, fever, leukocytosis, or acidosis (pH <7.3). Seek vascular surgical opinion regarding embolectomy or endarterectomy if embolic cause probable (e.g. patient in AF).

① Chronic radiation proctitis/colitis

This usually occurs following radiotherapy for cervical or prostate malignancy, since the field of radiation is adjacent to the recto-sigmoid colon. Chronic obliterative endarteritis causes chronic ischaemia, resulting in strictures and bleeding from telangiectatic vessels. Symptoms usually develop 9–12mo after radiotherapy, although may develop up to 20y later. Appearances at colonoscopy are characteristic, at which time thermal ablation using argon plasma coagulation is very effective at reducing frequency of bleeding (see 📖 p. 12). Two to three sessions are usually required to obliterate all vessels.

① Colonic vasculitis

Systemic vasculitides, such as PAN or SLE, often affect the GI tract, causing mesenteric ischaemia/infarction. Abdominal pain is common; rectal bleeding occurs in ~5%. ESR is raised. Other features of vasculitis are usually present (skin lesions, hypertension, mononeuritis multiplex in PAN; arthritis, glomerulonephritis, Raynaud's phenomenon in SLE). Treat the underlying condition with immunosuppression.

① Colonic angiodysplasia

Angiodysplasia (which technically should be called phlebectasia) are most commonly submucosal veins that lack smooth muscle; these are prone to bleeding (see Colour plate 13). They are a common cause of bleeding in patients with iron deficiency anaemia and usually located in the small intestine or proximal colon, but can present with low-volume rectal bleeding. Bleeding is more likely with concurrent coagulopathy, platelet dysfunction (e.g. uraemia, von Willebrand's disease, use of antiplatelet agents), or in the elderly. Re-bleeding occurs in 80%. They can be successfully obliterated endoscopically using argon plasma coagulation (see 📖 p. 12).

① Anastomotic bleeding

Occurs within 1mo of surgery, often following re-warfarinization or aspirin/clopidogrel use. Endoscopic therapy usually curtails bleeding.

☺ Aorto-enteric fistulation

This is an emergency. Suspect in any patient who has a known abdominal aortic aneurysm or aortic graft, presenting with severe rectal bleeding and hypotension. Request an immediate abdominal CT with contrast, which has very high sensitivity. Emergency diagnostic and therapeutic laparotomy is required in patients in whom there is a high index of suspicion, or in whom the degree of haemodynamic compromise renders them unsafe to delay for imaging studies.

① Rectal ulceration

Usually caused by repeated straining during defaecation, termed 'solitary rectal ulcer syndrome' (SRUS). Patients can present at any age and there is no gender difference. The incidence is ~1/100,000. A solitary rectal ulcer is seen endoscopically, and biopsies reveal characteristic features that confirm the diagnosis (particularly hypertrophy of the inner circular layer of the muscularis propria). Bleeding ulcers can be treated endoscopically, similarly to peptic ulcers (see 🕮 p. 12). Patients should be advised to avoid straining at stool, and try and open their bowels for no more than 5min, twice per day.

① Haemorrhoidal bleeding

This usually presents with painless, fresh rectal bleeding (see Colour plate 14). Anaemia is rare. The diagnosis is best made by proctoscopy. As haemorrhoids are common, all patients require at least a complete flexible sigmoidoscopy to exclude more proximal lesions. Treatment with band ligation or phenol injection is performed (for historical reasons) by the surgeons. Severe bleeding may require haemorrhoidectomy.

① Anal fissures

Presentation is characteristic with burning pain during defaecation associated with, at most, small-volume rectal bleeding. Anal sphincter spasm often makes digital rectal examination painful. Treatment with 0.4% topical GTN or topical diltiazem bd for 6wk is usually effective.

Co-morbidity and lower gastrointestinal bleeding

Inflammatory bowel disease

Bleeding in patients known to have IBD usually represents a flare of disease, although this is not always the case:

- Dysentery may result from infection with *Shigella*, *Campylobacter*, *Salmonella*, *Escherichia* (*E.*) *coli*, or *Entamoeba histolytica*. This occurs in <1% patients with relapses of IBD. However, stool cultures should routinely be performed to exclude an infective exacerbation.
- Similarly, *C. difficile*-associated diarrhoea is more common in patients with IBD and should be specifically excluded.
- Colon cancer occurs more commonly in patients with pan-colitis of >10y duration and can present with rectal bleeding following ulceration into a colonic arteriole.

Patients with a first presentation of IBD often present with rectal bleeding (more common in ulcerative colitis than Crohn's disease). Consider IBD in the following circumstances:

- Blood tests suggest inflammation ($\uparrow$CRP, ESR, leukocyte count, platelets; $\downarrow$albumin, Hb).
- Sub-acute history (weeks, not days).
- Family history of IBD.

Histology usually confirms the diagnosis. The management of IBD is described in Chapter 7.

HIV infection

See Chapter 12. Patients with a CD4 cell count <250 x 10^9/L are at risk of opportunistic pathogens, some of which can cause rectal bleeding. The commonest is CMV; others include HSV, *Salmonella*, *Yersinia*, *Shigella*, and *Campylobacter*. Kaposi's sarcoma causes rectal bleeding if located within the recto-sigmoid colon. Make sure the endoscopist is aware that samples need to be taken for both histology and viral PCR. Avoid placing biopsy forceps into formalin, which interferes with PCR reactions.

Infectious proctitis occurs in high-risk groups for sexually transmitted infection (sex workers, men who have sex with men (MSM)).

- In one survey of MSM with proctitis, gonorrhoea, *Chlamydia trachomatis* and HSV were each found in 10–20%. Syphilis was present in 1%.
- In 2005–6, an epidemic of lymphogranuloma venereum (caused by *Chlamydia*) occurred in promiscuous MSM, causing florid proctitis. Treatment is with doxycycline 100mg bd for 15d.
- At-risk patients should be referred for a sexual health screen.

Non-severe overt lower gastrointestinal bleeding

Likely causes are:
- Haemorrhoids. Painless, fresh bleeding associated with defaecation.
- Fissure. Painful defaecation.
- Left-sided colon polyps or cancer. Unlikely <50y unless strong family history. Cancer associated with change in bowel habit.
- Proctitis. Mucus, diarrhoea, urgency, and tenesmus.
- Rectal ulcers. Mucus, straining, tenesmus.

All patients need investigation. Request a colonoscopy in:
- Patients with a change in bowel habit of >3wk.
- Patients that required admission because of bleeding.
- Patients with 'alarm features' (see Box 2.1). These patients are more likely to have IBD or neoplasia.

In general, flexible sigmoidoscopy is reserved for young (<50–60y), stable patients with fresh outlet-type bleeding that is likely to be haemorrhoidal.

Acute lower gastrointestinal bleeding

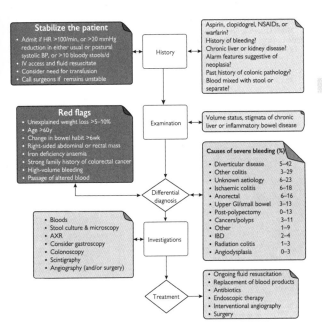

Stabilize the patient
- Admit if HR >100/min, or >20 mmHg reduction in either usual or postural systolic BP, or >10 bloody stools/d
- IV access and fluid resuscitate
- Consider need for transfusion
- Call surgeons if remains unstable

History

Aspirin, clopidogrel, NSAIDs, or warfarin?
History of bleeding?
Chronic liver or kidney disease?
Alarm features suggestive of neoplasia?
Past history of colonic pathology?
Blood mixed with stool or separate?

Red flags
- Unexplained weight loss >5–10%
- Age >60y
- Change in bowel habit >6wk
- Right-sided abdominal or rectal mass
- Iron deficiency anaemia
- Strong family history of colorectal cancer
- High-volume bleeding
- Passage of altered blood

Examination

Volume status, stigmata of chronic liver or inflammatory bowel disease

Causes of severe bleeding (%)
- Diverticular disease — 5–42
- Other colitis — 3–29
- Unknown aetiology — 6–23
- Ischaemic colitis — 6–18
- Anorectal — 6–16
- Upper GI/small bowel — 3–13
- Post-polypectomy — 0–13
- Cancers/polyps — 3–11
- Other — 1–9
- IBD — 2–4
- Radiation colitis — 1–3
- Angiodysplasia — 0–3

Differential diagnosis

- Bloods
- Stool culture & microscopy
- AXR
- Consider gastroscopy
- Colonoscopy
- Scintigraphy
- Angiography (and/or surgery)

Investigations

Treatment

- Ongoing fluid resuscitation
- Replacement of blood products
- Antibiotics
- Endoscopic therapy
- Interventional angiography
- Surgery

Further reading

Angtuaco TL, Reddy SK, Drapkin S, et al. (2001) The utility of urgent colonoscopy in the evaluation of acute lower gastroint©estinal tract bleeding: a 2-year experience from a single center. *Am J Gastroenterol* **96**: 1782–5.

Bloom S, Webster G, Marks D (2012) *Oxford Handbook of Gastroenterology and Hepatology*, 2e. Oxford University Press, Oxford.

Strate LL (2005) Lower GI bleeding: epidemiology and diagnosis. *Gastroenterol Clin North Am* **34**: 643–64

Severe iron deficiency anaemia

Implication of iron deficiency

In the developed world, the commonest cause of iron deficiency anaemia (IDA) and its prelude iron deficiency is menstrual blood loss. Worldwide, hookworm infection is prevalent and causes IDA in those with heavy parasite load. About 4% of men/post-menopausal women have iron deficiency, and 1–2% have related IDA. Iron deficiency rises to ~20% in pre-menopausal women (remainder often have considerably reduced iron stores).

In non-menstruating individuals, iron deficiency usually reflects gradual GI blood loss. As such, it is a marker for GI tract abnormalities, especially peptic ulceration and colonic malignancy (the latter found in 12%, especially with ferritin <10µg/L, LDH >250U/L, and in the elderly).

Causes of iron deficiency

Blood loss
- Menorrhagia.
- GI losses (benign or malignant).
- Persistent overt bleeding (e.g. recurrent epistaxis).
- Pregnancy, parturition.
- Post-menopausal bleeding (uterine malignancy).
- Post-surgical.
- Repeated blood donation.

Decreased iron absorption
- Low-iron diet (vegetarian).
- Malabsorption (suspect if refractory to oral iron replacement):
  - Atrophic or *Helicobacter (H.) pylori* gastritis.
  - Villous atrophy (coeliac disease, Whipple's disease, tropical sprue).
  - Bacterial overgrowth.
  - Foods (phytates in bran, oats, or rye; polyphenols in tea; soy).
  - Medication impairing iron absorption (calcium-containing antacids).

Rare causes
- Intravascular haemolysis with haemoglobinuria/siderinuria (paroxysmal nocturnal haemoglobinuria, prosthetic heart valves).
- Pulmonary haemosiderosis (e.g. Goodpasture's disease).
- Post-erythropoietin treatment in chronic renal disease.
- Gastric bypass surgery.
- Renal tract bleeding (including renal cell carcinoma).
- Congenital conditions causing defective absorption.

No diagnosis is made in ~20%.

Overt or occult bleeding

Patients with large-volume bleeding present acutely with symptoms and signs of haemodynamic compromise; there is usually insufficient time to develop iron deficiency. Small-volume, overt bleeding (e.g. chronic haemorrhoidal bleeding) can cause IDA. Normally, 1–2mg iron is absorbed daily, equivalent to 3–5mL whole blood. Iron stores are ~1g in males/post-menopausal women. Hence, persistent daily loss of >5mL blood leads to iron deficiency. Note that up to 100mL blood loss/d can still result in normal-looking stools.

Iron deficiency has been shown in those >65y to be a frequent marker for GI tract disease (Joosten et al., 1999). There is a lower frequency of abnormalities in younger patients with iron deficiency. Iron deficiency and mild IDA (Hb >10g/dL) are only investigated in menstruating females with another alarm symptom (e.g. weight loss, abdominal pain, change in bowel habit, rectal bleeding). Post-menopausal women and men of any age with iron deficiency require investigation unless there is a likely explanation and no alarm symptoms. Temporary iron deficiency is common following a prolonged gastroenteritic illness.

Diagnosing iron deficiency

Haematinics (iron studies, B12, red cell folate) and ferritin should be measured in any patient found to be anaemic. Iron studies and ferritin should be checked in those with red cell microcytosis. The MCV is usually normal in iron deficiency but can be between 70–80fL. In thalassaemia trait, Hb and MCV are usually ~11g/dL and <75fL, respectively, with normal or raised iron and normal or raised RBC count. Request Hb electrophoresis if likely (raised HbA2 with β-thalassaemia). Request haematology opinion to exclude sideroblastic anaemia if microcytic, normal iron stores, and thalassaemia excluded. Request B12, red cell folate, TFT, γGT, and a blood film in those with macrocytosis. It is very unusual to require bone marrow measurement of iron stores to diagnose IDA.

Iron indices in IDA typically demonstrate increased total iron binding capacity (TIBC, also known as transferrin), reduced serum iron, and reduced iron saturation. Note that pregnancy and OCP use increase TIBC, which can be misinterpreted as IDA. Ferritin below the normal range (in the absence of inflammation, infection, liver or malignant disease) is virtually pathognomonic for iron deficiency (<40ng/mL, 98% specific and 98% sensitive). Do not discount iron deficiency because of a normal TIBC, as this reflects transferrin synthesis by the liver, which can be impaired in chronic disease or inflammation.

Iron indices in anaemia of chronic disease (ACD) demonstrate reduced TIBC, reduced serum iron, and normal or low saturation. Often, the indices of ACD are misinterpreted as IDA; diagnose the former if ferritin >100ng/mL with saturation >20%.

Presentation and investigations

Emergency presentation
Rare due to haemodynamic compensation that occurs as Hb concentration falls. May arise with co-morbidity (e.g. angina with ischaemic heart disease, dyspnoea with left ventricular failure).

History and examination
- May be asymptomatic.
- Can present with:
  - Lethargy, weakness.
  - Dyspnoea, particularly exertional.
  - Headache.
  - Pica (in 32%; pica for ice more specific and seen in 28%).
  - Glossal pain, xerostoma.
  - Pruritus, restless leg syndrome.
- Beeturia (red urine after eating beetroot), although rare, is more common in iron deficiency, caused by increased GI absorption of betanin without systemic decolourization due to limited ferric ions.
- In pre-menstrual women, establish whether periods are heavy or light, and their duration.
- Ask about gastric and duodenal ulceration, *H. pylori* status, coeliac disease, chronic liver disease and portal hypertension, blood donation, and family history of bleeding diatheses (von Willebrand disease, hereditary haemorrhagic telangiectasia) and colonic neoplasia.
- Take a drug history, including use of over-the-counter medications (particularly aspirin and NSAIDs). Bisphosphonates and potassium salts also injure the gastric mucosa.

Examination may reveal:
- Conjunctival pallor.
- Atrophy of tongue papillae.
- Stomatitis.
- Alopecia.
- Tachycardia.
- Postural hypotension.
- Koilonychia, indicative of chronic, severe IDA (now rare).
- Mucocutaneous stigmata of GI disease: dermatitis herpetiformis, Peutz–Jegher lentigines, telangiectasia.
- Plummer–Vinson (≈ Patterson–Kelly) syndrome, now very rare; characterized by dysphagia due to an oesophageal web, atrophic glossitis, and IDA.

Investigations
- FBC. Anaemia, usually microcytic; can have normal MCV if dimorphic picture (look for elevated RDW); may be associated with mild thrombocytosis.
- U & E (renal impairment).
- LFT (hypoalbuminaemia).
- Haematinics (see Table 3.1).

- Blood film. RBCs microcytic and hypochromic. Target and pencil cells may be seen in severe anaemia.
- Anti-tissue transglutaminase (TTG) antibodies for coeliac disease.
- Screen for haemolysis (reticulocytes, LDH, haptoglobin, DAT).

Table 3.1 Interpretation of iron indices

Diagnosis	Iron	TIBC	IBS	Ferritin
Iron deficiency	↓	↑	↓	↓
ACD	↓	↓	↓	N/↑
Haemolytic anaemia	↑	N/↓	↑	↑
Sideroblastic anaemia	N/↑	N/↓	↑	↑

IBS, iron-binding saturation; N, normal.

Often, IDA is diagnosed incidentally when blood tests are performed for another reason. Once diagnosed, decide the following:

① Is inpatient care required?

Admit patients with haemodynamic compromise (HR >100/min without another explanation), those with end-organ ischaemic damage, and those with Hb <7g/dL. Have a lower threshold in the elderly or those with co-morbidity (especially heart disease). Provide blood transfusion to Hb >8g/dL.

Which investigations, and when should they occur?

Urgent, but not immediate, investigation is warranted, as some causes of IDA are serious. Perform within 2wk.

- Request gastroscopy and colonoscopy unless there is another clear cause for IDA. This should include D2 biopsies to look for coeliac disease unless anti-TTG known to be negative.
- In general, substitute CT colonography for colonoscopy in those >80y.
- There is no role for faecal occult blood testing, as consequences of false negative results are profound.
- If likely cause for anaemia discovered at gastroscopy, still proceed to lower GI investigation as concomitant disease occurs, especially in the elderly.
- Capsule endoscopy should be reserved for those in whom iron therapy is unable to maintain Hb >10g/dL, or in those in whom a significant small bowel lesion is suspected (e.g. weight loss, abdominal pain). Perform a prior patency capsule if Crohn's disease suspected (capsule retention 9%).
- Angiography and red cell scintigraphy are rarely helpful, as they lack sensitivity for bleeds <2mL/min. Contrast radiography similarly has low yield. Consider Meckel's scan in patients where no bleeding source is found.
- Check for microscopic haematuria (renal cell cancer causes ~1% IDA).
- Request echocardiogram in those with suspected valvular heart disease. Turbulent flow across stenosed valves shears von Willebrand

protein complexes, reducing the amount available to enable normal platelet function, resulting in ongoing bleeding from GI angiodysplasia.

Should all patients be investigated?

Pre-menopausal women do not require investigation unless amenorrhoeic or alarm symptoms present. Patients with documented, stable long-term (>3y) iron deficiency may not need investigation, especially if likely explanation present (e.g. aspirin use). Patients with a clear cause for iron deficiency and no alarm symptoms can defer investigation as long as iron deficiency does not recur following attempted correction of the underlying aetiology.

What to do with negative investigations?

Investigations should only be repeated if patients become transfusion-dependent or new alarm symptoms develop.

Treatment

There are two principles: prevent ongoing loss and replace iron.

Preventing iron loss

- Request dietetic assessment if dietary intake reduced.
- Treat malabsorption if present.
- Remove or ablate bleeding diathesis (e.g. surgery for malignant lesion, endoscopic therapy of angiodysplasia).
- Remove any predisposing factors (e.g. NSAIDs).
- If above not possible, try medical therapy (tranexamic acid 1g PO tds).

Iron replacement

- Provide non-enteric, coated oral iron (e.g. ferrous sulphate 200mg PO tds), taken with an empty stomach.
- Avoid concomitant antacids, milk, tea, or coffee.
- Ascorbic acid 250mg PO with each dose of iron will increase absorption.
- Elixirs are available and may lessen GI side effects that occur in ~10% (e.g. Sytron® 10mL in a small glass of orange juice PO 30min before breakfast, lunch, and supper).
- Provide iron for 6wk if wish to correct anaemia, and exclude ongoing losses (i.e. to be sure cause for blood loss resolved); or for 3mo if wish to replenish iron stores, although ability to exclude ongoing loss will be delayed.
- Confirm Hb increase (2–4g/dL after 3wk). If not, consider the following:
  - Poor compliance.
  - Poor iron absorption ('absorption test': >100µg/dL increment in fasting serum iron 4h post-ingestion of 325mg ferrous sulphate).
  - Incorrect diagnosis.
  - Net ongoing iron losses.
  - Coexistent ACD or renal impairment.

Provide IV therapy if:
- Oral treatment not tolerated or effective.
- Consider in patients with IBD (oral therapy may precipitate flare).
- In dialysis patients.
- When oral therapy provides inadequate replacement due to more rapid blood loss (e.g. if requiring blood transfusion more often than every 2wk).

IV formulations include Ferinject® and Monofer®. The latter allows up to a 5g/dL increment in Hb for a 70kg person following a single infusion; serious adverse events are infrequent and no test dose is required. Check FBC after 2–3wk to show appropriate increment in Hb (~1g/dL per wk). Check FBC after another 3wk, and FBC and iron studies at 3 and 6mo, to exclude recurrence of anaemia.

Use of anticoagulation and antiplatelet agents
- If possible, avoid using anticoagulants, NSAIDs, aspirin, or clopidogrel in patients found to have IDA until the cause has been established.
- Those with existing metallic heart valves or coronary artery stents require prior discussion with cardiology before discontinuing these medications.
- If antiplatelet agents are required, provide PPI cover (e.g. omeprazole 20mg PO bd) until gastroscopy performed; test for *H. pylori* first.
- Expedite investigations in those who urgently require antiplatelets (e.g. awaiting coronary angiography).

Anaemia of chronic disease

ACD is often confused with IDA. ACD is common in medical patients, characterized by reduction in TIBC as well as serum iron and saturation (saturation is normal in 20%). TIBC is normal or raised in IDA. However, some patients have a mixture of ACD and IDA; suspect if the TIBC is low, but serum iron and saturation are very low. A trial of iron therapy may be required to establish whether IDA is present, with a resultant increase in Hb. Evidence supports the use of erythropoietin in ACD patients with renal failure or chemotherapy-associated anaemia, providing iron stores are normal.

Severe iron deficiency anaemia

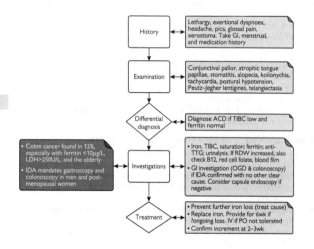

History ↔ Lethargy, exertional dyspnoea, headache, pica, glossal pain, xerostoma. Take GI, menstrual, and medication history

Examination ↔ Conjunctival pallor, atrophic tongue papillae, stomatitis, alopecia, koilonychia, tachycardia, postural hypotension, Peutz–Jegher lentigines, telangiectasia

Differential diagnosis ↔ Diagnose ACD if TIBC low and ferritin normal

Investigations ↔
- Iron, TIBC, saturation; ferritin; anti-TTG; urinalysis. If RDW increased, also check B12, red cell folate, blood film
- GI investigation (OGD & colonoscopy) if IDA confirmed with no other clear cause. Consider capsule endoscopy if negative

(left box) ↔
- Colon cancer found in 12%, especially with ferritin <10µg/L, LDH>250U/L, and the elderly
- IDA mandates gastroscopy and colonoscopy in men and post-menopausal women

Treatment ↔
- Prevent further iron loss (treat cause)
- Replace iron. Provide for 6wk if ?ongoing loss. IV if PO not tolerated
- Confirm increment at 2–3wk

Further reading

Joosten E, Ghesquiere B, Linthoudt H, *et al.* (1999) Upper and lower gastrointestinal evaluation of elderly inpatients who are iron deficient. *Am J Med* **107**: 24–9.

Severe vomiting

Pathophysiology

Vomiting is a reflex behaviour coordinated by the vomiting centre in the medulla oblongata (see Fig. 4.1). It may be triggered by afferent inputs from chemo- or mechano-receptors in the upper GI tract, by activation of the chemoreceptor trigger zone (located in the area postrema, adjacent to the fourth ventricle) or by inputs from vestibular centres. The area postrema is rich in dopamine receptors, and the vestibular centres in 5-hydroxytryptamine (5-HT) receptors; these are the targets of most anti-emetic medications.

Initiation of the vomiting reflex leads to a wave of reverse peristalsis, commencing in the middle of the small intestine. The pyloric sphincter and stomach relax to receive intestinal contents. Forceful contraction of abdominal muscles then elevates intra-abdominal pressure, driving gastric contents towards the oesophagus. Simultaneously, the lower oesophageal sphincter relaxes, and the gastric pylorus and antrum contract. Peripheral dopamine receptors play important roles in orchestrating these processes.

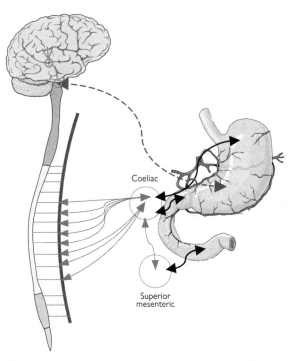

Fig. 4.1 Neurological control of the foregut. Sympathetic control of the foregut arises from the thoracic spinal cord. The sympathetic chain (light grey line) connects to the coeliac and superior mesenteric ganglia via the splanchnic nerves (dark grey arrows). Post-ganglionic fibres (black arrows) innervate the stomach, small bowel, and proximal colon. Efferent sympathetic nerves inhibit intestinal motility; afferent nerves transmit nociceptive stimuli. Parasympathetic stimulation increases GI motility, mediated by the vagus nerve. Afferent nerves (dashed arrows) synapse in the nucleus tractus solitarius in the medulla; thereafter, fibres travel to the area postrema chemoreceptor trigger zone). This connects with higher centres. Vomiting is initiated by efferent vagal nerve fibres. Reprinted from Medicine, 37, 2, Marcus Harbord, 'Nausea and vomiting', pp.115–118. Copyright 2009, with permission from Elsevier.

Clinical assessment

History
Ask about:
- *Duration.* Onset within hours (and up to 3d) usually suggests gastroenteritis, especially if associated diarrhoea.
- *Timing.* Early morning vomiting may occur in normal pregnancy, hyperemesis gravidarum, or raised intracranial pressure. Regurgitation of food contents during or immediately after a meal is usually due to oesophageal obstruction or motility disorders but may be psychogenic. Vomiting 30min to several hours after a meal may result from impaired gastric emptying, presence of a foodborne pre-formed toxin, small bowel obstruction, or biliary disease.
- *Nature of vomitus.* Recognizable food suggests oesophageal disease or gastric stasis. Bilious vomiting implies proximal bowel obstruction, and faeculent material distal small bowel or large intestinal obstruction. For investigation and management of haematemesis, see Chapter 1.
- *Force of expulsion.* Consider a CNS cause with projectile vomiting (often without nausea). In infants (but not adults), this frequently characterizes pyloric stenosis.
- *Distinguish vomiting from regurgitation.* Regurgitation refers to return of small amounts of food or secretions into the hypopharynx; it is effortless without the muscular activity that accompanies vomiting and may be associated with a sour taste in the mouth but not nausea. It occurs in obstructive and motility disorders of the oesophagus, gastro-oesophageal acid or alkaline reflux, and psychogenic disorders.
- *Pain.* The pain of peptic ulceration is typically epigastric and may be relieved by vomiting. Gastric ulcers classically cause pain at mealtimes and consequent weight loss due to food avoidance. Duodenal ulceration is associated with night-time pain and weight gain, as food intake stimulates neutralizing alkaline bicarbonate secretion. Severe RUQ/back pain may be caused by posterior duodenal ulceration, choledocholithiasis, pancreatitis, or pancreatic cancer. Central, colicky abdominal pain, associated with borborygmi and profuse bilious vomiting, suggests small bowel obstruction or infarction; vomiting due to large bowel obstruction occurs after absolute constipation and abdominal distension have developed. Consider non-GI causes, including ureteric colic, pyelonephritis, and pneumonia.
- *Associated symptoms.* Diarrhoea suggests an infective cause but rarely may be seen in patients with IBD or primary metabolic disturbances. Vomiting with constipation should prompt consideration of bowel obstruction: have a high index of suspicion in patients with colicky abdominal pain if not passing flatus. Severe constipation, in itself, can be a primary cause of vomiting. Headache may suggest a neurological cause: headache worse in the morning and on lying flat, sneezing, coughing, or straining is typical of raised intracranial pressure; there may be associated visual disturbance or focal neurological signs, and nausea may be absent.

- *Appetite.* Most patients with nausea and vomiting have reduced appetite. While appetite can be preserved in bowel obstruction, normal appetite should raise suspicion of a psychogenic cause.
- *Weight.* Weight gain suggests the absence of serious organic disease, although it may be seen in patients with duodenal ulceration or ascites.
- *Exacerbating and relieving factors.* Recent surgery or electrolyte disturbances can cause ileus and pseudo-obstruction.
- *Past medical history.* Previous surgery is important (may predispose to reduced gastric capacity, or bowel obstruction through herniae or intra-abdominal adhesions), as is a history of gallstones, coeliac disease, or IBD.
- *Drug history.* Common offenders include opiates, antibiotics, aspirin and NSAIDs, chemotherapeutic drugs, and digoxin toxicity.
- *Social factors.* Information regarding home, family, and work environments may be important in identifying a psychogenic cause; previous physical or sexual abuse constitute high risk.

Examination

Assess:
- *Volume status.* Look for evidence of dehydration (tachycardia, tachypnoea, postural or overt hypotension). Document weight.
- *Oral cavity.* Examine for dentition (tooth destruction often implies chronicity), stigmata of immunocompromise (candidiasis, oral hairy leukoplakia, Kaposi's sarcoma), and for peri-oral pigmentation (Peutz–Jegher).
- *Abdomen.* Determine whether there is any distension, tenderness, or peritonism. Listen for bowel sounds (tinkling in mechanical obstruction, absent in ileus) and a gastric succussion splash. Digital rectal examination is required in any patient in whom obstruction is suspected.
- *Fundoscopy.* Check for papilloedema and absence of retinal vein pulsation, as both suggest raised intracranial pressure (although their absence does not rule it out).
- Request bedside testing of capillary blood glucose and, in all women of childbearing potential, urinary β-HCG.

Differential diagnosis

- GI disorders:
  - Oesophageal pathology (stricture, achalasia, Chagas disease).
  - Impaired gastric emptying (gastric outlet obstruction, pyloric stenosis, gastroparesis, surgical reduction of gastric capacity).
  - Upper GI haemorrhage (see Chapter 1).
  - Acid or alkaline reflux disease.
  - Coeliac disease.
  - Food poisoning and gastroenteritis (see Chapter 6).
  - Intestinal obstruction or ileus (see Chapter 9).
  - Acute appendicitis.
- Hepatopancreatobiliary and urinary tract disease:
  - Gallstone disease (biliary colic, cholecystitis).
  - Pancreatitis, pancreatic cancer.
  - Acute liver failure.
  - Ureteric colic, UTI, pyelonephritis.
- Non-GI infections:
  - Pneumonia.
  - Septicaemia.
- Endocrine and metabolic disturbances:
  - Metabolic acidosis, including diabetic ketoacidosis.
  - Addison's disease.
  - Hyperthyroidism.
  - Hypercalcaemia.
- Neurological:
  - Raised intracranial pressure (space-occupying lesion, obstructive hydrocephalus, benign intracranial hypertension, cerebral venous sinus thrombosis).
  - CNS infection (meningitis, encephalitis).
  - Intracranial haemorrhage.
  - Migraine.
  - Vestibular (motion sickness, viral labyrinthitis, benign positional vertigo, Ménière's disease).
- Pregnancy-related vomiting:
  - Normal pregnancy (first trimester).
  - Hyperemesis gravidarum.
  - Pregnancy-related liver disease (see Chapter 19).
- Drug-induced:
  - Alcohol.
  - Antibiotics.
  - Aspirin, NSAIDs.
  - Centrally acting (opiates, digoxin, levodopa, chemotherapy).
- Functional and psychological disorders:
  - GI motility disorders.
  - Anorexia and bulimia nervosa.
  - Cyclical vomiting syndrome.
  - Somatoform and factitious disorders.

Investigation

These are guided by the differential diagnosis suggested by history and examination and may include:

- Blood tests:
  - FBC may demonstrate anaemia, which should be followed up with full haematinics. Iron deficiency found in gastritis, peptic ulceration, malignancy, or small intestinal disease (often also associated with folate or B12 deficiency). Raised MCV can correlate with alcohol misuse.
  - U & E contribute to assessment of hydration and risk of acute kidney injury. Severe vomiting can cause hyponatraemia and hypokalaemia. Consider Addison's disease in patients with hyponatraemia but elevated or 'inappropriately normal' K^+.
  - LFT, calcium, TFT, and amylase may reveal underlying aetiology.
  - In patients with elevated capillary blood glucose, check for urinary ketones, and perform VBG or ABG to measure pH to look for diabetic ketoacidosis.
  - In febrile patients, consider a broad septic screen, including blood cultures, as vomiting can be a sign of systemic infection.
- Imaging:
  - A plain abdominal X-ray should be requested if there is clinical suspicion of obstruction. If abnormal, follow up with CT.
  - US is the modality of choice for initial investigation of the liver and biliary tree.
  - Request a low-dose CT KUB if the history suggests ureteric colic.
  - In patients in whom intracranial pathology is suspected, the most appropriate initial scan is usually a contrast-enhanced CT (although if available, MRI avoids radiation risk, especially important in young patients). If this is normal, lumbar puncture, including measurement of opening pressure, may be required.
- Endoscopy and functional GI studies:
  - Upper GI endoscopy may help identify peptic ulceration or other mucosal disease but is a poor test of function.
  - Barium studies are better for assessment of upper GI stasis and obstruction. These may require follow-up with oesophageal function tests (manometry, pH) or gastric emptying scintigraphy.

General management

The following general principles apply:
- Several classes of anti-emetic are available for symptomatic relief.
- Where possible, identify the underlying cause and institute specific therapy.
- Avoid precipitants, including emetogenic drugs and alcohol.
- Correct volume depletion and electrolyte disturbances.
- Psychological input may be valuable in patients with functional disorders.

Anti-emetic medications

- Antihistamines:
  - Act on vestibular centres and the chemoreceptor trigger zone. Effective for management of general nausea and vomiting, treatment of motion sickness and primary vestibular disorders.
  - May cause sedation and anti-muscarinic side effects (dry eyes and mouth, tachycardia, urinary retention, and confusion in the elderly).
  - *Cyclizine* 50mg tds may be administered PO, SC, IM, or IV. Its physicochemical properties are compatible with a number of other medications useful for symptom control and, therefore, it is a useful drug if required for a syringe driver in palliative care medicine. Avoid in patients with severe heart failure. Be aware that IV administration is potentially addictive, and some patients develop cyclizine-seeking behaviours.
  - *Cinnarizine* 15–30mg PO tds is useful for treatment of motion sickness and vestibular disorders.
  - *Hyoscine hydrobromide* patches 1mg/72h may be used for prevention of motion sickness; apply 5–6h prior to journey.
- Dopamine antagonists:
  - Act centrally on D2 receptors in the chemoreceptor trigger zone and peripherally on those modulating motility in the GI tract. Extremely useful for treating nausea and vomiting associated with gastroparesis, and gastroduodenal and biliary disease, where peripheral prokinetic effects are particularly beneficial.
  - Adverse effects include acute dystonic reactions (including facial and skeletal muscle spasms), oculogyric crises (more common in the young and very old, may require procyclidine 5–10mg IM/IV to abort), Parkinsonism, hyperprolactinaemia, and (rarely) neuroleptic malignant syndrome.
  - Contraindicated in breastfeeding women, mechanical bowel obstruction, and phaeochromocytoma.
  - *Metoclopramide* 10mg PO/IM/IV tds. Parenteral formulations readily available.
  - *Domperidone* 10–20mg PO/PR tds has better side effect profile than metoclopramide, as it penetrates the blood-brain barrier poorly.
  - *Prochlorperazine* is a phenothiazine that is particularly effective for acute labyrinthitis and other vestibular disorders. Administer

20mg PO or 12.5mg IM for treatment of an acute attack, then 5–10mg PO bd/tds if further prevention required. Be aware, however, that long-term use in chronic vestibular disorders can impede adaptation.

- *Levomepromazine* 6–25mg PO/24h or 6.25mg SC bd is a useful second-line drug for chemotherapy-induced vomiting and in palliative care.

- Serotonin receptor antagonists:
  - Block 5-HT$_3$ receptor-dependent afferent impulses to the chemoreceptor trigger zone. Potent anti-emetics, particularly for post-operative and chemotherapy-induced nausea and vomiting. Also have specific role in the treatment of nausea and vomiting associated with carcinoid tumours.
  - Side effects include constipation, which may be severe (particularly in patients on concurrent opiates). Use with caution in patients with cardiac disease as may prolong QT interval. Contraindicated in severe liver impairment.
  - *Ondansetron* 4–8mg PO/SC/IM/IV tds is the routine dose. Can administer 16mg by slow IV injection 1h preoperatively.
  - *Granisetron* 2–9mg/24h PO/IV in divided doses.

- Drugs for specific indications:
  - *Lorazepam* 1–2mg PO/IV is effective for anticipatory nausea and vomiting in patients receiving chemotherapy.
  - *Dexamethasone* 4–8mg PO/IV is a useful anti-emetic to cover general anaesthesia, delayed nausea and vomiting associated with cytotoxic chemotherapy (continue for 3–5d), and for vomiting caused by raised intracranial pressure (particularly when there is substantial vasogenic oedema).
  - *Aprepitant* is a neurokinin (NK1) receptor antagonist, licensed as an adjunct to dexamethasone and 5-HT$_3$ receptor antagonists, for prevention of acute and delayed nausea and vomiting associated with chemotherapy or the post-operative period. Administer 125mg PO 1h prior to chemotherapy or 3h prior to surgery, then 80mg od for the next 2d.

① ⚙ ☠ Complications

Deleterious consequences of severe vomiting include:
- Volume depletion and electrolyte disturbance.
- Mucosal injury and bleeding (including Mallory–Weiss tears).
- Aspiration pneumonitis and pneumonia.
- Oesophageal rupture (Boerhaave's syndrome) (see Chapter 8).

ℹ️ **Other gastrointestinal causes of vomiting**

Gastroparesis

Nausea and vomiting may result from impaired gastric motility in the absence of mechanical obstruction or inflammation. Suspect gastroparesis in patients with symptoms shortly after eating, in whom endoscopy and barium studies are normal. Diagnosis is usually clinical, although scintigraphic gastric emptying studies remain the gold standard. Specialist centres occasionally perform antroduodenal motility tests or electrogastrography to confirm slowed muscular activity, but these are not routine in clinical practice. Diabetes is the commonest cause: ~25% of insulin-dependent patients with coexistent peripheral neuropathy have upper GI symptoms suggestive of autonomic involvement, and up to 50% of all diabetic patients demonstrate delayed emptying on scintigraphy.

Treatment involves:
- Dietary measures: small, frequent meals and maintenance of hydration.
- Tight glycaemic control.
- Prokinetic agents (taken 15–30min before meals):
  - Metoclopramide 10mg PO tds or domperidone 10–20mg PO tds.
  - Erythromycin 250mg PO tds.
- Cholinergic agonists and anticholinesterases are occasionally trialled on an individual patient basis but not widely used. The 5-HT$_4$ receptor antagonist prucalopride is currently under evaluation.
- NJ or jejunostomy tubes are occasionally required.
- Surgical insertion of a gastric pacemaker has been shown to improve symptoms in up to 50% patients with intractable vomiting.

ℹ️ **Gastric outlet obstruction**

Gastric outlet obstruction can result from benign stricturing disease or malignancy. Symptoms include nausea, vomiting, early satiety, weight loss, and epigastric pain on eating. A succussion splash may be elicited on physical examination. Electrolyte disturbances can be profound, with hypokalaemic hypochloraemic metabolic alkalosis (gastric HCl loss results in compensatory renal $NaHCO_3$ and $KHCO_3$ loss). Causes include:
- Benign:
  - Peptic ulcer disease.
  - Gastric polyps.
  - Caustic stricture.
  - Pyloric stenosis (usually due to peptic ulcer disease or gastric cancer in adults; hypertrophy is rare, in contrast to infants).
  - TB.
  - Crohn's disease.
  - Amyloidosis.
  - Duodenal webs.
  - Gallstones (Bouveret's syndrome).
  - Pancreatic pseudocyst.
  - Foreign body or bezoar.

- Malignant:
  - Gastric adenocarcinoma (including linitis plastica).
  - Pancreatic carcinoma.
  - Ampullary or duodenal adenocarcinoma, cholangiocarcinoma.
  - Lymphoma.
  - GIST.

The diagnosis may be established by barium contrast study, but CT is more useful as it can reveal extrinsic obstructing lesions. OGD can be diagnostic (allowing direct visualization of an obstructing lesion and tissue sampling for histology) and therapeutic (placing a stent or feeding tube), but often requires a prolonged fast ± gastric decompression via a wide-bore nasal tube.

Management includes:
- Correction of fluid and electrolyte imbalances.
- NG intubation to decompress stomach if very distended.
- Maintenance of nutrition (may require NJ tube, PEJ, or PN).
- Acid suppression with PPI and/or H_2 receptor blocker.
- Endoscopic balloon dilatation. Caution in malignant strictures as higher risk of perforation. Effective in pyloric stenosis for short-term relief, although recurrence in ~80% unless additional therapy provided (PPI for peptic ulcer disease; stenting in malignant disease).
- Surgical antrectomy, pyloroplasty, or gastrojejunostomy for definitive correction. Pyloromyotomy may be attempted in pyloric stenosis.

⊙ Gastroenteritis
See Chapter 6.

⚙ Bowel obstruction
See Chapter 9.

Vomiting in pregnancy

Nausea and vomiting are common in normal pregnancy, occurring in 50–90% and 22–55%, respectively. Symptoms most frequently commence in the first trimester between wk 6–8, peak during wk 9, and settle by wk 12. Although often known as 'morning sickness', symptoms may persist throughout the day. Most cases are self-limiting and require no specific investigation. Mild symptoms respond to reassurance, maintenance of oral hydration, and dietary change (small regular meals, avoid food triggers).

⊙ Hyperemesis gravidarum
Occurs in 0.3–2% of pregnancies and characterized by intractable vomiting and ketosis. It is more common in multiple pregnancies. Dehydration can be severe, and women may lose >5% of their pre-pregnancy weight. Electrolyte disturbances can be life-threatening and include hyponatraemia, hypokalaemia, and hypochloraemic metabolic alkalosis. Substantially reduced dietary intake confers risk of Wernicke's encephalopathy. Women

who are severely dehydrated and ketotic need to be assessed in hospital.
Management involves:
• Fluid replacement. Normal saline is the most appropriate initial fluid;
  starting with glucose solutions risks worsening hyponatraemia and
  precipitating Wernicke's encephalopathy.
• Electrolyte replacement. U & E should be monitored once or twice
  daily, depending on severity of derangement. Hyponatraemia is almost
  always due to upper GI losses and should correct with IV replacement.
  Hypokalaemia should be treated by adding 40mmol KCl to each litre
  of fluid until plasma concentrations are restored to normal.
• Re-check urinary ketones daily.
• Thiamine supplementation. Should be administered routinely to all
  women admitted for prolonged vomiting. Prescribe oral thiamine
  100mg bd if able to tolerate by mouth; otherwise Pabrinex® IV.
• Anti-emetics. See 'Anti-emetics in pregnant women', 📖 p. 56.
• Thromboprophylaxis. Pregnancy and dehydration both increase risk
  of venous thromboembolic disease; prophylactic doses of LMWH and
  thromboembolic stockings are appropriate.
• Nutritional support. Usually not required, but rarely TPN has been
  needed in prolonged, refractory cases.
• Pregnancy outcomes are usually unaffected, although there is a risk of
  fetal growth restriction if malnutrition is profound.

Other causes of severe vomiting in pregnancy

Nausea and vomiting may result from the same conditions that affect non-
pregnant women. Also consider whether they are manifestations of:
• UTI.
• Molar pregnancy.
• Pre-eclampsia (check BP, urine for protein).
• Pregnancy-associated liver disease (see Chapter 19).

Anti-emetics in pregnant women

There are substantial data showing that most anti-emetics are safe in pregnancy but little evidence that any is superior:
• Cyclizine, metoclopramide, and prochlorperazine have been
  extensively used and are appropriate first-line agents.
• 5-HT$_3$ receptor antagonists, such as ondansetron, are effective.
  Teratogenicity is not generally recognized, although there is less
  experience with these agents.
• PPIs and H$_2$ blockers are useful adjuncts in women with dyspepsia.
• Ginger root and acupressure are effective for nausea and vomiting in
  normal pregnancy, but there is no convincing evidence in hyperemesis.
• Pyridoxine 20mg PO tds ameliorates nausea and vomiting, both in
  normal pregnancy and hyperemesis gravidarum.
• Steroids (hydrocortisone 100mg IV bd) may improve symptoms but
  should be limited to intractable cases.

① **Nausea and vomiting in the cancer patient**

Over 50% of patients with advanced cancer experience nausea and vomiting. In 80%, this is due to one of the following:

- Intestinal obstruction. In advanced disease, clinical signs can be masked by multiple intra-abdominal malignant adhesions. Abdominal distension may be minimal and bowel sounds can be normal, and some patients present with diarrhoea rather than constipation.
- Gastric stasis. Dysmotility can arise as a side effect of medication (particularly opioids and anti-muscarinics), electrolyte disturbance, or autonomic or visceral neuropathy. Neuropathy may result from spinal cord compression, bulky retroperitoneal disease, adenocarcinoma of the pancreatic head, or paraneoplastic phenomena.
- Drugs (see 'Differential diagnosis', 📖 p. 50).
- Biochemical abnormalities (particularly hypercalcaemia).
- Cerebral metastases or primary tumours elevating intracranial pressure.

In general, treatment is directed at correcting reversible causes (e.g. modifying medication, draining ascites, and treating hypercalcaemia). However, these should be guided by patient wishes, and active interventions may not be appropriate for individuals who are dying.

Surgery for bowel obstruction is reasonable if there is an easily reversible cause (such as post-operative adhesions or a single discrete neoplastic obstruction) and the patient has good performance status. It is contraindicated if previous laparotomy findings preclude the prospect of successful intervention, or in the presence of diffuse intra-abdominal carcinomatosis or massive ascites that re-accumulates rapidly following paracentesis.

The approach to anti-emetic therapy is similar to that described in 'General management' (see 📖 p. 52). Non-drug measures (making sure the patient is not assailed by food odours, advising small frequent portions at mealtimes, and acupressure) can all improve symptom burden. In the palliative patient, medications should usually be administered orally or subcutaneously. In individuals able to request symptom control medication targeted to when they need it, prescribe 'as required' (PRN) initially to quantify daily requirements. These can then be converted into regular dosing or long-acting preparations if symptoms are expected to be protracted or irreversible. For patients requiring regular doses of subcutaneous medication, consider setting up a syringe driver containing the total daily dose running over 24h to minimize peaks and troughs of efficacy. The following may help target anti-emetics more effectively:

- Prokinetics (domperidone, metoclopramide, haloperidol) are particularly useful for patients with gastritis, gastric stasis, or functional bowel obstruction. They may worsen symptoms in mechanical bowel obstruction.
- Haloperidol 1.5–3mg PO/SC bd is helpful for chemical causes of nausea and vomiting, including drug side effects, renal failure, and hypercalcaemia. Avoid if risk of seizures.

- Antihistamine medications (such as cyclizine) are useful for patients with mechanical bowel obstruction, raised intracranial pressure, or motion sickness. Hyoscine butylbromide 20mg PO/SC qds prn or 80–160mg/24h as a SC/IV infusion in palliative care relieves colicky abdominal pain. Avoid using antihistamines with anti-muscarinic properties (such as cyclizine) concurrent with drugs for prokinetic effect, as the former block the final common pathway through which prokinetics act.
- 5-HT$_3$ receptor antagonists (such as ondansetron) are very effective for chemotherapy- and radiotherapy-related nausea and vomiting, but may cause profound constipation.
- If there is little or no benefit with the initial anti-emetic regime despite dose optimization, consider whether the presumed cause of symptoms is correct. If not, change to a more appropriate first-line drug. Otherwise, add in another first-line agent.
- If optimal control is still not achieved, consider use of levomepromazine 6–12.5mg PO/SC bd–qds or dexamethasone 8–16mg PO/SC bd (avoid giving at bedtime, reduce dose if possible after 7d, and co-administer a PPI or H$_2$ receptor antagonist for gastroprotection).
- See 'General management' (📖 p. 52) for specific roles of lorazepam and aprepitant in anticipatory and post-exposure nausea and vomiting, respectively, for patients receiving highly emetogenic chemotherapy.

① Cyclical vomiting syndrome

Cyclical vomiting syndrome is a chronic functional disorder of unknown aetiology. It is characterized by paroxysmal, recurrent episodes of intense unremitting nausea and vomiting lasting hours to days. The patient is symptom-free in the intervening periods. It typically affects children (peak age 2–7y old) and resolves in adolescence; however, it can occur in adults. There is considerable interindividual variability but, within individuals, attacks are usually stereotyped; 75% occur at characteristic times of the day (usually night or early morning). NASPGHAN propose the following criteria for diagnosis, all of which must be present:
- At least five episodes in total, or at least three episodes over 6mo.
- Episodic attacks of intense nausea and vomiting lasting 1h–10d, occurring at least 1wk apart.
- Stereotypical pattern and symptoms in the individual patient.
- Vomiting during episodes at least four times/h.
- Return to baseline health between episodes.
- Not attributable to another disorder.

Abdominal pain is present in 80%, and may mimic the acute abdomen or dyspepsia, leading to unnecessary investigation or even surgery. A trigger is identifiable in 80% of cases, including infection (40%, particularly chronic sinusitis), psychological stress (35%), foods (especially chocolate, cheese, and monosodium glutamate), physical exhaustion, sleep deprivation, and menstruation. There is an association with migraine and chronic cannabis use.

The goal of investigation is exclusion of other organic pathologies. It is usually appropriate to perform upper GI endoscopy with D2 biopsies, and an upper GI contrast study. Consider an MRI head to rule out space-occupying lesions, vestibular testing, and endocrine and metabolic causes.

Treatment

A 'prevent-abort-support' approach to management is advocated. Most guidance is based on open-label trials or expert opinion.

- *Prevention.* Advise patients to avoid known precipitants. Anti-migraine drugs (such as pizotifen) as well as propranolol, amitriptyline, erythromycin, and pyridoxine have some evidence of efficacy. Cyproheptadine 2mg bd/tds is the first-line agent in children under 5y.
- *Abort acute attacks.* Replace fluids, correct electrolytes, and prescribe standard anti-emetics. Glucose solutions provide superior symptom relief, possibly by truncating ketosis, but monitor U & E due to risk of hyponatraemia. Lorazepam 0.5–1mg PO/IV or sumatriptan 50mg PO/6mg SC/10–20mg intranasal may be helpful. There are isolated reports of using aprepitant for severe recalcitrant cases.
- *Support.* Appreciate that symptom burden for these patients is highly disruptive to their personal and family lives. Consultation with a sympathetic gastroenterologist reduces attack frequency by up to 70%. Direct the patient towards the Cyclical Vomiting Syndrome Association and their website (see ℘ http://www.cvsa.org.uk/).

Severe vomiting

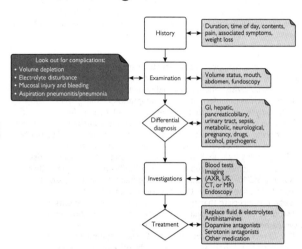

Severe acute diarrhoea

Definition and physiology of severe diarrhoea

Formally refers to passage of >250g stool/24h. From a practical perspective, better defined as an increase of three or more watery stools/day for up to 2wk. Stool consistency can be judged using the Bristol scale (Lewis and Heaton, 1997); type 7 refers to completely liquid faeces.

About 10L of fluid passes through the small bowel per day. Most is resorbed via Na^+/glucose transporters. Only 1.5L enters the colon, with 200–300mg/d passed as stool. Normal gut transit time is 12–48h; this decreases (i.e. speeds up) during infection.

Small bowel diarrhoea is often high-volume and can be foul-smelling. Some small bowel pathogens interfere with gut motility rather than fluid resorption, producing cramping, bloating, and weight loss. Bacterial pathogens that infect the colon are often invasive, producing frequent, low-volume bloody diarrhoea and fever. Tenesmus suggests proctitis.

Aetiology of severe diarrhoea

Predominantly infective (see Chapter 6). Common pathogens, their incubation times, and sites of disease are shown in Table 5.1. More than 50% are viral, 30% unknown, and <10% bacterial (although *C. difficile* is a common cause of hospital outbreaks). Be aware that systemic sepsis can also manifest with acute diarrhoea.

Table 5.1 Infectious causes of diarrhoea

Organism	Site	Incubation
Enteroadhesive *E. coli*	S	8–18h
Enterotoxigenic *E. coli*	S	16–72h
Enterohaemorrhagic *E. coli*	L	72–120h
Salmonella	S + L	16–72h
Shigella	L	16–72h
Campylobacter	L + S	16–72h
Norovirus	S	16–72h
Adenovirus	S	10d
Giardia lamblia	Proximal S	1–2wk
Strongyloides stercoralis	S	1wk–y
Entamoeba histolytica	L	1–3wk
Cryptosporidium	S	1–2wk

S, small bowel; L, large bowel.

Initial assessment of severe diarrhoea

History

- Define duration, and stool frequency and consistency. Ask whether blood is present and, if so, whether this is bright red, maroon, or melaena.
- Clarify whether nocturnal diarrhoea also present. Suggests infective, inflammatory, or secretory cause.
- Determine relationship to oral intake (may suggest malabsorption).
- Ask about recent food intake (restaurants, airplanes, cruise ships) and whether companions affected.
- Ask about nausea and vomiting (pre-formed toxins, small intestinal pathogens), fever (invasive organisms), and presence and location of any abdominal pain. Pale stools, bloating, and weight loss suggest small bowel aetiology.
- Inquire about co-morbidities (renal, cardiovascular, IBD, HIV).
- Recent antibiotic use, hospitalization, and achlorhydria (pernicious anaemia, *H. pylori* infection, PPI use) predispose to *C. difficile* infection.
- Inquire about ill contacts and contact with potentially infected water.
- Establish travel history. This broadens range of exposure to infectious pathogens. Also be aware that malaria can present as a gastroenteritic illness and should, therefore, be excluded in patients returning from endemic areas.

Examination

Assess fluid status. Dehydration is suggested by any of: HR >100/min, systolic BP <100mmHg (or postural drop >20/10mmHg), reduced skin turgor, or sunken eyes. Abdominal tenderness is common, but guarding suggests peritoneal involvement (in which case request surgical review). Fever suggests invasive disease (bacterial or viral). Look for evidence of malnutrition and weigh the patient.

Investigations

- Blood tests: FBC, U & E, LFT, calcium, PO_4^{3-}, Mg^{++}, CRP.
- Stool for microscopy and culture, viral PCR, and *C. difficile* assay. Make sure the stool pot is labelled and sealed!
- Erect CXR and AXR (to look for perforation and toxic megacolon, respectively) in patients with guarding or the frail/elderly.
- Sigmoidoscopy can be useful in certain patients, e.g. to diagnose IBD.

Indications for flexible sigmoidoscopy

- Immunocompromise.
- Suspected ischaemic colitis.
- Suspected IBD.
- Severe diarrhoea persisting for >5d.

Who to admit?

- Haemodynamic compromise.
- Severe abdominal pain.
- Profuse, bloody diarrhoea.
- Temperature >38.5°C (invasive disease).

Have a lower threshold to admit elderly patients, or those with significant co-morbidity, immunocompromise, or IBD.

Management of severe diarrhoea

Fluid resuscitation

The cornerstone of management is fluid resuscitation and electrolyte replacement:

- In most patients, this is best achieved orally, with oral rehydration solution (ORS). Commercial preparations (e.g. Dioralyte®) contain less salt than recommended, so advise adding salt to food. In an emergency, make up ORS by adding a half teaspoon salt, half teaspoon baking soda ($NaHCO_3$), and four tablespoons sugar to 1L of clean water.
- Obtain IV access if the enteral route is not available or insufficient to meet hydration requirements. Estimate fluid deficit, ongoing fluid losses, and insensible losses (~500mL/24h, higher if febrile). Infuse 0.9% saline (± KCl, see 'Electrolyte replacement', 📖 p. 64) at a rate dependent on the degree of dehydration; ≥4L/d is usually necessary. Switch to ORS as soon as possible.
- Review fluid balance twice daily. Avoid overloading patients with cardiac disease (listen for lung crepitations).
- Provide thromboprophylaxis to patients who are dehydrated and bedbound with low-dose LMWH and compression stockings.

Electrolyte replacement

- Provide electrolytes as guided by plasma level. Monitor K^+, Mg^{++}, Na^+, calcium, and PO_4^{3-}.
- Daily K^+ requirement is ~60mmol. Patients with severe diarrhoea may need twice this for 2–3d (a fall in plasma K^+ concentration of 1mmol/L ≈ 200mmol reduction in total body K^+). Vomiting will lead to severe hypokalaemia due to aldosterone secretion, causing H^+/K^+ exchange in the kidneys. Oral K^+ is usually sufficient if K^+ >3mmol/L; use an effervescent preparation (Slow-K® and Sando-K® contain 8mmol and 12mmol K^+, respectively). Never prescribe K^+ replacement for >3d without checking serum levels.
- Hypomagnesaemia (<0.6mmol/L) may prevent correction of hypokalaemia due to renal ion exchange; if so, provide two doses of 8mmol (≈2g) magnesium sulphate IV over 1h, then 6mmol magnesium glycerophosphate PO qds until plasma levels stable.

Antibiotics

Use of antimicrobial agents is discussed in Chapter 6. Indications include:
- Persistent (>3d) community-acquired diarrhoea with systemic symptoms.
- Confirmed enteropathogenic *E. coli*, *Shigella*, or *C. difficile* infection.
- Traveller's diarrhoea.
- Proven parasitic infection.

Avoid if suspected or confirmed enterohaemorrhagic *E. coli* (e.g. *E. coli* O157:H7; risk of precipitating haemolytic uraemic syndrome (HUS)) or non-typhoidal *Salmonella* (prolongs carriage).

Loperamide

Used to prevent diarrhoea when inconvenient, e.g. travelling. Dose 2mg after each loose bowel action (maximum 16mg). Can mask fluid losses and said to contribute to colon dilatation in severe colitis (although little evidence for this). Contraindicated in enterohaemorrhagic *E. coli*. Not usually used in hospital for acute diarrhoea unless active infection/inflammation excluded.

Probiotics

Preparations containing ~10 billion cfu/d *Lactobacillus-* or *Saccharomyces boulardii* reduce diarrhoea duration by 1d if commenced within 48h of symptom onset (Allen *et al.*, 2010). Avoid *Saccharomyces* in immunocompromised patients, as fatal cases of septicaemia reported.

Nutrition

Encourage patients to eat. Food intake assists fluid absorption and enterocyte repair. Initially, recommend plain food, added salt, and reduced dairy produce (secondary lactose intolerance common).

Outcomes

In most cases, symptoms settle within 2–3d. Discharge patients once liquid stool resolving, fever and inflammatory markers decreasing, haemodynamic compromise resolved, and oral intake re-established. Advise patients with *Salmonella* or *Campylobacter* to avoid preparing non-cooked food for 4wk (20–50% secrete organisms at 2wk). No routine follow-up is required, although several post-infective sequelae can occur:
- *Guillain–Barré syndrome.* Occurs after 1–2wk in 1:3,000 patients. Particularly associated with *C. jejuni* infection.
- *Reactive arthritis.* Occurs 1–6wk later in 1–2% of patients with bacterial diarrhoea.
- *Secondary lactose intolerance.* May persist for months.
- *IBD.* Incidence increases from 3/10,000 to 7/10,000 in the year following infection.
- *Post-infective irritable bowel.* Occurs in ~3%, tends to last few months.

Special situations

The returning traveller

Travellers' diarrhoea is usually caused by viruses or enterotoxigenic *E. coli*. Laboratories do not routinely screen for these, as they cause self-limiting illness. The preferred empirical treatment is rifaximin 200mg PO tds for 3d. If not available, a single dose of ciprofloxacin 500mg or azithromycin 500mg reduces duration of diarrhoea from 3d to 2d.

For investigation and treatment of specific pathogens, see Chapter 6.

Antibiotic-associated diarrhoea

Reduction in commensal flora with antibiotic use increases intra-colonic carbohydrate (producing osmotic diarrhoea) and reduces intra-colonic short-chain fatty acids (that normally nourish the colonocyte). Diarrhoea improves with reduced oral intake and antibiotic cessation. Probiotics are protective, but it is still unclear whether they effectively improve symptoms once diarrhoea has already developed.

For management of *C. difficile* infection, see 📖 p. 68.

The patient with HIV

Opportunistic infections occur when CD4 count is suppressed:

See Chapter 12. Up to 50% of cases are due to highly active anti-retroviral treatment (HAART), especially ritonavir and nelfinavir (particularly likely if HAART medication recently changed and there are no additional symptoms). Many of the remainder are due to non-HIV specific causes, with increased prevalence of *C. difficile* reported. Giardia and sexually transmitted causes more common in men who have sex with men (MSM). Opportunistic infections occur when CD4 count is suppressed:

- CD4 <200/mm³. Suspect cryptosporidiosis or HIV enteropathy.
- CD4 <100/mm³. Suspect viral causes (CMV and HSV), fungi (microsporidia), helminths (*Strongyloides*), protozoa (coccidia), mycobacteria (*M. tuberculosis*, *M. avium* complex), or neoplasia (lymphoma, Kaposi's sarcoma).
- Symptoms may flare as part of an immune reconstitution inflammatory syndrome (IRIS) when HAART introduced.
- IBD severity tends to improve in patients with lower CD4 counts.

Management of specific conditions is detailed in Chapter 12. Involve the HIV team early, especially if CD4 count suppressed. Request sigmoidoscopy with biopsies if symptoms persist >5d, and gastroduodenoscopy with mid-duodenal biopsies if small bowel likely infected. Request dietetic review if patient malnourished.

All patients should be counselled about strict hand hygiene and avoiding unsafe sexual practices to prevent faeco-oral transmission (including autoinfection). Patients on HAART may require therapeutic drug monitoring if associated malabsorption whilst diarrhoea present.

Specific therapies depend on the causative organism, often requiring more prolonged treatment and, in some cases, secondary prophylaxis.

ⓘ Patients known or thought to have inflammatory bowel disease

See Chapter 7. It can be difficult to distinguish between infective diarrhoea and a flare/new presentation of IBD, and sometimes both occur simultaneously. Up to 10% of patients with a presumed flare have positive stool cultures or *C. difficile* infection (latter three times more likely in IBD). Infective diarrhoea is suggested by:

• Rapid onset of symptoms (days rather than weeks).
• Cramping abdominal pain with fever.
• Symptoms improving within 1wk.

Send stool samples in all patients for bacterial culture and *C. difficile* antigen and toxin, and to parasitology for ova, cysts, and parasites if appropriate travel history. Blood inflammatory markers (WCC, CRP, ESR) do not distinguish infective from inflammatory diarrhoea but do correlate with severity. Toxic dilatation (see Fig. 5.1) (transverse colon diameter >6cm on AXR) is more common in IBD than infective colitis: inform senior physician and surgical team if present, as may require emergency colectomy.

Rigid sigmoidoscopy in A & E can exclude a flare of ulcerative proctitis/colitis (mucosa appears normal), but will not differentiate IBD from bacillary dysentery. The rectum may be normal in Crohn's disease. Consider taking a rectal biopsy using *flexible* biopsy forceps at the same time if flexible sigmoidoscopy unavailable within 24h. If stool cultures are non-contributory and symptoms persist or worsen, request flexible sigmoidoscopy. Histology can usually differentiate between a flare of IBD and infective colitis, although crypt architecture is typically preserved in novel acute IBD, which can cause uncertainty.

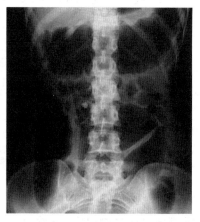

Fig. 5.1 Toxic megacolon.

The treatment of IBD is detailed in Chapter 7; involve a gastroenterologist early in management. Provide ciprofloxacin 500mg PO bd and metronidazole 400mg PO tds for 5d if steroids required and infective colitis has not been satisfactorily excluded.

① *Clostridium difficile*-associated diarrhoea

C. difficile-associated diarrhoea (CDAD) is a major cause of in-hospital morbidity and mortality due to enterotoxin and cytotoxin production. *C. difficile* is carried by 2–3% of the healthy population and 25% of nursing home residents. Modern PCR-based techniques diagnose carriage. Its frequency has increased 20-fold over the past 10y. Reduced IgG and IgA-mediated immunity can be demonstrated in ~40%. Risk factors include old age, chronic hospitalization, recurrent antibiotic or PPI use, achlorhydria, immunocompromise, and tube feeding. More severe disease occurs in the elderly and those with renal impairment. The 027/B1/NAP1 strain (first described in the UK in 2003) is associated with more severe outbreaks (60% of cases in a London-wide outbreak in 2008), and can cause disease in healthy, young adults. It produces 20-fold more toxin, often causing disease in patients without risk factors, and may be more common following ciprofloxacin use. Mortality with this strain is ~10%.

The spectrum of *C. difficile*-associated disease includes:
- *Diarrhoea.* Usually watery but not bloody, and sometimes accompanied by lower abdominal cramps. *C. difficile* toxins can be detected in stool samples in ~80% of those in whom toxin production is causing diarrhoea. Endoscopy is usually normal.
- *Colitis.* Most common clinical manifestation. Patients usually have fever, malaise, abdominal pain, and high-volume watery diarrhoea, sometimes with a trace of blood. Leukocytosis is common. On sigmoidoscopy, patchy erythematous colitis is seen without pseudomembranes.
- *Pseudomembranous colitis* (see Colour plate 15). Systemic illness with severe bloody diarrhoea, abdominal pain and tenderness, and fever. Hypoalbuminaemia can result from protein losses.
- *Fulminant colitis.* Affects up to 3% of patients in some series. Presents with paralytic ileus and toxic megacolon (which may progress to perforation).

Investigations
- Send stool for *C. difficile* analysis. PCR detects presence of organism and merely reflects carriage of inactive spores; therefore, in general, do not request unless patient has diarrhoea. Toxin assay detects presence of toxin A and/or toxin B, which cause inflammation in those immunologically susceptible (i.e. the 60% of individuals who do not secrete IgA against *C. difficile*.).
- Toxin assays are 95% specific but only 70–90% sensitive, so treat regardless if high suspicion of CDAD. PCR more sensitive (>95%).
- Cell culture provides the gold standard but is only available in reference laboratories.
- If patients are *C. difficile* PCR-positive but toxin-negative, this is likely asymptomatic carriage or early infection. Only treat if diarrhoea present (but re-send test if still symptomatic after 1wk). Otherwise, expectant management is reasonable.

- Flexible sigmoidoscopy and biopsy may demonstrate pseudomembranes and typical histological appearances, but often classic changes occur proximal to the sigmoid colon.
- Request AXR, VBG and lactate if ≥2 severity markers present (see Box 5.1).
- Monitor FBC, U & E, and Mg^{++} regularly.
- Serial AXR (±CT) and surgical review necessary in patients with fulminant colitis: suspect if several severity markers present, especially if lactate above normal range.

☼ Box 5.1 Markers of severity of CDAD

- Age >60y.
- WCC >15 × 10^9/L.
- Temperature >38°C.
- Albumin <25g/L.
- Hypotension/tachycardia.
- Oliguria/GFR <40mL/min.
- Ileus (may mask fluid losses).*
- Stools >10/d.*
- Dilatation on AXR.*
- Abdominal distension/tenderness.

* Markers suggestive of fulminant colitis.

Treatment

Infection control is paramount. Isolate patients in a side room with barrier nursing. Avoid fomite spore transfer (keep all medical notes and charts outside).

- Prescribe metronidazole 400mg PO tds for 10–14d in patients without severity markers. Can use metronidazole 500mg IV tds in patients who are nil-by-mouth, or have an ileus or severe malabsorption, but otherwise this is less effective than oral therapy.
- Prescribe vancomycin 125mg PO qds in severe or relapsed disease (Drekonja et al., 2011). Short-term cure rates ~95%. Consider using first-line in elderly.
- Escalate therapy in patients with multiple relapses. Involve microbiologist in these decisions, as there are little data to guide choice of therapy. Duration guided by symptoms. Options include:
  - Vancomycin 500mg PO qds, tapering over 6wk.
  - Vancomycin 125mg PO qds + metronidazole 400mg PO tds.
  - Fidaxomicin 200mg PO bd.
  - Nitazoxanide 500mg PO bd.
  - Teicoplanin 100mg PO bd (Nelson et al., 2011).
  - Rifaximin 400mg PO tds.
  - Vancomycin enemas 500mg PR qds.
  - Faecal transfer therapy, by NG/NJ tube or enemas.
- Evidence for probiotics in CDAD is mixed. Although individual positive trials have been reported, the overall recommendation (Pillai and Nelson, 2008) is that, overall, there is insufficient evidence to justify

their use in disease treatment or prevention. Only one randomized trial demonstrated efficacy, evaluating *Saccharomyces boulardii* 250mg PO qds for 4wk in addition to standard antibiotics (McFarland *et al.*, 1994).
• Colectomy may be necessary in patients with fulminant colitis and, occasionally, in patients with intractable severe disease.

Overall, 10–25% of patients relapse after one course of therapy; up to two-thirds of these have a further relapse. Relapse rates are not dependent on the initial antibiotic used; 10% patients with a first recurrence have poor outcome (colectomy, megacolon, perforation, or death within 30d). Reduction in antibiotic use, with restrictive prescribing policies, is the most effective means of preventing high-population rates of CDAD.

☼ *E. coli* 0157:H7 and 0104:H4

Enterohaemorrhagic *E. coli* species cause severe gastroenteritis, of which E0157:H7 is the most important serotype. Bloody diarrhoea, leukocytosis, and severe abdominal pain occur 3–4d following ingestion of undercooked meat or unpasteurized milk. Fever is often mild. Shiga-like toxin causes HUS (acute kidney injury, thrombocytopaenia, and microangiopathic haemolytic anaemia with schistocytes on blood film) in 5%. Of these, ~25% develop neurological complications and 5% die. Treatment is supportive. Public health measures (including source and contact tracing) should be initiated immediately to limit spread. Antibiotics can worsen HUS and should be avoided.

A novel strain of *E. coli* 0104:H4, arising through acquisition of genes encoding shiga toxins by a previously enteroaggregative organism, caused a serious outbreak of foodborne illness in Europe in 2011. This was associated with an unusually high rate of HUS.

☼ Ischaemic enteritis and colitis

Acute small bowel ischaemia (see 📖 pp. 143–6) presents with diarrhoea and severe peri-umbilical abdominal pain. Nausea and vomiting are common. Physical examination findings are initially mild. VBG may show lactic acidosis. If the diagnosis is suspected:
• Request urgent contrast abdominal CT and surgical review.
• Doppler US can demonstrate vascular insufficiency of the coeliac trunk or superior mesenteric artery.
• Angiography with thrombolysis diagnostic and therapeutic.

Colonic ischaemia usually presents with rectal bleeding (see 📖 pp. 146–7). Usually due to hypotension followed by arteriolar spasm rather than arterial embolus or thrombosis. Diagnosis is typically made on contrast CT (shows thumb-printing, mural thickening, loss of haustration, and intramural gas), although appearances overlap with severe IBD and diverticulitis. Colonoscopy with biopsies can be diagnostic, although this is inadvisable if the bowel wall is necrotic.

Optimal management of ischaemic colitis has yet to be determined. In the absence of peritonitis, patients should be managed conservatively with bowel rest, broad-spectrum antibiotics, IV fluid and electrolyte replacement, and TPN. In patients with peritonitis, laparotomy is mandated with segmental resection or total colectomy, depending on intraoperative findings (Diaz Nieto *et al.*, 2011).

Factitious diarrhoea

This is rare and should only be diagnosed once organic disease has been excluded. Suspect if multiple normal investigations. More common in women. Individuals who abuse laxatives can generally be categorized into four groups: patients with an eating disorder (largest group) who use as a method of weight control; those who believe daily bowel movement is essential for good health (normal range actually between every 3d to three times daily); professional athletes in sports with set weight limits; and patients who are malingering for secondary gain (Roerig et al., 2010). Can usually be investigated as an outpatient.

- Send 20mL urine for laxative screen (bisacodyl, senna, dantron), and stool for castor oil.
- Request osmolality, Na^+, K^+, and Mg^{++} on *fresh* stool:
  - Stool osmolality < plasma osmolality (280–300mOsmol/kg) is diagnostic of water or urine contamination. Consider measuring stool urea or creatinine to confirm latter.
  - If >300mOsmol/kg, calculate osmolar gap:

    Osmolar gap = serum osmolality $- 2 \times$ (stool $[Na^+ + K^+]$)

  - If osmolar gap >50mOsmol/kg, suspect magnesium (stool Mg^{++} would be >45mmol/L), sorbitol, or lactulose intake.
  - If osmolar gap <50mOsmol/kg, this is likely due to fermentation products.
- A metabolic alkalosis occurs, as HCO_3^- secretion into the renal tubule is inhibited by low serum Cl^- and K^+ caused by laxative use; hence, venous HCO_3^- is raised in factitious (but not infective) diarrhoea.
- Lower GI endoscopy may show melanosis coli, a non-pathological reversible pigmentation of the colon, associated with anthraquinone use (senna, co-danthramer).

Complications of laxative abuse

- Electrolyte disturbances. Particularly hypokalaemia and hyponatraemia due to GI losses. Hypermagnesaemia associated with large doses of Mg^{++}-containing laxatives can present with paralysis.
- Chronic bowel motility dysfunction.
- Renal failure. Multifactorial. Due to a combination of volume depletion, hypokalaemia, rhabdomyolysis, hyperuricaemia, nephrolithiasis, and direct nephrotoxicity.

Management

The goal of treatment is to stop laxative misuse. This includes identifying:
- Motivation for laxative use.
- Beliefs regarding their effects on body weight.
- Beliefs regarding normal bowel function.

In patients who have been misusing laxatives chronically, drugs should be slowly weaned. In the first instance, stop stimulant laxatives, and replace them with fibre and osmotic supplements to establish normal bowel movements. Advise on appropriate dietary changes and the importance of oral hydration. Refer patients with an underlying psychiatric disturbance to team with expertise in its management.

The patient with severe leukopaenia

Patients undergoing bone marrow transplantation often present with diarrhoea, with or without bleeding. Exclude standard pathogens and *C. difficile* infection. Flexible sigmoidoscopy with biopsies usually required to exclude graft-versus-host disease or CMV colitis.

Typhlitis is a necrotizing enterocolitis, usually involving the caecum. It affects profoundly immunocompromised patients (5% of patients with haematological malignancies, or patients treated with high-dose chemotherapy for solid tumours). It is characterized by transmural inflammation of the bowel wall, thought to be caused by an acute mucosal injury due to cytotoxic drugs followed by secondary infection. Consider if WCC $<0.5 \times 10^9/L$. Presents with diarrhoea, right iliac fossa pain, and fever; rectal bleeding may occur. If suspected, request urgent abdominal CT scan (confirms diagnosis and excludes appendicitis); also take blood cultures. Treat with bowel rest, NG aspiration, IV fluid and nutritional replacement, and broad-spectrum antibacterial and anti-fungal medication. Consider G-CSF if neutropaenic. Surgery indicated if peritonitis. Mortality has been reported as high as 40–50%, though likely lower with modern care.

First presentation of chronic diarrhoea

Chronic diarrhoeal diseases may initially present as an acute illness. Be alert, therefore, for these conditions (see Box 5.2) if symptoms persist.

Box 5.2 Common causes of chronic diarrhoea

- Coeliac disease.
- Diverticular disease.
- Lactose intolerance.
- Hyperthyroidism.
- Medication-related.
- Adenocarcinoma.
- IBD.
- Exocrine pancreatic insufficiency.
- Bacterial overgrowth.
- Bile salt malabsorption.
- Following ischaemic colitis.
- Neuroendocrine tumour (carcinoid, VIPoma, gastrinoma).

Severe acute diarrhoea

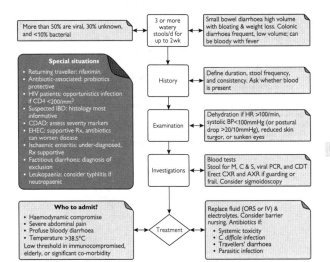

3 or more watery stools/d for up to 2wk

More than 50% are viral, 30% unknown, and <10% bacterial

Small bowel diarrhoea high volume with bloating & weight loss. Colonic diarrhoea frequent, low volume; can be bloody with fever

Special situations
- Returning traveller: rifaximin.
- Antibiotic-associated: probiotics protective
- HIV patients: opportunistics infection if CD4 <200/mm³
- Suspected IBD: histology most informative
- CDAD: assess severity markers
- EHEC: supportive Rx, antibiotics can worsen disease
- Ischaemic enteritis: under-diagnosed, Rx supportive
- Factitious diarrhoea: diagnosis of exclusion
- Leukopaenia: consider typhlitis if neutropaenic

History

Define duration, stool frequency, and consistency. Ask whether blood is present

Examination

Dehydration if HR >100/min, systolic BP<100mmHg (or postural drop >20/10mmHg), reduced skin turgor, or sunken eyes

Investigations

Blood tests
Stool for M, C & S, viral PCR, and CDT
Erect CXR and AXR if guarding or frail. Consider sigmoidoscopy

Who to admit?
- Haemodynamic compromise
- Severe abdominal pain
- Profuse bloody diarrhoea
- Temperature >38.5°C
Low threshold in immunocompromised, elderly, or significant co-morbidity

Treatment

Replace fluid (ORS or IV) & electrolytes. Consider barrier nursing. Antibiotics if:
- Systemic toxicity
- C. difficile infection
- Travellers' diarrhoea
- Parasitic infection

Further reading

Allen SJ, Martinez EG, Gregorio GV, et al. (2010) Probiotics for treating acute infectious diarrhoea. *Cochrane Database Syst Rev* **11**: CD003048.

Diaz Nieto R, Varcada M, Ogunbiyi OA, et al. (2011) Systematic review on the treatment of ischaemic colitis. *Colorectal Dis* **13**: 744–7.

Drekonja DM, Butler M, MacDonald R, et al. (2011) Comparative effectiveness of Clostridium difficile treatments: a systematic review. *Ann Intern Med* **155**: 839–47.

Lewis SJ, Heaton KW (1997) Stool form scale as a useful guide to intestinal transit time. *Scand J Gastroenterol* **32**: 920–4.

McFarland LV, Surawicz CM, Greenberg RN, et al. (1994) A randomized placebo-controlled trial of Saccharomyces boulardii in combination with standard antibiotics for Clostridium difficile disease. *JAMA* **271**: 1913–18.

Nelson RL, Kelsey P, Leeman H, et al. (2011) Antibiotic treatment for Clostridium difficile-associated diarrhea in adults. *Cochrane Database Syst Rev* **9**: CD004610.

Pillai A, Nelson R (2008) Probiotics for treatment of Clostridium difficile-associated colitis in adults. *Cochrane Database Syst Rev* **1**: CD004611.

Roerig JL, Steffen KJ, Mitchell JE, et al. (2010) Laxative abuse: epidemiology, diagnosis and management. *Drugs* **70**: 1487–503.

Chapter 6

Gastroenteritis

Community-acquired gastroenteritis

Acute diarrhoea and vomiting are most frequently infectious in origin. In immunocompetent individuals, illness is typically self-limiting, with no intervention required beyond oral rehydration. If symptoms persist beyond 14d, they are classified as persistent, and often non-infectious or parasitic. Diarrhoea may be generated through osmotic, secretory or inflammatory mechanisms, or by increased motility. Infectious agents can elicit disease through any of these by mucosal adherence and invasion, or enterotoxin production.

Clinical presentation

Symptoms and risk factors guide the range of potential pathogens and threshold for active treatment. Ask about:

History

- Age. Very young and elderly at greatest risk.
- Duration and rapidity of onset of illness.
- Vomiting. Implies proximal bowel involvement. Also consider bowel obstruction.
- Presence and location of abdominal pain. Cramping is particularly prominent in *Campylobacter* infection. May also be caused by electrolyte disturbance. In patients >50y old, consider the possibility of bowel ischaemia.
- Stool frequency and volume. Quantify number of stools passed/24h and number overnight (correlates with inflammatory diarrhoea).
- Stool character. Bulky faeces that float suggest small bowel malabsorption. Copious 'rice water' stools characteristic of cholera.
- Presence of blood in stool and tenesmus. Predicts lower GI pathology and proctitis, respectively.
- Systemic symptoms or fever suggest invasive disease or bacteraemia.
- Past medical and drug histories for:
  - Increased susceptibility. Diseases and medications causing achlorhydria elevate risk, as does immunocompromise. The latter also broadens the spectrum of pathogens (see Chapter 12). Recent use of antibiotics, and recent or recurrent hospitalization predispose to *C. difficile*.
  - Differential diagnosis. Other medical conditions and drugs can cause acute diarrhoea (see 'Differential diagnosis', 📖 pp. 77–8).
- Contact with potentially infected food or water, including shellfish, raw or undercooked meat, or reheated rice.
- Unwell contacts.
- Travel history. Modifies range of pathogens and antibiotic sensitivities (see 'Travellers' diarrhoea', 📖 p. 84).
- Social history. Food poisoning and infectious bloody diarrhoea are notifiable diseases. Contact tracing may be required, particularly if the patient is a food handler. Sexual history important if oro-anal intercourse practised.

Examination

Goal is principally to exclude other diagnoses and assess degree of dehydration (measure pulse, BP and postural drop, and capillary refill time). The abdomen should be examined for masses, peritonism, or distorted bowel sounds. Perform digital rectal examination to determine presence of blood or mucus in the stool.

Causes of infectious diarrhoea and vomiting

Most cases (50–70%) are viral, with the majority of the remainder bacterial. They can be subdivided into those in which vomiting is the predominant feature (often due to ingestion of a pre-formed toxin or spores) and those causing non-bloody or bloody diarrhoea (see Table 6.1). Small bowel involvement is suggested by high-volume, watery stool and mid-abdominal pain; faecal blood is rare. Large bowel involvement manifests as lower abdominal pain with tenesmus and mucoid or bloody diarrhoea.

Differential diagnosis

- Toxin ingestion. Symptoms usually within few hours of ingestion; many toxins not destroyed by heat:
  - Seafood. Reef-dwelling tropical fish ingest algae that produce a heat-stable neurotoxin called ciguatera. The fish do not taste or appear unusual. It is common in certain parts of the world, accounting for more than half of fish-borne food poisoning in the USA. GI, neurologic and, occasionally, cardiovascular symptoms occur. Treatment is supportive. Scombroid toxin is another common cause of seafood-borne gastroenteritis after consumption of contaminated dark meat fish (such as tuna, mahi-mahi, and mackerel). Bacteria grow in improperly stored fish, then decarboxylate histidine in the fish to histamine that produces an anaphylactoid reaction within 1h. Fish may taste bubbly or peppery. Treat with antihistamine and supportive care; consider β_2 agonists, or even adrenaline, if bronchospasm.
  - Mushrooms. Amatoxins are found in a variety of poisonous mushrooms (including *Amanita phalloides*). Typically, gastroenteritis occurs 6–24h post-ingestion, then apparent recovery followed by fulminant hepatic and multisystem organ failure (at 48–72h). If suspected, give activated charcoal and seek specialist advice.
  - Acute heavy metal poisoning. Arsenic (look for garlic smell to breath and prolonged QTc), lead (acute toxicity causes colicky abdominal pain rather than typical gastroenteritis).
- GI diseases:
  - Irritable bowel syndrome.*
  - Coeliac disease.*
  - IBD.*
  - Intestinal obstruction.
  - Motility disturbance, including severe gastroparesis.*
  - Acute appendicitis (particularly in children).
  - Food intolerance.*
  - Pancreatic insufficiency.*

- Radiation enteritis.*
- Whipple's disease.*
- Endocrine diseases:
  - Hyperthyroidism, thyrotoxicosis.*
    - Diabetic ketoacidosis
  - Addison's disease.*
- Secretory tumours:
  - Carcinoids, VIPoma, medullary thyroid carcinoma.*
- Drugs:
  - Laxative abuse, magnesium.*
  - Antibiotics.
  - Chemotherapy.
  - Colchicine, quinidine.
- Non-GI infection:
  - Sepsis, toxic shock syndrome, malaria.
- Factitious diarrhoea.*

* Unlikely to present as gastroenteritis as chronic symptoms usually predominate.

Table 6.1 Microbial causes of diarrhoea and vomiting

Vomiting	Non-bloody diarrhoea	Bloody diarrhoea
Staphylococcus aureus	Viral gastroenteritis	Campylobacter
Bacillus cereus	Salmonella	Shigella
Clostridium perfringens	E. coli (ETEC, EPEC)	Salmonella
	Vibrio	E. coli (EHEC, EIEC)
	C. difficile	Yersinia
	Giardia lamblia	Entamoeba histolytica
	Strongyloides	Schistosoma
	Coccidia	Trichuris trichura

EHEC, enterohaemorrhagic E. coli; EIEC, enteroinvasive E. coli; EPEC, enteropathogenic E. coli;
ETEC, enterotoxigenic E. coli.

Investigation
Diagnosis is usually clinical, but the following reduce threshold for investigation:
- Duration >2wk.
- Systemic upset.
- Tenesmus or bloody diarrhoea.
- Outbreak suggesting food poisoning.
- Ingestion of raw shellfish.
- Recent antibiotic usage.
- Men who have sex with men (MSM).
- Immunocompromise.

Blood tests

FBC may be normal, but WCC is usually elevated with *Salmonella*, and normal or low with left shift with *Shigella*. Eosinophilia may indicate helminth infection. U & E help assess dehydration and electrolyte losses. Fever or systemic symptoms should prompt blood cultures (and malaria film if appropriate travel history). VBG is helpful if severely dehydrated or septic to risk-stratify and guide adequacy of fluid replacement; high lactate should also prompt consideration of bowel ischaemia.

Imaging

Plain AXR is useful in appropriate clinical scenarios to exclude toxic mega-colon (see Fig. 5.1) or bowel obstruction. Diffuse intestinal inflammation may also be evident as mucosal oedema with 'thumb-printing'.

Stool microscopy and culture

Microscopy for faecal leukocytes is typically positive with *Shigella*, *Campylobacter*, and enteroinvasive and enterohaemorrhagic *E. coli*; variable in *Salmonella*, *Yersinia*, and *C. difficile*; and negative in cholera, enterotoxigenic *E. coli*, viral infection, and giardiasis. Routine microscopy and acid-fast staining can often detect oocysts in parasitic infection. Electron microscopy or PCR are required to diagnose microsporidia or viruses.

Stool should not be routinely cultured: only 2% of samples are positive, mixed infections are common, single cultures are insufficient for some pathogens, and results often take too long to alter management. In practice, culture should be limited to:

- Investigation of potential outbreaks and disease surveillance.
- History requires exclusion of a pathogen for which specific antibiotics would be indicated, particularly parasitic infection.
- Non-infectious aetiology suspected.
- Clinical condition severe enough to require hospital admission.
- The features outlined above under 'Investigation', 🕮 p. 78.

Special tests

Serological and/or ELISA tests may be indicated in potential tropical infections (see 'Parasitic infections', 🕮 pp. 86–8). Send stool for *C. difficile* toxin if recent antibiotic use or hospitalization; many centres now use a PCR test, which is very sensitive (97%) and specific (93%), rather than enzyme immunoassay tests for the toxin (sensitivity 60–95%). A compatible clinical history of diarrhoea is needed if using the PCR test to differentiate those with colitis from carriers. Endoscopy ± biopsy indicated if symptoms persistent and diagnosis not achieved by other means.

Principles of therapy

The mainstay of treatment is replacement of fluid and electrolyte losses, ideally orally. This is most effectively provided as oral rehydration salts with glucose dissolved in water: the WHO solution contains 90mEq/L sodium, 2g/dL glucose, 20mEq/L potassium, and 80 mEq/L chloride. IV fluids are indicated in patients with intractable vomiting or severe intra-vascular depletion (as recognized by resting tachycardia and hypotension or postural BP drop). *Source isolate or barrier nurse if in hospital to prevent nosocomial transmission.*

There is no benefit to fasting, although eating can be uncomfortable and further stimulate defaecation. Dairy products should be avoided, as transient lactose intolerant is common. Alcohol, caffeine, and carbonated drinks may worsen symptoms.

Antimotility agents provide symptomatic relief, but they should be avoided in acute severe colitis as there is risk of precipitating megacolon. They may also prolong shedding of infectious organisms. Loperamide 2–4mg PRN (qds max) is the drug of choice if (absolutely) required.

When to give antibiotics

Antibiotics are indicated in:

- Community-acquired diarrhoea with >4 stools/d for >3d with at least one of: abdominal pain, fever, rectal bleeding, vomiting, myalgia, or severe headache. In most cases, empirical therapy with a fluoroquinolone (ciprofloxacin 500mg PO bd for 3d) is appropriate (use currently not advised in pregnant women or children as risk of arthropathy, although this is based on animal studies).
- Confirmed *Shigella*, enteropathogenic *E. coli*, or *C. difficile* infection. Antibiotics should be avoided in enterohaemorrhagic *E. coli* infection due to risk of precipitating HUS, and in uncomplicated *Salmonella* to prevent prolonging shedding of viable organisms in the stool.
- Travellers' diarrhoea (see 🕮 p. 84). Antibiotics shorten duration.
- Proven parasitic infection. Empirical treatment is sometimes appropriate for suspected giardiasis if the history is highly suggestive.

ⓘ **Complications**

- Dehydration.
- Electrolyte imbalance, particularly hypokalaemia.
- Sepsis.
- Anaemia.
- Renal failure, most commonly due to volume depletion but occasionally HUS associated with enterohaemorrhagic *E. coli* 0157, *Campylobacter*, or *Shigella*.
- Reactive arthritis, Reiter's syndrome.
- Guillain–Barré syndrome (0.03% risk in 2mo after *Campylobacter*).
- Post-infectious irritable bowel syndrome (in up to 28%).
- Temporary post-infectious lactose intolerance.

Specific pathogens

Specific microbial aetiologies may be suspected on the basis of clinical presentation, or confirmed on laboratory testing. This section covers those most frequently encountered. Parasitic infections are considered separately (see 📖 p. 86).

Food poisoning due to ingested bacterial toxin or spores

Staphylococcus aureus causes severe vomiting due to ingestion of a pre-formed toxin, 2–6h after exposure. *Bacillus (B.) cereus* and *Clostridium (C.) perfringens* cause symptoms following spore ingestion. *B. cereus* spores are commonly acquired from eating reheated rice and, as such, cases are often associated with takeaway food. The incubation period is 1–6h, and symptoms include diarrhoea and vomiting. *C. perfringens* spores are mostly acquired from cooked poultry that has subsequently been cooled but not properly reheated. The incubation period is 8–24h, and patients present with abdominal cramps and diarrhoea; vomiting is less common. Treatment is supportive.

Viral gastroenteritis

Multiple viruses cause diarrhoea and vomiting, transmitted by the faeco-oral route. Particularly important are:

- Rotavirus. Commonest cause in children. Incubation period is 24–72h. Vaccination is now available.
- Norovirus. Acquisition often nosocomial; hospital inpatients and nursing home residents are at high risk. May also be ingested from shellfish contaminated with faeces. Presents with sudden onset nausea and vomiting, followed later by diarrhoea; headache, fever, and myalgia occur in 50%. Highly infectious: faeco-oral transmission can even be aerosolized when patients vomit or flush a toilet containing contaminated stool. Most cases resolve spontaneously within 36h.
- Adenovirus. Presents with watery diarrhoea and vomiting, often accompanied by respiratory symptoms and low-grade fever. Incubation period is 7d and virus shed for up to 2 wk.

Other common viral causes include calicivirus, astrovirus, parvovirus, and coronavirus. Diagnosis is by PCR or electron microscopy of vomitus or stool; this is rarely done but may be helpful in hospital for outbreak monitoring and to guide infection control measures. Treatment is supportive.

① *Escherichia coli*

GI infection from *E. coli* can result from eating undercooked meat or unwashed salads and vegetables. Incubation period is 12–72h. Enteric *E. coli* are classified on the basis of serological and virulence properties:

- Enterotoxigenic (ETEC). Commonest cause of bacterial diarrhoea in children, and travellers' diarrhoea worldwide. Toxins cause increased secretion of fluid and electrolytes.
- Enteropathogenic (EPEC). Similar clinical presentation to ETEC but mediates diarrhoea through intestinal epithelial cell disruption.
- Enteroinvasive (EIEC). Causes a syndrome reminiscent of shigellosis (see 'Shigella', 📖 p. 82), with high fever and profuse bloody diarrhoea.

- Enterohaemorrhagic (EHEC). Presents with bloody diarrhoea, typically in the absence of fever. Includes strain 0157:H7, which causes HUS. See also Chapter 5, 📖 p. 70.

E. coli are often sensitive to fluoroquinolones; ciprofloxacin 500mg PO bd for 3d is usually sufficient. However, antibiotic resistance is an increasing problem, so be guided by sensitivities.

① *Salmonella*

Salmonella species can be divided into those causing enteric fever (*S. typhi* and *S. paratyphi*) or gastroenteritis (of which multiple subspecies are recognized, with *S. enterica* and *S. typhimurium* the most common). Acquisition is similar to *E. coli*. Outbreaks have previously been attributable to contaminated eggs; an association with pet reptiles is also well described. Incubation period is 6–36h. Patients present with nausea, vomiting, abdominal cramps, and diarrhoea. The latter is frequently non-bloody, although severe colitis can develop with dysentery and risk of toxic megacolon and perforation. Median duration of illness is 3–4d, and antibiotics are not usually required (and indeed may prolong faecal shedding of infectious organisms). If disease is severe or the patient immunocompromised, ciprofloxacin 500mg PO bd for 10–14d is appropriate.

① *Campylobacter*

This is usually acquired from contaminated animal meat, most frequently undercooked chicken. Horizontal person-to-person transmission is also common. Two principal subspecies are responsible for human disease: *C. jejuni* and *C. coli*. The incubation period is slightly longer than those of *E. coli* and *Salmonella* at 48–96h. Patients present with a 24h prodrome of fatigue and myalgia, followed by nausea, abdominal pain with severe cramps (often identified as the least bearable feature of the illness), and diarrhoea (frequently bloody).

Due to extensive antibiotic use in poultry husbandry, there is now widespread resistance to ciprofloxacin. Macrolides are the first-line antimicrobial agents if required; indications are similar to those for *Salmonella*. Erythromycin 500mg PO bd for 7d (not well tolerated if vomiting) or azithromycin 500mg PO od for 3d are effective. Guillain–Barré syndrome is recognized as a post-infective complication.

① *Shigella*

Shigella is acquired by faeco-oral transmission from contaminated dairy products or water. Infection through oro-anal intercourse is also well recognized. *Shigella* is highly contagious (1000-fold more than *Salmonella*), and outbreaks occur. Four serogroups cause disease (in decreasing order of severity): *S. dysenteriae*, *S. flexneri*, *S. boydii*, and *S. sonnei*. Incubation period is 24–48h, and disease manifests with a toxigenic phase of fever, followed by lower abdominal pain and severe bloody diarrhoea with tenesmus. Illness may be self-limiting but, if severe or the patient is immunocompromised, antibiotic therapy with ciprofloxacin 500mg PO bd or ampicillin 500mg PO tds for 5d hastens recovery. Use of antimotility agents in patients with dysentery is not encouraged due to risk of precipitating toxic megacolon. Post-infectious reactive arthritis and Reiter's syndrome are recognized.

⊙ Yersinia enterocolitica

Yersinia is a less common cause of gastroenteritis, usually acquired from dairy products. Bacteria invade the small bowel epithelium overlying Peyer's patches and generate terminal ileal inflammation that can mimic Crohn's disease. The incubation period is 48–144h, and patients present with fever, lower abdominal pain, and diarrhoea (usually bloody). Extra-intestinal manifestations include erythema nodosum and erythema multi-forme. Treatment is with ciprofloxacin 500mg PO bd or co-trimoxazole 960mg PO bd for 5d in mild infections, or ceftriaxone 1–2g IV od for 5–7d in severe infection.

⊙ Vibrio species

Several species of Vibrio are pathogenic. V. cholerae is acquired from fae-cally contaminated food or water in an endemic area. The incubation period is 2–144h. It infects the small intestine where cholera toxin causes increased intracellular cAMP production and drives secretion of water, Na^+, K^+. HCO_3^-, and Cl^-. Clinically, this manifests with characteristic large-volume 'rice water' stools. Management focuses on fluid and elec-trolyte replacement, best achieved with ORS. Antibiotics are not usually required, although tetracyclines (doxycycline 200mg PO first dose fol-lowed by 100mg PO od for 7d) accelerate recovery in severe disease or immunocompromised individuals; these are contraindicated in pregnancy.

V. parahaemolyticus and V. vulnificus are acquired from raw seafood and cause gastroenteritis; the incubation period is 24–48h. V. vulnificus infec-tions may occur as part of an outbreak (common in warm climates); they are often severe (mortality is 33%) and may be associated with bullous dermatitis. Illness due to V. parahaemolyticus is typically self-limiting and does not require specific treatment. Given the potential severity of V. vul-nificus infection, a course of doxycycline (200mg PO first dose followed by 100mg PO od for 7d) is recommended if this organism is identified.

① Clostridium difficile-associated diarrhoea

C. difficile is a Gram-positive, spore-forming anaerobe that causes diar-rhoea via exotoxin production. Acquisition is most often nosocomial, with carriage rates as high as 30% in those recurrently hospitalized or resident in nursing homes. Community-acquired cases have been reported, espe-cially with the highly virulent strain (NAP1). The principal risk is recent use of broad-spectrum antibiotics. Although clindamycin was classically reported to confer greatest susceptibility, co-amoxiclav, cephalosporins, and ciprofloxacin are now the principal offenders. C. difficile infection can also underlie exacerbations of IBD.

Clinical features range from asymptomatic carriage to severe colitis (see also 📖 p. 68). In symptomatic individuals, diarrhoea and abdominal cramps usually occur within the first week of acquisition but can be delayed up to

6wk. Fulminant disease presents with fever, nausea, tachycardia, tenderness, guarding, abdominal distension, and reduced bowel sounds.

Stool should be sent for PCR ± toxin assay. If only the former is positive this represents asymptomatic carriage, early infection, or a false negative toxin result. Antibiotics are indicated if the patient has diarrhoea. If the diagnosis is not clear, sigmoidoscopy reveals characteristic yellow-white raised plaques (pseudomembranous colitis; see Colour plate 15) which on biopsy, have 'summit lesions' (outpourings of pus from surface micro-ulcerations). Proctoscopy is not sufficient, as the rectum is spared in 30%. In severe cases, request a plain AXR to look for toxic megacolon. If present, this requires follow-up with CT, VBG (raised lactate associated with need for surgery), and surgical consult due to risk of perforation.

There is no proven benefit in treating asymptomatic carriers. First-line antimicrobial therapy for *C. difficile*-associated diarrhoea consists of metronidazole 400mg PO tds for 10–14d. If there is subsequent recurrence or disease is severe or fulminant, vancomycin 125mg PO qds for 10–14d is appropriate. Avoid antimotility agents, such as loperamide, due to risk of precipitating toxic megacolon. Relapse occurs in 10–25% following a first treatment and 30–60% with subsequent treatment courses. There is some evidence this is reduced by use of probiotics (*Saccharomyces* 1g/d for 4wk).

Travellers' diarrhoea

Diarrhoea in travellers is usually mild and self-limiting. Symptoms usually start within 5–15d of arrival abroad and may be accompanied by malaise, anorexia, and abdominal cramps, with or without nausea and vomiting. One-third have fever. Investigation and treatment are required if associated with bloody diarrhoea, significant systemic upset, or persistence after returning home.

Risk factors
- Achlorhydria.
- Immunosuppression.
- Underlying bowel disease.
- Travel on cruise ships.
- Failure to observe basic hygiene.
- Exposure to contaminated food or water.

Aetiological agents
E. coli (mainly ETEC) and *Shigella* are the most common in Africa and the Middle East; *Campylobacter* predominates in Asia. Up to 30% are viral. Other bacteria (including *Aeromonas*, *Plesiomonas*, and *Vibrio* species) are less common. Parasitic causes are considered in 'Parasitic infections' (see 📖 p. 86); *Giardia* is responsible for ~5%, and amoebiasis should be considered if diarrhoea is bloody. Note that diarrhoea can be prominent in malaria; send a blood film for anyone who has travelled to a high-risk zone.

Treatment and prophylaxis

Unlike community-acquired gastroenteritis, it is often appropriate to provide antibiotics; rifaximin 200mg PO tds for 3d is the preferred empiric choice. Treatment is otherwise according to likely causal organism and follows the guidelines in 'Specific pathogens' (see 📖 pp. 81–3). If rifaximin is not available, ciprofloxacin 500mg PO (single dose) is the second-line agent, apart from for travellers to Asia where azithromycin 500mg PO (single dose) may be more effective given widespread fluoroquinolone resistance. Travellers should be advised to ensure adequate hydration, preferably with oral rehydration salts.

A number of measures are proven to reduce risk of contracting travellers' diarrhoea. These include:

- Hand washing.
- Avoid shellfish in any unregulated environment, areas of recent outbreak, or for any person with liver disease.
- Avoid raw or undercooked eggs and poultry.
- Wash all fruits and vegetables in bottled water prior to consumption.
- Stick to hot foods and beverages (make sure they arrive 'steaming' hot), acid foods (citrus), dry foods, and carbonated drinks.
- Avoid non-bottled water, ice, unpeeled raw fruits, raw vegetables, unpasteurized milk or dairy products, and street food.

At present, routine antibiotic chemoprophylaxis is not recommended because of concerns about side effects and emerging resistance. It is reasonable, however, to provide this to:

- Short-term travellers who will spend <1wk in an endemic area and whose schedules would be severely disrupted by infection.
- Patients with an underlying bowel disorder.
- Immunocompromised individuals.

Tropical sprue

This is a malabsorptive disease that develops during or after travel to the tropics. It is characterized by acquired small intestinal villous atrophy and is presumed infective in origin. Symptoms include diarrhoea or steatorrhoea, epigastric bloating, nausea, early satiety, fatigue, and weight loss; blood tests may confirm malabsorption. Diagnosis is through endoscopy and biopsy, alongside exclusion of other causes (particularly coeliac disease, giardiasis, and strongyloidiasis). Treatment is with doxycycline 100mg PO od and folic acid 5mg PO od for 3–6mo.

Parasitic infections

Protozoal and helminthic infections are more common in the returning traveller and individuals born or resident in endemic areas. Consider in patients from these backgrounds or those with unexplained persistent diarrhoea.

Giardiasis

Giardia lamblia is acquired by faeco-oral transmission of oocysts. It most frequently occurs via contaminated water, although may be person-to-person or venereal. Incubation period is 7–10d. *Giardia* primarily infects the small bowel. Symptoms include non-bloody diarrhoea, fatigue, epigastric bloating, early satiety, nausea, belching and flatus (often described as sulphurous), and (in the longer term) weight loss. Fever and systemic symptoms are rare.

Diagnosis is usually made on stool microscopy, looking for *Giardia* cysts or trophozoites. Their excretion is variable, so send multiple samples; a single stool examination has sensitivity of 50–70%, which rises to >90% with three examinations. Stool ELISA is also available. If these are negative, but clinical suspicion remains high, a course of empiric treatment is reasonable. If unsuccessful or symptoms recur, upper GI endoscopy with D2 biopsies should be undertaken, which may demonstrate the organism or alternative diagnoses.

Treatment is with metronidazole 400mg PO tds for 10d or tinidazole 2g single dose PO on d1 and d5; advise patients to avoid alcohol until 4d after the last dose.

Strongyloides stercoralis

Nematode endemic in tropical areas, with a global distribution. Penetrates skin after contact with contaminated soil, which may be associated with rash (larva currens) at the entry point. Larvae then migrate to the respiratory tract, where they can be expectorated and swallowed. They subsequently mature in the small intestine, and eggs are excreted into faeces; these then establish a cycle of auto-infection through re-entry into the body via peri-anal skin.

The incubation period is ~3wk. GI symptoms may arise at this point, but latency can be prolonged (even years or decades). Many individuals are asymptomatic and, in some, symptoms only manifest when there is a second precipitating event causing immunocompromise. Symptoms are similar to giardiasis, including bulky loose (but non-bloody) stool, epigastric bloating, nausea, and early satiety. There may occasionally be wheeze and cough, depending on respiratory tract parasite burden. Peripheral blood tests usually demonstrate eosinophilia.

Diagnosis may be achieved by stool microscopy (although up to 70% of samples are negative) or peripheral blood serology (sensitivity 85%). Sensitivity of stool microscopy is improved by charcoal culture. Occasionally, upper GI endoscopy with duodenal biopsy is required to demonstrate the worm. Check HTLV-1 serology in patients of Caribbean, South American, West African, or Japanese origin, as co-infection enhances disease severity.

The most effective treatment is ivermectin 200μg/kg stat dose PO. Albendazole 400mg PO od for 3d is an alternative.

① Amoebic dysentery

Entamoeba histolytica is acquired from faecally contaminated food and water, most frequently from exposure in developing countries (but cases in industrialized societies are also seen). Incubation period highly variable (latency may range to months), as is severity of presentation (asymptomatic to fulminant colitis). When present, symptoms include lower abdominal pain, bloody diarrhoea (in 95%), and tenesmus.

Diagnosis is usually made by stool microscopy. Routine samples may identify cysts, although these are not distinguishable on morphological grounds from non-pathogenic *Entamoeba dispar* or *Entamoeba coli* (90% cysts are non-pathogenic); follow-up stool antigen testing can help clarify. Haemophagocytic trophozoites are pathognomonic but can only be demonstrated on fresh stool samples processed immediately. Ensure these are delivered directly once produced by the patient, and call the lab to let them know they are on their way! Peripheral blood immunofluorescence antibody testing (IFAT) is available but can be negative in early disease. Flexible sigmoidoscopy and biopsy may be required to demonstrate the organism and exclude other causes of inflammatory colitis.

Treatment is with tinidazole 2g PO od for 3d or metronidazole 400mg PO tds for 5d; advise patients to avoid alcohol until 4d after the last dose. These are active against the pathogenic trophozoites. Intestinal cyst carriage subsequently needs to be eliminated with diloxanide furoate 500mg PO tds for 10d.

The management of amoebic liver abscess is detailed in Chapter 17.

Schistosomiasis

Trematode infection acquired from skin penetration of cercariae in contaminated water; intermediate host is the freshwater snail. Four species cause intestinal schistosomiasis: *Schistosoma (S.) mansoni* and *S. intercalatum* in Africa, South America, the Caribbean, and Middle East; and *S. japonicum* and *S. mekongi* in South East Asia. *S. haematobium* causes urinary tract pathology. Incubation period is 3–6wk, as worms migrate from the skin to GI tract where they then mature into the adult form; however, symptoms may only manifest on a chronic basis.

Many patients are asymptomatic or diagnosed following investigation for subclinical anaemia or malnutrition. At the more severe end of the spectrum, intestinal schistosomiasis manifests with recurrent episodes of abdominal pain and bloody diarrhoea, and hepatosplenomegaly. Diagnosis is by stool microscopy for eggs and peripheral blood serology (which can remain positive for years after successful treatment); sigmoidoscopy and biopsy are rarely required.

Patients may also present with an acute illness (Katayama fever), generated by an immunological response to the helminth migratory phase soon after acquisition. This typically manifests as urticaria, fever, and wheeze but may have associated abdominal pain, vomiting, and diarrhoea. Peripheral blood eosinophilia is usually present (but settles in the chronic phase). Katayama fever remains principally a clinical diagnosis; serology is negative at this stage, and the parasite has yet to migrate to its target organ. Confirmatory serology and stool microscopy should be delayed until 3mo after exposure.

Treatment of chronic schistosomiasis is with praziquantel 20mg/kg PO; provide two doses to be taken 4–6h apart after food. Nausea and vomiting are common side effects, and patients may prefer to take medication in the evening. Katayama fever is an allergic reaction, treated with steroids (prednisolone 20–40mg PO od, dose dependent on severity). Praziquantel is only effective against adult schistosomes and, therefore, most appropriately delayed until 3mo after exposure.

Trichuris trichiura

Roundworm principally acquired in Asia but to a lesser extent in Africa and South America. Transmitted via ingestion of eggs, usually from faecally contaminated food. Incubation period may be prolonged (worms live up to 5y). Light infestations are usually asymptomatic, with heavier infestations presenting with mucoid or bloody diarrhoea and iron deficiency anaemia; patients occasionally develop rectal prolapse. Diagnosis is based on stool microscopy for eggs and peripheral blood serology; there is frequently associated peripheral blood eosinophilia. The worm may be visualized on endoscopy, but this is rarely necessary. Treatment is with albendazole 400mg PO bd for 3d (contraindicated in pregnant women and infants); mebendazole 500mg PO bd for 3d is an alternative.

Coccidia

Obligate intracellular parasites, acquired from ingestion of contaminated water. Those causing human disease include *Cryptosporidium parvum*, *Cyclospora cayetanensis*, *Isospora belli*, and microsporidia. Incubation period is approximately 1wk. In immunocompetent adults, they usually cause mild, self-limiting illness (mean duration 2wk), characterized by watery diarrhoea, abdominal cramps, and mucus in the stool. In the young or immunocompromised, this can be protracted and/or severe. Diagnosis is made on stool electron microscopy. Treatment is principally supportive. There is no well-established antimicrobial therapy for *Cryptosporidium*. Co-trimoxazole 960mg PO bd for 7d may be effective in severe cases of *Cyclospora* or *Isospora*; increase dosing frequency to qds in immunocompromised patients. Severe cases of microsporidia can be treated with albendazole 400mg PO bd, with duration dependent on response.

Potential pitfalls

The following are the commonest errors in the emergency diagnosis and management of gastroenteritis:

- Underestimating the extent of dehydration and electrolyte losses.
- Missing diagnoses of:
  - Sepsis.
  - Bowel obstruction.
  - Appendicitis (particularly in children).
  - Immunocompromise.
  - *C. difficile*.
  - Toxic megacolon.
  - HUS.
- Complications from inappropriate use of antimotility agents.

Gastroenteritis

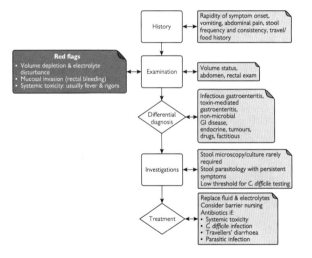

Complications of inflammatory bowel disease

Description of ulcerative colitis and Crohn's disease

Ulcerative colitis (UC) causes chronic inflammation of the rectum (proctitis) and colon (colitis). Caused by environmental triggers (possibly NSAIDs, infections, stress) in genetically susceptible hosts. Lifetime risk ~0.1% (1–2% if affected first-degree relative). Onset at any age, with bimodal distribution (15–30y and 50–70y). Presents with diarrhoea and rectal bleeding, followed by periods of remission and relapse. At any time, ~25% of patients are well (taking no medication), while two-thirds have mild disease requiring simple therapies (Odes *et al.*, 2010). Extra-intestinal symptoms occur in the minority (see Box 7.1). Diagnosis is made by flexible sigmoidoscopy or colonoscopy, with biopsies showing characteristic features of chronic/ inflammation. Long-term treatment is usually with mesalazine, orally and or topically per rectum. Severe flares require steroids, hospital admission and, occasionally, colectomy. A 2.5-fold increased risk of colon cancer after 10y of extensive colitis mandates colonoscopic surveillance. Patients with only rectosigmoiditis do not have increased susceptibility, while those with concomitant primary sclerosing cholangitis (PSC) have substantially elevated risk, requiring annual colonoscopy from diagnosis.

Crohn's disease (CD) is a relapsing-remitting chronic inflammatory disorder that principally affects the ileocaecum (40% of patients), small bowel (30%), and/or colon (30%). It is believed to be caused by environmental triggers in genetically susceptible individuals. Lifetime risk is 0.1% (3–5% if affected first-degree relative). Age of onset similar to UC. Crohn's ileitis presents with abdominal pain and malabsorption; Crohn's colitis with diarrhoea and rectal bleeding. Peri-anal disease (skin tags, abscesses and fistulae; 25% of patients) and extra-intestinal features (see Box 7.1) may be present. Diagnosis is established using a combination of endoscopy, histology, and radiology. 5-aminosalicylate drugs are largely ineffective, so most patients receive the steroid-sparing agents azathioprine or mercaptopurine. Anti-TNF therapy (e.g. infliximab or adalimumab) are used in steroid-dependent or persistently active disease. Patients with CD pan-colitis have increased risk of colorectal carcinoma similar to UC and require intermittent surveillance 10y after diagnosis.

An iPad enabled comprehensive algorithmic description of the management of IBD, based on ECCO guidelines, can be found at: ℘ http://ipad.prorenata.net/

Box 7.1 Extra-intestinal features of IBD

- Aphthous ulcers.*
- Clubbing.
- Erythema nodosum (10%).*
- Pyoderma gangrenosum.*
- Uveitis (5%).*
- Enteropathic arthritis (20%); principally affects large joints.*
- Ankylosing spondylitis. In HLA-B27 positive patients.
- Sclerosing cholangitis.

* Features associated with active IBD; lifetime risk in parentheses.

Initial assessment of the patient with suspected IBD

History

Consider IBD in patients with >10d diarrhoea. Rectal bleeding is more suggestive of UC and abdominal pain of CD.

- Fresh bleeding occurs due to rectosigmoiditis. Darker blood loss suggests more proximal disease. Anaemia may be present. Most patients with severe UC bleed, compared to only 40% with colitis due to CD.
- Frequent diarrhoea (defined as an increase of 3+ loose stools daily) is usual in patients with IBD colitis. Ask specifically about nocturnal diarrhoea as suggests an inflammatory cause.
- Proctitis presents with urgency and tenesmus, rectal mucus, and bleeding. These also occur in patients with:
  - Rectal cancer.
  - Infectious proctitis (Neisseria (N.) gonorrhoeae, syphilis, lymphogranuloma venereum, Herpes simplex).
  - Solitary rectal ulcer syndrome (SRUS). Arises in anxious patients who strain excessively during defaecation, causing a fold of rectal mucosa to prolapse and ulcerate. Presents with lower abdominal pain before and during defaecation. Advise avoidance of straining and bowel opening for no more than 5min, twice per day.
- Lower abdominal pain occurs in CD but also diverticulitis (usually left-sided, associated with rectal bleeding) and colorectal malignancy.
- Lethargy is common in both IBD and malignancy.
- Ask about family history.
- Weight loss >5% body weight is more suggestive of malignancy, although can occur with severe IBD.
- Ask about NSAID and antibiotic use, which can exacerbate colitis. Ask about risk factors for vascular disease (ischaemic colitis, mesenteric angina; see Chapter 9). Take a travel history.
- Determine smoking history (exacerbates CD, protective in UC).

Examination

Examination may reveal a mass (particularly RIF) and/or abdominal discomfort in CD (also found in patients with malignancy, appendix mass, or diverticular abscess). Abdominal pain or guarding in suspected UC suggests fulminant colitis with serosal involvement. Patients with severe UC are often dehydrated and may be anaemic. Peri-anal abnormalities (fistulae, skin tags, anal fissure) are strongly associated with CD, although can occur with UC. Examine for extra-intestinal manifestations of IBD, many of which correlate with disease activity.

Investigations

Most patients with chronic rectal bleeding or diarrhoea can have outpatient investigation. Criteria for admission are given in Box 7.2. Investigations depend on symptoms and disease type (UC or CD) and include:

- Blood tests:
  - FBC. Look for anaemia, microcytosis (suggestive of chronic blood loss), leukocytosis, and thrombocytosis (active inflammation).
  - ESR and CRP. Both raised in inflammation, although lower sensitivity for small bowel disease. CRP quicker to respond (half-life 19h).
  - Check iron studies. Low TIBC with low iron and iron saturation more suggestive of chronic disease than iron deficiency.
  - Vitamin B12 may be low in patients with terminal ileal CD.
  - Exclude renal impairment and electrolyte disturbances. Check calcium, Mg^{++}, and LFT (albumin <20g/L predictive of poor surgical outcome.
- Stool tests. Send one sample for microscopy and culture if diarrhoea, and two samples for *C. difficile* (which is related to 5% of IBD flares; see Chapter 6). Often these samples are overlooked, so liaise with the nurses to make sure they are collected, the pot sealed and labelled properly, and safely delivered to the laboratory. Request 3 sequential days of stool analysis for ova, cysts, and parasites in high-risk populations or those who have travelled to the developing world in the previous 3mo.
- Radiology:
  - Request AXR if severe UC or obstruction suspected, or in the frail or elderly. Do not request indiscriminately as provides 4mo of background radiation. Colonic dilatation (transverse colon >6cm) occurs in fulminant colitis (and, occasionally, infectious colitis). Rate of diameter change rather than absolute value more prognostic. Mandates daily AXR, at least twice daily clinical assessment, and NGT for gaseous decompression. Recommend rolling supine to prone position every 2h to redistribute intestinal gas.
  - CT with oral and IV contrast (and surgical opinion) should be obtained in those with abdominal guarding.
  - If CD is suspected, request a small bowel follow-through in patients over 65y, and MR follow-through in younger patients (avoids radiation risk). Also request pelvic MRI in those with peri-anal disease.
- Small bowel US in expert hands is valuable in the diagnosis and monitoring of ileocaecal CD.
- Capsule endoscopy can be used to diagnose CD but requires prior patency capsule to identify those in whom the procedure should be avoided (9% capsule obstruction in CD).

---

① Box 7.2 Criteria for admission to hospital

- Too frail for outpatient investigation.
- Hypovolaemia (postural hypotension).
- Severe or fulminant colitis (present in 10% of flares).
- Severe abdominal pain.
- Profuse bloody diarrhoea (>5 bloody stools/d).
- Temperature >38°C (invasive disease).

Have a lower threshold in the elderly or immunocompromised.

- All patients with IBD should have baseline bone densitometry.
- Endoscopy:
  - Flexible sigmoidoscopy should be the first endoscopic investigation in active UC, as it is quick and safe, provides a diagnosis, and excludes alternative diagnoses (e.g. CMV colitis).
  - Colonoscopy can be performed following remission to exclude more proximal pathology.
  - Consider air contrast CT in patients >80y or those with significant co-morbidity.
  - Barium enema has lower diagnostic yield than colonoscopy or air contrast CT scan and should not be requested.
  - Patients with Crohn's colitis should be similarly investigated. Request flexible sigmoidoscopy to exclude rectal involvement in those presenting with peri-anal CD.

Indications for urgent flexible sigmoidoscopy

- Immunocompromise.
- Suspected ischaemic colitis.
- Suspected new diagnosis of IBD.
- Severe diarrhoea persisting for >5d.
- Patients requiring admission to hospital.

Flare of IBD or infection?

It can be difficult to distinguish between infective diarrhoea and a flare or new presentation of IBD, and sometimes both occur simultaneously. Up to 10% of patients with a presumed flare have positive stool cultures or *C. difficile* infection (latter three times more likely in IBD). Diagnosis is made based on history, stool samples, endoscopic appearances, duration of illness, and histology. Infective diarrhoea suggested if rapid onset of symptoms (days rather than weeks), cramping abdominal pain, and fever in a patient with UC, and symptomatic improvement within 1wk. Infective colitis is not more common in patients treated with anti-TNF drugs.

- Blood tests do not distinguish between infective and inflammatory diarrhoea but do correlate with disease severity.
- Toxic dilatation is more common in IBD than infective colitis. Inform senior physician and surgical team if present as may require colectomy.
- Rigid sigmoidoscopy in the Emergency Department can exclude a flare of ulcerative proctitis/colitis (mucosa appears normal). The mucosa can be inflamed in either IBD or bacillary dysentery; the rectum may be normal in CD. Consider taking a rectal biopsy using *flexible* biopsy forceps at the same time if flexible sigmoidoscopy unavailable within 24h.
- If stool cultures are non-contributory and symptoms persist or worsen, request urgent flexible sigmoidoscopy. Histology can usually differentiate between a flare of IBD and infective colitis, as crypt architecture is preserved in the latter (although this may also be normal in the first few weeks of IBD).

Metronidazole 400mg PO tds and ciprofloxacin 500mg PO bd for 5d can be provided if steroids are deemed necessary before infective colitis has been excluded by stool analysis; also provide metronidazole if amoebic colitis suspected until histology and microscopy available.

If patients deteriorate following introduction or escalation of immunosuppression, consider a diagnosis of CMV colitis. Review histology for presence of inclusion bodies (pathognomonic but sensitivity only 25–60%) and request CMV immunohistochemistry. Responds to ganciclovir 5mg/kg IV bd or valganciclovir 900mg PO bd for 14d.

Assessing disease severity

Truelove and Witt's classification of UC severity (Table 7.1)

Table 7.1 Truelove and Witt's classification

Activity	Mild	Severe
Bloody stools/d	<4	>6
Temperature (°C)	Afebrile	>37.8
HR (beats/min)	Normal	>90
Hb (g/dL)	>11	<10.5
ESR (mm/h)	<20	>30

Reproduced from *British Medical Journal*, S. C. Truelove, 'Cortisone in Ulcerative Colitis', 2, pp. 1041–1047, Copyright 1955, with permission from BMJ Publishing Group Ltd.

Severe colitis is defined as 6 or more bloody stools/d with at least one of the other factors. Score should be calculated daily. Fulminant disease describes a subset of patients with severe colitis who additionally have anorexia and abdominal pain, and are at risk of progressing to toxic megacolon and colonic perforation. Stool frequency >8/d or CRP >45mg/L on d3 of admission predicts 85% likelihood of colectomy during the admission.

Modified Baron score to assess severity at sigmoidoscopy (Table 7.2)

Table 7.2 Modified Baron score

Mild	Moderate	Severe
Erythema and decreased vascular pattern	Marked erythema; loss of vascular pattern; friable mucosa	Spontaneous bleeding and ulceration

From The New England Journal of Medicine, Schroeder *et al.*, 'Coated Oral 5-Aminosalicylic Acid Therapy for Mildly to Moderately Active Ulcerative Colitis', 317, 26, pp. 1625–1629. Copyright © 1987, Massachusetts Medical Society. Reprinted with permission from Massachusetts Medical Society.

Harvey–Bradshaw activity index (Box 7.3)

> **Box 7.3 Harvey–Bradshaw activity index for Crohn's disease**
> - Wellbeing in previous 24h:
>   - Very well ≈ 0.
>   - Slightly below par ≈ 1.
>   - Poor ≈ 2.
>   - Very poor ≈ 3.
>   - Terrible ≈ 4.
> - Abdominal pain in previous 24h:
>   - None ≈ 0.
>   - Mild ≈ 1.
>   - Moderate ≈ 2.
>   - Severe ≈ 3.
> - Number of liquid stools in past 24h. Score 1 per motion.
> - Presence of abdominal mass:
>   - None ≈ 0.
>   - Dubious ≈ 1.
>   - Definite ≈ 2.
>   - Definite + tender ≈ 3.
> - Extra-intestinal manifestations. One point each for arthralgia, iritis, erythema nodosum, pyoderma gangrenosum, aphthous ulcers, anal fissure, new fistula, and abscess.
>
> A score <5 implies remission; 5–7 mild, and 8–16 moderate disease; >16 indicates a severe flare. The Harvey–Bradshaw score provides equivalent stratification to the Crohn's disease activity index (CDAI), but is much easier to use. Reprinted from *The Lancet*, 315, 8167, R.F. Harvey and J.M. Bradshaw, 'A simple index of Crohn's disease', p. 514, Copyright 1980, with permission from Elsevier.

Management of ulcerative colitis

Proctitis

Nocturnal 1g mesalazine suppositories promote sustained remission in >75% by 3wk. Provide as topical enema if poor response (e.g. Salofalk® 2g). Long-term treatment required following second relapse. Topical steroids (e.g. Predfoam®) less effective but useful addition in patients with poor response. Oral therapy less effective than topical therapy.

Left-sided colitis

Nocturnal topical mesalazine enemas for 28d more effective than topical steroid enemas. Latter may be added in refractory disease, in which case consider budesonide enemas to minimize side effects. Oral mesalazine up to 4.8g/d for 1–2mo enables remission in 43% and overall improvement in 70% by 6wk. Addition of topical to oral therapy provides further advantage. Beclometasone m/r, a non-absorbed steroid, at a dose of 5mg PO od can be used in those with mild-to-moderate disease who do not tolerate mesalazine. Prednisolone (40mg PO od for 2wk, then taper by 5mg each 5–7d), with adjunctive calcium/vitamin D, may be required if moderate or severe disease does not respond by 1–2wk despite above therapies. Thiopurines (azathioprine at least 2mg/kg PO od or mercaptopurine 1–1.5mg/kg/d) used as steroid-sparing agents in those receiving >2 courses of steroids in any 1y. Maintenance therapy (e.g. mesalazine 1.6g/d) advocated following remission.

Extensive colitis

Oral mesalazine ± topical therapy is used in mild-to-moderate disease (see Colour plate 16). Persistent troublesome symptoms are usually treated with steroids (for regime, see 'Left-sided colitis', 📖 p. 97), with a number needed to treat of 3 (as one-third would improve anyway and one-third are steroid-refractory (see 📖 p. 97).

☼ Severe and fulminant colitis

- Hydrocortisone 100mg IV qds or methylprednisolone 20mg IV tds, usually for 5d.
- Supplementary IV fluid replacement if dehydrated (e.g. 1L 0.9% saline over 12h, then 1L 5% glucose over 12h, each with 40mmol KCl).
- Correct electrolytes daily (Na$^+$, K$^+$, Mg^{++}, calcium, PO$_4^{3-}$).
- LMWH thromboprophylaxis (patients with severe colitis have >30 relative risk of venous thromboembolism).
- Withhold mesalazine. Stop if flare coincided with introduction as occasionally exacerbates colitis.
- Stool chart (often preferable if patient completes).
- IV ciprofloxacin + metronidazole if fulminant disease (requires surgical review, medical review twice daily). Remember signs attenuated by steroids.
- Daily AXR until improving. NGT if colonic dilatation.
- Consider topical therapy at 72h if tenesmus/urgency.
- If no response at 3–5d, consider second-line agents:
  - Ciclosporin 2mg/kg/d IV, then oral preparation for up to 3mo; 80% respond initially.
  - Infliximab 5mg/kg IV at 0, 2, and 6wk. As of 2012, there has been one comparative trial that demonstrated equivalent outcomes between infliximab and ciclosporin. A multicentre UK study (CONSTRUCT) to assess this further is ongoing.
  - Adverse effects prevent the use of these agents concurrently or sequentially outside of clinical trials.
  - Protocols for using these agents can be found at: see 🖰 http://www.ibdqip.co.uk/.
  - ~20% of thiopurine naive, and 40% of non-naive patients require colectomy within 1y.
- ~30% of patients are steroid-refractory, requiring second-line agents during their admission. A similar number are steroid-dependent and will subsequently require a steroid-sparing agent.
- The lifetime risk of colectomy in UC is ~10%, but up to 30% in extensive UC. ~10% of those admitted with severe UC have a colectomy during the admission.

Antibiotics
There is no role for antibiotics to treat a UC flare other than that specified here (see 'Severe and fulminant colitis', 📖 p. 98).

Loperamide
Can be used in mild disease, particularly to allow uninterrupted sleep. Avoid in severe disease, as anecdotal reports suggest may precipitate colonic dilatation.

Probiotics
E. coli Nissle 1917 has been shown to be equipotent to mesalazine in mild UC. VSL#3 (a preparation of eight bacteria) 3g od is effective in prophylaxis and treatment of pouchitis.

Nutrition
There are no diets that precipitate or treat flares in UC. Patients should take a balanced, low-residue diet when symptomatic. Dietetic advice is helpful. Anecdotal opinion has advocated the specific carbohydrate diet (see 🖰 http://www.ccfa.org/about/news/scd). If patients have had poor nutrition for >1wk, enteral supplements may be required. TPN has no role other than as an adjunct to surgery in some patients.

Proximal constipation
Check for build-up of stool above the level of inflammation with AXR if colitis does not seem to be improving. Advise increased dietary fibre and initiate an osmotic laxative (e.g. macrogol).

Surgery
Indications for surgery
- Fulminant colitis and rapidly dilating colon or ileus.
- Non-responsive fulminant colitis despite 72h medical therapy.
- Non-responsive severe colitis despite 7–10d medical therapy, including second-line agents.
- Moderate-to-severe colitis despite maximal medical therapy.
- Multifocal colonic dysplasia or malignancy.

Types of operation
- Proctocolectomy with permanent (Brooke) ileostomy.
- Proctocolectomy with continent ileostomy (Koch pouch).
- Abdominal colectomy with ileorectal anastomosis (rarely performed).
- Colectomy, mucosal proctectomy, and ileal pouch anal anastomosis (IPAA).
- Colectomy and stapled ileal pouch distal rectal anastomosis
- Subtotal colectomy, ileostomy, and rectal mucous fistula/rectal closure is the procedure of choice in toxic/fulminant disease.

Preoperative preparation
- Optimize medical status. Correct anaemia, fluid depletion, electrolytes, coagulopathy, and nutrition. Consider 48h preoperative TPN in patients whose symptoms worsen with enteral nutrition.
- Stop steroids or taper (if possible) to, at least, a dose equivalent of prednisolone 10mg daily. Patients with possible adrenal

suppression should undergo low-dose ACTH (Synacthen®) test preoperatively, as they may need peri-operative steroid cover. Other immunosuppressants can be continued, although anti-TNF agents increase risk of pelvic anastomotic infection and, therefore, mandate a three-stage IPAA.
- Assess liver function and reserve in patients with PSC.
- Provide patient information and ensure stoma nurse review.

Factors to consider at discharge
- Measure TPMT level so that a thiopurine can be more safely provided in the future if needed.
- Check serological immunity for hepatitis A and B, and pneumococcus and varicella zoster, ideally before immunosuppression started. Arrange for any vaccinations to occur soon after stopping steroids (as diminished levels of immunity are stimulated in those taking thiopurines).
- Remind patients they need annual influenza vaccinations.
- Restart mesalazine 2.4g PO od at discharge.
- Consider providing topical therapy once steroid course finished if persistent symptoms.
- Provide contact details in case of relapse.
- Arrange virtual follow-up (telephone or email) within 2wk and outpatient follow-up at 8wk.
- Plan to perform bone density scan and colonoscopy if required once patient in remission.
- Provide absence from work certificate for at least 10d; rest and avoidance of stress are important treatments.
- Remind the patient that compliance with therapy is often reduced in chronic illness, but that it has been shown to significantly improve response rates in IBD.
- Advise patient to avoid NSAIDs and excess alcohol.

Management of Crohn's disease

The history, examination, and investigation of patients with CD have been described (see 📖 p. 93). The principles of managing patients with CD are broadly similar to UC.

Crohn's colitis and ileitis
- Mild colitis may respond to sulfasalazine or steroids.
- Moderate disease is an indication for an immunomodulator (thiopurine or methotrexate).
- Severe disease should be treated with an anti-TNF agent and thiopurine.
  - Before starting a thiopurine, know the TPMT level (reduce doses if low activity and avoid if no activity). One regime is to provide azathioprine 50mg PO od for 1wk, and, if tolerated, increase to 2–2.5mg/kg/d.
  - Before starting anti-TNF therapy, exclude HBV (check HBsAg and HBcAb), HCV, HIV and TB (IFN-γ release assay and CXR), and exclude urine and stool infections. Infliximab is given as a 5mg/kg

infusion over 2h at 0, 2, and 6wk. Adalimumab is given as a 160mg SC injection at wk 0, 80mg at wk2, and then 40mg every 2wk.

- Methotrexate is a suitable alternative to a thiopurine, given as a 25mg dose IM weekly for 12wk, then 15mg weekly IM (in practice, often PO) give folic acid 5mg PO 2d after each dose.
- An alternative to the therapies above is an exclusive polymeric diet, although the efficacy is less than that of steroid therapy (55% compared to 65% response rate). Some find it unpalatable. Semi-polymeric diets (50% low residue, 50% polymeric supplements) can be provided for several weeks following symptom resolution.

- Localized ileocaecal disease should be similarly treated, although use budesonide 9mg PO od for 2mo, then 3mg for 1 further month, instead of sulfasalazine.
- There is some benefit in treating colonic disease with antibiotics: metronidazole ± ciprofloxacin, or rifaximin 800mg PO bd for 12wk (Prantera et al., 2012).
- Loperamide may be useful in the absence of extensive colitis.
- Colesevelam 1.25g PO bd should be given as a therapeutic trial to those with ileal disease and diarrhoea as a screen for bile salt malabsorption. Advise patients to avoid ingesting other medication 1h before or 4h after this drug. Diagnosis can be confirmed by 23-seleno-25-homotaurocholic acid (SeHCAT) radionuclide study.
- Lactose intolerance is common in those with ileal disease.
- Indications for surgery are similar to UC (see 📖 p. 99) but also include stenotic disease not amenable to endoscopic dilation (i.e. >4cm long).

☼ Small bowel obstruction

- Usually subacute and non-strangulating.
- Treat with bowel rest, NGT, and IV fluids.
- Obtain imaging, ideally small bowel protocol MR study (see Fig. 7.1).
- Determine whether active or fibrotic disease is the cause of obstruction (possibly with associated food impaction), or adhesions:
  - Active disease is usually found in context of raised blood (CRP, ESR) and stool (calprotectin) inflammatory markers. Mucosal contrast enhancement is seen on small bowel MRI. Treat medically with parenteral glucocorticoids.
  - Surgery is required for fibrotic disease (stricturoplasty) or patients with evidence of bowel infarction (lactic acidosis, abdominal pain, reduced bowel sounds). Liaise closely with colorectal surgical team.
  - Assess and correct nutritional status (see Chapter 10).

Post-operative therapy for ileocolonic Crohn's disease

- Stop smoking.
- Recommend lifelong prophylactic medical therapy.
- Mesalazine 4g PO od for at least 3mo (not needed beyond 3mo in conjunction with thiopurine therapy).
- Metronidazole 400mg PO bd for 3mo, though often poorly tolerated.
- Thiopurine if adverse prognostic features:
  - Age <30y.
  - Fistulating disease.
  - Extensive resection or second resection.

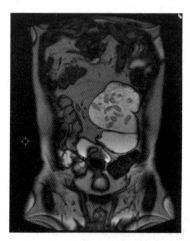

Fig. 7.1 MRI showing food debris in dilated jejunum due to Crohn's disease stricture.

- Consider anti-TNF therapy if surgery occurred despite use of a thiopurine.

① **Crohn's disease masses**
- Obtain cross-sectional imaging to define the degree of inflammation and exclude intra-abdominal abscess:
  - Small abscesses/inflammatory masses managed with antibiotics.
  - Liquid abscesses can be drained percutaneously, although up to 50% eventually require surgery.
  - Do not provide steroids or anti-TNF whilst abscesses >1cm diameter *in situ*.
  - Surgery indicated if peritonitis or if mass persists following drainage. Rectus sheath and psoas abscesses require surgery.
  - Assess and correct nutritional status (see Chapter 10).
- Could it be TB?
  - Non-specific abdominal pain in 80%.
  - Abdominal radiology cannot discriminate from CD; abnormal CXR in <50%.
  - Aphthous ulcers with normal adjacent mucosa suggest CD. Inflammation surrounding circumferential ulcers or a deformed ileocaecal valve appearing like a fish mouth suggestive of TB.
  - Deep endoscopic biopsies for histology, PCR, and culture required (granulomas of TB submucosal, unlike CD).
  - PCR of biopsy specimens provides results within 48h.
  - Have a low threshold for anti-tuberculosis therapy in those in whom TB is suspected, especially if from an endemic region.

Response to therapy usually within 2wk; if does not occur, consider laparoscopy to exclude actinomycosis, amoebiasis, *Yersinia enterocolitica*, lymphoma, and adenocarcinoma.

Enteral fistulae

May be between loops of bowel (entero-enteric), between bowel and another hollow organ (entero-vesical, entero-vaginal), or between bowel and skin (entero-cutaneous). Peri-anal fistulae occur in 20% (see 'Peri-anal disease' 📖 p. 103), and other enteral fistulae in 15%; ~50% associated with internal strictures.

- Internal fistulae may be asymptomatic. Symptoms depend on the degree of bypassed bowel. Ileosigmoid is the commonest entero-enteric fistula and presents with diarrhoea, weight loss, and pain. Suspect an entero-vesical fistula with pneumaturia, faecaluria, and recurrent UTIs.
- Investigation requires cross-sectional imaging, usually MRI. Therapy is usually surgical once nutritional state optimized and sepsis temporarily treated. Outcomes are poorer with vaginal fistulae.
- There are no controlled trial data of medical therapy other than infliximab (ACCENT II); closure was seen in 45% of 25 patients with recto-vaginal fistulae.

Peri-anal disease

- Peri-anal abscesses develop in 50% of patients with peri-anal CD. Present with pain, especially on sitting. Occasionally there are associated constitutional symptoms or drainage of pus. Examination may reveal erythema.
- Mainstay of therapy is drainage of contained sepsis.
- Request urgent MR pelvis and EUA by an experienced surgeon for seton insertion.
- Start metronidazole 400mg PO tds.
- Request flexible sigmoidoscopy to exclude luminal disease; treat if present, as peri-anal disease usually persists if active proctitis.
- Simple, low fistulae treated with metronidazole, seton, or possibly fistulotomy.
- Complex fistulae (see Fig. 7.2) treated with metronidazole, a non-cutting seton, and a thiopurine ± anti-TNF.
- Assess and correct nutritional status (see Chapter 10).

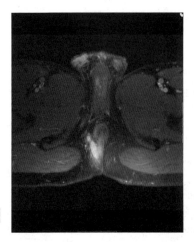

Fig. 7.2 Anal intersphincteric fistula due to Crohn's disease.

Special situations

The returning traveller
Infections in patients with IBD and dysentery can be missed. Screen patients with bloody diarrhoea returning from the developing world for tropical infections, particularly amoebiasis (see Chapter 6).

The patient with HIV
See Chapter 12.

① The pregnant patient
- The course of IBD is unaffected by pregnancy.
- One-third relapse during pregnancy, similar to non-pregnant patients.
- Active disease at conception often remains active.
- There is a slight increase in low birthweight and preterm deliveries in patients with IBD (more in CD and in those with active disease at conception).
- Active peri-anal CD is a relative indication for Caesarian section.
- Flexible sigmoidoscopy is safe in pregnancy.
- IBD medication is safe in pregnancy with the following caveats:
  - Avoid ciprofloxacin.
  - Breastfeed at least 4h after ingesting thiopurines.
  - Avoid methotrexate.
  - Ideally, avoid anti-TNF drugs beyond second trimester (26wk); they can be provided to nursing mothers if absolutely necessary.
- Liaise with the obstetric team.

Complications of medical therapy

Steroids

- Side effects common and usually dose-dependent, especially skin thinning, purpura, Cushingoid appearance, hyperglycaemia, hypertension, insomnia, and weight gain.
- Cataracts occur after 1y. Glaucoma precipitated in susceptible patients.
- Osteonecrosis, osteoporosis, and myopathy occur. Recommend weight-bearing exercise and supplement calcium/vitamin D. Provide bisphosphonate (e.g. alendronate 70mg PO weekly) if treating for >3mo or providing >7.5mg prednisolone/d to high-risk patients (>65y, previous fragility fracture). Monitor with bone densitometry.
- Gastric irritation occurs in those taking concomitant NSAIDs. Provide protection (e.g. omeprazole 20mg PO od).
- Immunosuppression increases risk of infection. Avoid live vaccines.

Metronidazole

- Significant side effects rare. Commonest are GI, especially nausea and metallic taste.
- Peripheral neuropathy occurs in up to 50% with chronic use.

5-aminosalicylates

- Side effects mild and rare; headache and GI upset most common.
- Hypersensitivity reaction are rare (pancreatitis, pneumonitis) but preclude continuation of therapy.
- Acute interstitial nephritis in 0.25%/patient-year; check U & E at 6wk, 6mo, and annually thereafter.
- May cause aplastic anaemia, agranulocytosis, or thrombocytopaenia.
- Sulfasalazine associated with Stevens–Johnson syndrome and oligospermia.

Thiopurines

- 10% do not tolerate therapy:
  - Allergic reaction (fever, rash, arthropathy; 2.5%).
  - Bone marrow suppression (1.5%).
  - Pancreatitis (1.5%).
  - Nausea (1.5%).
- TPMT levels guide dosing.
- Check FBC, U & E, LFT, and CRP weekly for 4wk, fortnightly for 2mo, then every 2–3mo.
- Mild rise in transaminases in 5%. Responds to dose reduction. Stop if bilirubin rises and no other explanation.
- Lymphoma increased from 0.2 to 0.9/1000 patient-years whilst patients take therapy.
- Increased risk of non-melanoma skin cancer. Advise use of high-factor sunscreen.
- Avoid in EBV-naive patients (risk of lymphoma at seroconversion).
- Avoid live vaccines.

Methotrexate
- Not tolerated by 15%.
- Nausea, vomiting, abnormal LFT, headache, and rash most common side effects.
- Teratogenic, so men and women must avoid if trying to conceive. Crosses into breast milk.
- Hepatoxicity reported but too rare to require surveillance biopsies. More likely following cumulative ingestion >4g.
- Extensively protein-bound: can be displaced by aspirin and NSAIDs.
- Avoid in EBV-naive patients.
- Avoid live vaccines.

Ciclosporin
- Main toxicities are renal and neurological:
  - Nephrotoxicity acute (reversible) or chronic (irreversible).
  - Causes tremor, headache, and paraesthesia.
- Other side effects include:
  - Hypertension.
  - Hyperkalaemia.
  - Gingival hypertrophy.
- Increased risk of cutaneous squamous cell carcinoma.

Anti-TNF
- Injection site, and acute or delayed hypersensitivity infusion reactions.
- Neutropaenia.
- Infections. Increased risk of serious and unusual infections, and TB. Avoid food-borne infections (e.g. *Listeria*). Treat intercurrent hepatitis B. Avoid live vaccines. Give PCP prophylaxis if intercurrent steroid use.
- Demyelinating disease. Association unclear, but stop drug immediately if occurs.
- Avoid in patients with heart failure.
- Cutaneous reactions, including psoriasis.
- Malignancy. Risks similar to azathioprine (see 'Thiopurines' p. 105).
- Autoimmunity.

Complications of inflammatory bowel disease

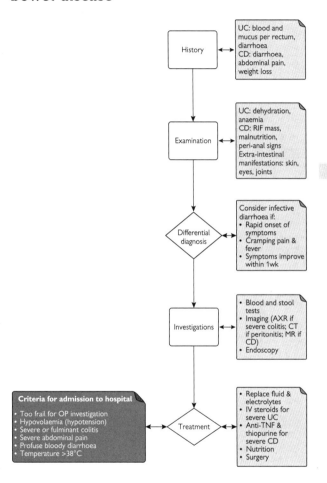

History
UC: blood and mucus per rectum, diarrhoea
CD: diarrhoea, abdominal pain, weight loss

Examination
UC: dehydration, anaemia
CD: RIF mass, malnutrition, peri-anal signs
Extra-intestinal manifestations: skin, eyes, joints

Differential diagnosis
Consider infective diarrhoea if:
• Rapid onset of symptoms
• Cramping pain & fever
• Symptoms improve within 1wk

Investigations
• Blood and stool tests
• Imaging (AXR if severe colitis; CT if peritonitis; MR if CD)
• Endoscopy

Treatment
• Replace fluid & electrolytes
• IV steroids for severe UC
• Anti-TNF & thiopurine for severe CD
• Nutrition
• Surgery

Criteria for admission to hospital
• Too frail for OP investigation
• Hypovolaemia (hypotension)
• Severe or fulminant colitis
• Severe abdominal pain
• Profuse bloody diarrhoea
• Temperature >38°C

Further reading

Odes S, Vardi H, Friger M, et al. (2010) Clinical and economic outcomes in a population-based European cohort of 948 ulcerative colitis and Crohn's disease patients by Markov analysis. *Aliment Pharmacol Ther* **31**: 735–44.

Prantera C, Lochs H, Grimaldi M, et al. (2011) Rifaximin-extended intestinal release induces remission in patients with moderately active Crohn's disease. *Gastroenterology* **142**: 473–481.e4.

Acute thoracic pain and dysphagia

Differential diagnosis of acute thoracic pain

The approach to acute thoracic pain should be to rapidly identify potentially life-threatening causes, then consider other sources.

☠ Immediately life-threatening

- Acute coronary syndrome.
- Aortic dissection.
- Tension pneumothorax.
- Pulmonary embolism.
- Oesophageal rupture.

① Other causes

- GI:
  - Oesophagitis.
  - Oesophageal motility disorders.
  - Food impaction.
  - Ingestion of hot or cold liquids.
  - Peptic ulcer disease (see Chapter 9).
  - Pancreatitis.
  - Cholecystitis.
- Cardiac:
  - Pericarditis.
  - Myocarditis.
  - Cardiac syndrome X (angina, positive ETT, normal angiogram).
  - Valvular heart disease.
- Respiratory:
  - Pneumonia.
  - Empyema.
  - Pleurisy.
- Musculoskeletal:
  - Muscular.
  - Costochondritis (Tietze's syndrome).
  - Inflammatory arthritides.
  - Costovertebral joint dysfunction syndrome.
  - Rib fracture.
  - Bone metastases.
  - Thoracic vertebral disc herniation.
- Neurological:
  - Herpes zoster.
  - Cervical spondylosis.
- Other:
  - Sickle cell crisis.
  - Da Costa's syndrome (left submammary stabbing pain, usually associated with anxiety).
  - Psychogenic.

① **Oesophagitis**

Oesophageal inflammation usually results from chemical injury to the mucosa, secondary to reflux of acid and pepsin from the stomach. Although reflux is common (10% in Western societies), it does not cause harm in the majority of individuals, as irritants are rapidly removed by peristalsis. Fewer than 5% of patients with reflux have demonstrable oesophagitis, although this rises to 50% in those with severe symptoms.

Risk factors for reflux disease

- Obesity.
- Cigarette smoking.
- Alcohol.
- Caffeine.
- Fatty or spicy foods.
- Pregnancy.
- Spinal cord injury.
- *H. pylori* eradication. Infection protective against reflux due to associated gastric atrophy reducing stomach acid.

Rare causes of oesophagitis

- Medication-induced oesophagitis:
  - High risk: NSAIDs, slow-release KCl, tetracycline, quinidine, bisphosphonates.
  - Medium risk: other antibiotics, ferrous sulphate.
  - Low risk: ascorbic acid, mexiletine, slow-release theophylline, captopril, phenytoin, zidovudine.
  - Chemotherapy (can cause mucositis directly, from neurological injury disrupting motility, or due to immune suppression): dactinomycin, bleomycin, cytarabine, daunorubicin, 5-fluorouracil, methotrexate, vincristine.
  - Sclerosant for treatment of oesophageal varices.
- Immunocompromise (see Chapter 12):
  - Candida.
  - Herpesviridae (CMV, HSV, VZV).
- Radiation:
  - 30Gy: retrosternal burning and odynophagia.
  - 40Gy: mucosal erythema.
  - 50Gy: significant oesophagitis.
  - 60Gy: severe oesophagitis with strictures, perforation, and fistulation. This dose can be used to treat oesophageal SCC.
- Caustic injury (see 📖 p. 123).
- Systemic disorders:
  - Epidermolysis bullosa, pemphigus vulgaris.
  - Stevens–Johnson syndrome.
  - Collagen vascular diseases (especially scleroderma), sarcoidosis.
  - Crohn's disease, Behçet's disease.
  - Eosinophilic oesophagitis.
  - Metastatic malignant disease.
  - Graft-versus-host disease.

Clinical presentation

The most common symptoms are heartburn, waterbrash, and non-specific retrosternal discomfort. Enquire about dysphagia, odynophagia, anorexia, weight loss, haematemesis, melaena, and significant cough or wheeze. Take a thorough drug history, including use of over-the-counter medications.

Examination is generally normal but should include the oral cavity for ulcers or candidiasis; consider rectal examination for occult blood loss. In patients with a suggestive history, look for signs of immunosuppression or dermatological manifestations of systemic disease.

Investigation

In general, FBC to detect microcytic anaemia is sufficient. ECG and troponin should be performed if there is any possibility that pain might arise from an acute coronary syndrome. *Always consider a cardiac cause of chest pain.* Diagnostic tests for underlying diseases should be guided by the history and examination findings.

Routine radiography is not indicated unless complications are suspected. A barium swallow study is first-line if dysphagia is the primary complaint and a proximal lesion, complex stricture, or achalasia is suspected. Otherwise, OGD should be performed, especially in patients who present with haematemesis, melaena, or suspected acute oesophageal obstruction; those aged >50 with new onset symptoms; and those with an abdominal mass, significant anaemia, or pain refractory to repeated trials of medication. The Los Angeles grading system for oesophagitis is often used (see Table 8.1).

Management

- Lifestyle measures. Avoid large meals and provocative foods (including alcohol and caffeine), stop smoking, and lose weight. Elevate the head of the bed (increasing the number of pillows alone is not recommended, as angulation of the body may increase intra-abdominal pressure). If symptoms are medication-related, advise to take pills with plenty of water.
- Antacids. May abort episodes but of no prophylactic value.
- PPI (e.g. omeprazole 20mg od for 4–8wk). If response satisfactory, maintain and titrate to symptoms. If recalcitrant, then consider repeat endoscopy, twice daily PPI, or surgery if severe or complicated.
- Dietician review if oral intake compromised.

Complications

Typically limited to those with severe oesophagitis.
- Bleeding. Rarely life-threatening unless from a deep ulcer associated with columnar metaplasia (Barrett's oesophagus).
- Benign stricturing.
- Barrett's oesophagus with malignant transformation.
- Perforation and mediastinitis.
- Weight loss, volume depletion.
- Laryngitis, bronchospasm, aspiration pneumonitis/pneumonia.

Table 8.1 Los Angeles grading system for oesophagitis

Grade	Findings
A	Mucosal break <5mm in length
B	Mucosal break >5mm
C	Mucosal break continuous between >2 mucosal folds
D	Mucosal break >75% of oesophageal circumference

Oesophageal spasm

This can be subdivided into two clinical entities: diffuse oesophageal spasm (in which contractions are uncoordinated) and nutcracker oesophagus (in which they are coordinated but excessive). The aetiology is not known, and contractions occur in the absence of any demonstrable structural stenosis.

Both syndromes may present with episodic central, crushing chest pain that can be very difficult to differentiate from cardiac ischaemia on the basis of history alone. They are accompanied by intermittent dysphagia in two-thirds of patients and may be associated with regurgitation or globus. Relationship to food intake is inconsistent.

Investigation

Blood tests are generally unhelpful, although a screen for diabetes causing neuropathy is useful. Barium swallow may demonstrate a corkscrew oesophagus; however, as the abnormalities are sporadic, they are frequently not present at the time of investigation. It can also rule out obstructing lesions (the most frequently missed is a Schatzki ring). Endoscopy has the advantage of excluding oesophagitis. Cardiac studies should be performed if there is any suspicion of an ischaemic cause of chest pain.

Oesophageal manometry is the gold standard and reveals intermittent, simultaneous, prolonged contractions interspersed with normal peristalsis. 24h ambulatory pH monitoring improves sensitivity for revealing abnormalities. The diagnosis can be one of exclusion.

Management

Usually no specific treatment is required beyond reassurance and simple analgesia. In patients with recurrent and uncontrolled pain, calcium channel blockers and nitrates have been used; these reduce amplitude of contractions, although this does not always translate into meaningful reductions in symptoms. Anecdotal reports suggest endoscopic dilatation can be effective. Surgery (myotomy or oesophagectomy) is very rarely appropriate and is restricted to patients with frequent and severe pain that limits normal daily activities; myotomy may also worsen the pain of nutcracker oesophagus by increasing reflux.

① Mallory–Weiss tear

Syndrome of oesophageal injury limited to the mucosa and usually induced by vigorous straining during an episode of vomiting (regardless of aetiology). Accounts for 10–15% of haematemesis in adults, with a peak incidence in the fifth and sixth decades. It is rare in children. In women of childbearing age, the most common cause is hyperemesis gravidarum.

Patients present with haematemesis, and up to 10% also have melaena. This is more common in the elderly taking antiplatelets or anticoagulants. Lightheadedness or syncope may indicate significant volume depletion. History is usually characteristic and examination unremarkable, although the latter should include assessment of intravascular volume. Haemorrhage is usually minor, although can be substantial enough to cause a postural BP drop in up to 40% and shock in 10% in some case series.

Investigation

FBC is useful to evaluate the extent of blood loss, and U & E the degree of volume loss. Clotting screen should be performed if coagulopathy suspected. All women of childbearing potential should have a pregnancy test.

Endoscopy is diagnostic and can be therapeutic. It may not be required if the diagnosis is likely and haemodynamic parameters remain stable. It characteristically shows a linear laceration at the gastro-oesophageal junction, and should be performed within 24h to maximize diagnostic sensitivity. After this time, the appearance of the tear changes: between 48–72h, the most common finding is a mucosal cleft with surrounding erythema and, by 96h, the mucosa has usually healed completely.

Management

In 80–90% of patients, haemorrhage stops spontaneously and re-bleeding is rare. Monitor intravascular volume and stabilize if significant hypovolaemia; correct coagulopathy if present (see Chapter 1). Uncontrolled haemorrhage usually responds to endoscopic injection, clipping, or electrocoagulation. Surgery is very rarely required in the event of a bleeding artery at the base of a tear.

☠ Oesophageal rupture

Spontaneous rupture (Boerhaave's syndrome)

Spontaneous oesophageal rupture (Boerhaave's syndrome, first described in 1724 after a Dutch admiral died following a gluttonous feast) is caused by straining against a closed glottis during vomiting. Rupture most commonly occurs in the left lower third of the oesophagus, followed by the right middle third. Subsequent discharge of gastric contents into the thorax causes mediastinitis, manifesting as severe chest pain and shock.

Diagnosis is often clinical, and Meckler's triad of vomiting, lower thoracic pain, and subcutaneous emphysema is characteristic. CXR may reveal pneumothorax, pneumomediastinum, unilateral pleural effusion (usually left-sided), and subcutaneous emphysema; these may, however, only become apparent several hours after injury. The V-sign of Naclerio is specific, although has low sensitivity (~20%): it describes the presence of radiolucent streaks of air dissecting the fascial planes between the heart and outlining the hemidiaphragms.

Management involves aggressive resuscitation, NBM, and intensive care involvement. Surgical repair is usually necessary, though if not possible consider endoscopic placement of a covered stent. Conservative treatment requires radiologically placed NGT drainage and IV nutrition. Antibiotic cover improves outcome and usually involves a cephalosporin with metronidazole; anti-fungal cover should be added in the event of non-resolving mediastinitis. Mortality is ~15% if treatment is initiated early although, if delayed >24h, it rises to >90%.

Iatrogenic perforation

Iatrogenic oesophageal perforation often follows dilatation for oesophageal strictures or achalasia, or malposition of a Sengstaken® balloon. Rupture is strongly suggested by the development of chest or epigastric pain directly after instrumentation, particularly in association with dyspnoea. Pneumothorax and surgical emphysema are diagnostic.

If perforation is suspected, request an immediate CXR. This should be repeated within a few hours if initially normal; also obtain a gastrograffin swallow ± CT chest (see Fig. 8.1). Broad-spectrum antibiotics should be given on suspicion, as these minimize the risk of mediastinitis. Prompt surgical review is recommended, although minor injuries can be managed conservatively with antibiotics, radiologically placed NGT drainage, and IV nutrition.

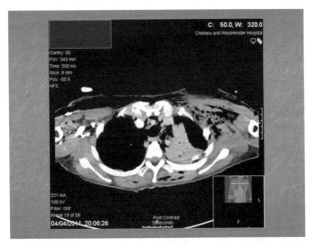

Fig. 8.1 Surgical emphysema and pneumonia following oesophageal rupture.

① Dysphagia

Difficulty whilst eating or drinking involves disruption of the swallowing process, which may encompass the oral, pharyngeal, or oesophageal phases as well as their neurological coordination. Patients may complain of difficulty in initiating the swallow, the sensation of food sticking in the oesophagus, coughing or choking with swallowing, sialorrhoea, nasal regurgitation, or a change in quality of phonation. Progressive dysphagia, initially only to solids, is more common in malignant or benign strictures, whereas dysmotility often causes intermittent symptoms. Complications include weight loss, alteration of dietary habits to compensate for dysphagia, and recurrent chest infections.

Examination should include cranial nerve function (particularly V and VII–XII) and inspection of the mouth, with assessment of jaw closure, dentition, and mastication. Presence of impaired cognitive state, dysphonia, and dysarthria all increase risk of associated dysphagia. Pharyngeal elevation can be assessed by palpating the larynx during swallowing, and gag reflex should be tested (although its absence does not necessarily result in impaired swallowing). Bedside swallow can be performed with 50mL water, observing for at least 1min for cough, wet or hoarse voice, and sialorrhoea.

Investigations should include FBC and TFT as well as basic nutritional assessment by measuring serum total protein and albumin. Haematinics should be checked in the anaemic patient. CXR is indicated if pneumonia secondary to aspiration is suspected.

Videofluoroscopy or modified barium swallow remain the gold standard for assessment of the global swallowing process. Fibreoptic transnasal laryngoscopy is useful in a cooperative patient to characterize the pharyngeal phase, looking particularly for premature bolus loss, laryngeal penetration, tracheal aspiration, and pharyngeal residue. Laryngeal EMG can be performed if a myopathic process is suspected.

Upper GI endoscopy is sensitive for detecting oesophageal (but not pharyngeal) intra-luminal and mucosal causes of obstruction, and manometry is usually diagnostic if achalasia is suspected. If these are negative, CT may be used to detect submucosal or extramural oesophageal lesions. CT/MRI of the head is also helpful if a neurological aetiology is suspected.

Specific causes of dysphagia

Achalasia

Absent or incomplete relaxation of the lower oesophageal sphincter, with impaired peristalsis. Pathogenesis relates to degeneration of inhibitory interneurons in the myenteric plexus. Incidence 1/100,000. Can affect all ages, although most frequently diagnosed in early adulthood. The same syndrome can be seen in South American trypanosomiasis (Chagas disease), infiltration of the oesophagus (neoplastic or amyloidosis, termed pseudo-achalasia), or as a paraneoplastic phenomenon.

Classically presents with dysphagia to both solids and liquids from time of onset. Often delay of months to years between symptom onset and diagnosis. Regurgitation is prominent and consists of bland-tasting material due to absence of stomach acid contamination. Often associated with

cramping chest pain and weight loss. There is increased risk of developing oesophageal SCC (16–28-fold, although some studies report no risk in
those treated; national societies do not advocate endoscopic surveillance).

Radiology may reveal an air-fluid level behind the heart on plain CXR,
and barium swallow a dilated oesophagus with reduced peristalsis; both
may be normal. The most sensitive method of diagnosis remains oesophageal manometry. Upper GI endoscopy with biopsy is important to exclude
malignancy and is performed before manometry.

Treatment is aimed at relaxing or forcefully dilating the lower oesophageal sphincter. This may be achieved medically with calcium channel blockers or nitrates, although these are short-acting and do not lead to sustained
symptom relief. Quadrantic intra-sphincteric injection with 25 units of
botulinum toxin is effective but needs to be repeated every 6–12mo.
Mechanical disruption through oesophageal dilatation (see 'Oesophageal
dilatation', 📖 p. 119) or surgical myotomy are the mainstays of long-term
treatment. A second endoscopic dilation is required in 25–50% of patients
within 5y. Oesophagomyotomy is usually performed laparoscopically or
thoracoscopically; it is effective in >90% of cases. Recurrence in symptoms
occurs in 50% of patients by 10y. Ultimately, the choice of endoscopic
or surgical myotomy depends on local expertise. Both are associated
with significant post-operative reflux disease in 5–10%, and most patients
require long-term acid suppression.

Schatzki ring

A short luminal stenosis at the gastro-oesophageal junction consisting
of both mucosa and submucosal tissue (see Colour plate 17). Although
present in ~10% of the adult population on barium swallow or OGD, they
rarely cause symptoms. The aetiology is unknown but assumed to be a
congenital anatomical variant or due to acid exposure. They may present
with intermittent dysphagia to solids, particularly meat ('steakhouse syndrome'). Sensitive diagnosis can only be achieved by asking an expert radiologist to specifically look for this condition. Endoscopy is more sensitive.
Specific treatment consists of disrupting the ring by endoscopic dilatation,
diathermy, or laser, although an OGD in itself often treats the stenosis
merely by passing the scope through the ring. Recurrence post-dilatation
lessened with acid suppression.

Oesophageal diverticula

Occur frequently in patients with systemic sclerosis, in which they are
characteristically multiple with wide lumens. Otherwise, they are usually
secondary to motility disorders and arise in the mid- to distal oesophagus. They are rarely symptomatic but can cause dysphagia and regurgitation. Unless symptoms are disabling, they may be managed expectantly.
Otherwise, surgical clipping is indicated, although post-operative leakage
is common if resected.

Zenker's diverticula are rare anatomical causes of dysphagia. They are
outpouchings through cricopharyngeus, not to be confused with a pharyngeal pouches, occurring principally in the elderly population. Diverticula
may be asymptomatic or lead to a classical presentation of dysphagia and
regurgitation of undigested food, aspiration, and halitosis. Barium swallow is diagnostic; symptomatic patients most commonly have a posterior

midline pouch >2cm diameter and superior to the cricopharyngeus muscle. Endoscopy is required to exclude malignancy. Small asymptomatic lesions require no further action. In the presence of significant symptoms, surgical myotomy is the treatment of choice, particularly for large diverticula in those <50y. Flexible or rigid endoscopic diverticulostomy and myotomy are preferable in those at high risk for surgery.

Extrinsic compression

Relatively common cause of dysphagia. The main culprit is malignant mediastinal adenopathy, although other causative lesions include primary tumours, massive cardiomegaly, an ectatic or aneurysmal aorta, pronounced kyphosis, or a congenital vascular abnormality such as an aberrant right subclavian artery. Barium swallow and endoscopy typically show relatively long distances of constriction with variable luminal calibre; the oesophageal mucosa appears normal. Treatment is both symptomatic and of the primary lesion. Dilatation may temporarily relieve symptoms, although may be short-lived due to elastic recoil of the oesophageal wall.

Intrinsic oesophageal strictures

See Colour plate 18. Causes include:
- Oesophageal malignancy. Discuss in multidisciplinary meetings to consider therapeutic or palliative surgery, radiotherapy, chemotherapy, and/or stenting.
- Acid reflux.
- Caustic injury.
- Post-variceal sclerotherapy or band ligation.
- Chemotherapy/radiotherapy.

Treatment relies on endoscopic dilatation (see 'Oesophageal dilatation', 📖 p. 119), healing oesophagitis if present, and minimizing recurrence. Maintenance PPI therapy is recommended.

Neurological causes

Dysphagia may result from neurological lesions at different levels. The differential includes:
- Stroke.
- Traumatic brain injury.
- Parkinson's disease.
- Motor neuron disease, multiple systems atrophy (Shy-Drager syndrome).
- Multiple sclerosis.
- Head and neck surgery.
- Cervical spondylosis.
- Motor peripheral neuropathies.
- Myopathies and myositis.
- Myasthenia gravis.
- Old age. Associated with increased risk of loss of coordination of swallowing mechanism.

Management

Multidisciplinary assessment, including a dietician and speech and language therapist, is essential. The primary aims are minimization of risks of dehydration, malnutrition, and aspiration. Depending on the magnitude and nature of the defect, restriction of oral intake to thickened fluids or puréed foods may be necessary. Swallowing exercises can be helpful, and extra care needs to be paid to dental hygiene. In patients in whom oral nutrition is likely to be non-transient, longer-term NG or PEG feeding may be appropriate. Specific treatment depends on the cause of dysphagia.

Oesophageal dilatation

The goals of dilatation are to alleviate symptoms, permit oral nutrition, and reduce risk of aspiration. Indications include benign peptic strictures, caustic strictures, oesophageal tumours, Schatzki rings, and achalasia. Dilatation should ideally be performed as a planned procedure, following radiological and endoscopic investigation, to assess the nature of the problem and the risk of complications.

The only absolute contraindication is oesophageal perforation. Relative contraindications include recent perforation or oesophageal surgery, pharyngeal or cervical deformity, presence of a large thoracic aortic aneurysm, severe cardiac or respiratory disease, and anticoagulation or coagulopathy. There is also an increased risk of complications in patients with an angulated stricture, oesophageal diverticulum, hiatus hernia, or previous radiotherapy. Concurrent radiotherapy or simultaneous mucosal biopsies are not contraindications.

Patients should be fasted 4–6h prior to the procedure. Any coagulopathy should be corrected. Patients on a heparin infusion should have this stopped for 4–6h before and after dilatation. Premedication IV opioid is appropriate. Antibiotic prophylaxis remains the subject of much debate. It was previously recommended for patients with prosthetic heart valves, previous infective endocarditis, synthetic vascular grafting within the past year, or systemic-pulmonary shunts. NICE, however, no longer supports their routine use in these patients, except in those with severe neutropaenia.

Dilatation should be performed by a skilled endoscopist, with two assistants present ± radiological guidance. Surgical support should be available in the event of a large or uncontrolled perforation. Both push (wire-guided) and balloon dilators are currently used; trials suggest little difference between the two. Target luminal diameter varies according to the nature of the stricture:

- Benign peptic strictures: 13–15mm.
- Malignant strictures: sufficient to facilitate stent insertion. Avoid large-calibre dilators.
- Schatzki ring: 16–20mm.
- Achalasia: 30–40mm. The aim is to forcibly disrupt the sphincter.

The lumen should be dilated by ~3mm at each dilatation, except achalasia that requires one prolonged dilatation. Therefore, multiple dilations may be required. The procedure should ideally be guided: endoscopy and radiology are both suitable and, sometimes, combined. Biopsies should be obtained if the nature of the stricture remains unclassified.

Complications occur in 2–6%, with a mortality of 1%. Written consent detailing these risks is essential. The major complication is perforation, which is particularly prevalent following dilatation of malignant strictures.

Regular routine observations and general examination are required post-procedure. Once sedation has worn off, patients can be allowed to drink water. Perforation should be suspected if a patient develops tachypnoea, tachycardia, fever, persistent chest pain, or subcutaneous emphysema, any of which should prompt cessation of oral intake as well as a CXR ± contrast study and a CT. Other complications include bleeding, aspiration, reflux (treated with PPI), and failure to relieve symptoms.

Odynophagia

Refers to oesophageal pain felt within 15s of swallowing. Causes include:
• Food impaction at sites of oesophageal stenosis or spasm.
• Oesophagitis (see 'Oesophagitis', 📖 p. 111).
• Ingestion of hot liquids or alcohol. May cause pain in an otherwise normal oesophagus.

Foreign bodies

May be swallowed accidentally or intentionally. Objects ingested differ between children and adults, and within certain subgroups of adult patients. Most cases present acutely, although chronic foreign bodies may present with an oesophageal or intestinal perforation, or with secondary infection of surrounding tissues in the throat, neck, or mediastinum.

Most patients have a clear history of ingestion. The nature of the foreign body and time since intake guide management. The presence of structural abnormalities, absent dentition or use of dentures, alcohol intake, or motor disturbances of the GI tract increase the probability of entrapment. Patients are usually able to accurately localize objects in the upper oesophagus as the oropharynx is well innervated, but below this localization is poor. Complete oesophageal obstruction is usually accompanied by significant sialorrhoea. Foreign bodies in the stomach are usually asymptomatic but may present with non-specific symptoms of fever, vomiting, and vague abdominal pain. Physical examination is typically not helpful but should be aimed at assessing risk of airway compromise and presence of complications.
• Children. Typically ingest everyday objects picked up and placed into the mouth such as coins, buttons, marbles, and crayons. The most frequent site of entrapment is at the upper oesophageal sphincter (75%).
• Adults. The commonest foreign bodies are food boluses, chicken or fish bones, and dentures. The majority lodge at the lower oesophageal sphincter (70%).
• Psychiatric patients. Often swallow multiple or bizarre objects, the most dangerous of which are irregularly shaped sharps (see Fig. 8.2) (e.g. open safety pins) and batteries. May also present with bezoars.
• Prisoners. May also swallow multiple or unusual objects, and drugs. Body packing refers to swallowing multiple wraps of drug (usually double-wrapped) for illicit transfer. This contrasts to stuffing, which

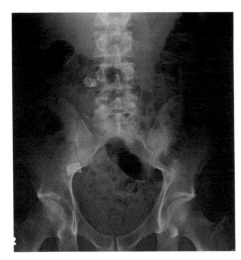

Fig. 8.2 Ingested razors passing through the GI tract.

is an attempt to elude arrest by swallowing packages in current possession. The latter has increased risk of contents leakage.

Once a foreign body has reached the stomach, it has a >90% chance of uncomplicated passage. In the small and large bowel, the only structural impediment normally is the ileocaecal valve. Rarely, a Meckel's diverticulum may provide another site of entrapment.

Management
Depends on the stability of the patient, the nature of the object ingested, and the presence of complications.

① *Stable patients*
Plain radiographs should be ordered for all patients with known or suspected radio-opaque foreign body ingestion. For non-opaque objects, plain radiography rarely influences management and often delays CT or endoscopy. For small children, a mouth-to-anus radiograph is appropriate; in older children and adults, PA and lateral CXRs provide better localization. Significant non-opaque foreign bodies include:

- Bones. Only 20–50% of endoscopically proven bones are visible on plain films.
- Toothpicks. These have a particularly high incidence of complications.
- Aluminium tabs from carbonated drink cans.

Non-opaque foreign bodies may be revealed by barium swallow, although this is not useful for detecting objects in the stomach or small intestine and contraindicated in suspected perforation. CT is the imaging modality of choice with a sensitivity of 80–100%; it is also useful for detecting perforation or abscesses. In cooperative patients with a suspected oropharyngeal foreign body, indirect laryngoscopy or fibreoptic nasopharyngoscopy may be both diagnostic and therapeutic. If the history is clear, it is appropriate to proceed straight to endoscopy without prior CT.

Perform emergency endoscopy if complete dysphagia (indicated by sialorrhoea), following disc or button battery ingestion since severe oesophageal necrosis can occur if ruptured, or if sharp, pointed objects are in the oesophagus. Perform endoscopy within 24h if non-obstructive objects lie in the oesophagus, if sharp objects or objects >6cm lie in the stomach or duodenum, or if objects are magnetic. Non-urgent endoscopy is indicated following ingestion of blunt objects >2.5cm diameter, coins that remain in the stomach >24h, batteries that remain in the stomach >48h, and all other blunt objects that remain in the intestine for >1wk. Lower the threshold for endoscopic removal in children. Consider use of an overtube to enable safe removal.

Alternatives approaches include use of a 12–16G Foley catheter to advance oesophageal foreign bodies into the stomach, or pharmacological relaxation of the lower oesophageal sphincter. The latter is achieved using glucagon 1–2mg IV in adults or 0.02–0.03mg/kg in children (not to exceed 0.5mg), followed by ingestion of a carbonated beverage. Nitrates and calcium channel blockers have also been reported to work but risk hypotension and are ineffective in patients with structural abnormalities. These methods should only be attempted by those experienced in their use, with back-up endoscopic facilities in the event of failure or complications.

In patients who have an entrapped food bolus, a meat tenderizer is sometimes advocated; this should not be administered to anyone with possible obstruction at the lower oesophageal sphincter, as it risks necrosis of the oesophageal wall.

Body packers should be admitted for regular observations, with specific monitoring for obstruction, perforation, and signs of drug toxicity. The latter indicates packet rupture and mandates resuscitation and surgical review. Endoscopic removal should be performed by highly competent endoscopists to prevent packet rupture.

☼ Unstable patients

Includes any patient with airway compromise, drooling, inability to tolerate fluids, evidence of sepsis, perforation or active bleeding, or those who have swallowed button batteries. Airway management is the priority followed by urgent endoscopy with removal of objects in the oesophagus, or fibreoptic nasopharyngoscopy if an oropharyngeal foreign body is suspected. Access to a suction catheter is important, as secretions are problematic.

If button barriers have been swallowed and progressed into the stomach, they can be allowed to pass but must be monitored radiographically for the next 24–48h to detect disruption. Thereafter, if they remain in the stomach, endoscopic removal is indicated.

Complications

• Mural abrasion and laceration.
• Haemorrhage.

- Oesophageal necrosis (particularly with button batteries).
- Intestinal puncture.
- Abscess formation, soft tissue infection.
- Perforation.
- Pneumomediastinum, pneumothorax.
- Mediastinitis.
- Pericarditis, cardiac tamponade.
- Fistulation.
- Vascular injury.

Follow-up

Adults with a resolved oesophageal foreign body should undergo radio-logical and/or endoscopic investigation when recovered; a substantial pro-portion possess underlying structural abnormalities, including malignancy. In children, resolved foreign bodies need no further follow-up.

Occasionally, patients present with a history of possible foreign body ingestion and entrapment. If they are stable and diagnostic work-up is negative, they can be discharged with analgesia and advice to re-present if still symptomatic after 24h. If the latter occurs, patients should undergo endoscopy.

:☠: Caustic injury

Strong acids and alkalis damage the oesophagus and are present at high concentrations in household cleaning and maintenance fluids. Laryngeal and gastric injuries may overshadow those to the oesophagus. Alkaline solutions tend to lack the unpleasant taste of acids and are, therefore, often consumed in greater quantities. They also tend to cause deeper injuries, as acids often form superficial coagulants that limit penetration.

The severity and extent of injuries do not correlate well with estimated volumes of ingestion. Approximately 50% of patients with a history of ingestion have no significant injury. Airway protection is the first prior-ity. Oesophageal injury causes odynophagia, dysphagia, and haematemesis. Prompt endoscopy is usually safe but needs to be performed very carefully, as there is high risk of perforation if extensive necrosis has developed. It most frequently reveals patchy mucosal erythema and oedema with small haemorrhagic ulcers. Extensive circumferential ulceration with grey or black areas of necrosis suggests transmural injury and poor prognosis.

Patients should be closely observed for signs of perforation. Those at high risk should have an NGT (ideally inserted under direct vision due to risk of perforation) and prophylactic broad-spectrum antibiotic cover. Use of steroids is controversial and probably unhelpful.

Oesophageal stricture is the principal short-term risk and a predictable consequence of severe injury. It is not preventable by prophylactic dilata-tion. Contrast radiography should be performed after 2–3wk to screen for stenosis, then at 3-monthly intervals thereafter for 1y. Early detection allows early therapeutic dilatation when its impact is greatest. The most concerning long-term complication is oesophageal carcinoma, with mean occurrence 40y after injury. The risk is >1,000 times greater than that of the general population.

Acute thoracic pain and dysphagia

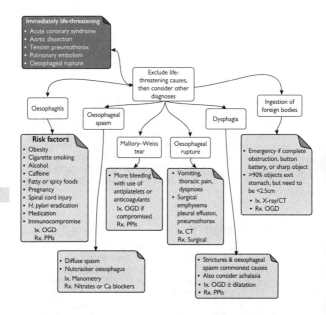

Immediately life-threatening
- Acute coronary syndrome
- Aortic dissection
- Tension pneumothorax
- Pulmonary embolism
- Oesophageal rupture

Exclude life-threatening causes, then consider other diagnoses

Oesophagitis

Oesophageal spasm

Dysphagia

Ingestion of foreign bodies

Risk factors
- Obesity
- Cigarette smoking
- Alcohol
- Caffeine
- Fatty or spicy foods
- Pregnancy
- Spinal cord injury
- H. pylori eradication
- Medication
- Immunocompromise
  Ix. OGD
  Rx. PPIs

Mallory–Weiss tear

- More bleeding with use of antiplatelets or anticoagulants
  Ix. OGD if compromised
  Rx. PPIs

Oesophageal rupture

- Vomiting, thoracic pain, dyspnoea
- Surgical emphysema pleural effusion, pneumothorax
  Ix. CT
  Rx. Surgical

- Emergency if complete obstruction, button battery, or sharp object
- >90% objects exit stomach, but need to be <2.5cm
  Ix. X-ray/CT
  Rx. OGD

- Diffuse spasm
- Nutcracker oesophagus
  Ix. Manometry
  Rx. Nitrates or Ca blockers

- Strictures & oesophageal spasm commonest causes
- Also consider achalasia
  Ix. OGD ± dilatation
  Rx. PPIs

Acute abdominal pain

Differential diagnosis

Table 9.1 shows the main differential diagnoses of acute abdominal pain, according to site of presentation. Overlap between sites is common. Generalized abdominal pain may be caused by peritonitis or medical disorders. Ensure a pregnancy test is performed in all women of childbearing potential.

Table 9.1 Causes of acute abdominal pain

Site/mechanism	Cause
Epigastric	Peptic ulcer, acute cholecystitis, oesophageal perforation, MI, myocarditis, pericarditis, aortic dissection
Right hypochondrium	Cholecystitis, hepatitis, peptic ulcer, right basal pneumonia, PE, Fitz–Hugh–Curtis syndrome
Left hypochondrium	Pancreatitis, peptic ulcer, splenic rupture, left basal pneumonia, PE
Peri-umbilical	Small bowel obstruction, early appendicitis, mesenteric ischaemia, aortic aneurysm, testicular torsion
Loin	Pyelonephritis, ureteric colic
Right iliac fossa	Appendicitis, large bowel obstruction, Crohn's disease, caecal perforation, psoas abscess, Meckel's diverticulitis, ectopic pregnancy, ovarian abscess, ovarian cyst rupture, salpingitis
Left iliac fossa	Diverticulitis, large bowel obstruction, colonic perforation, IBD, ectopic pregnancy, ovarian abscess, ovarian cyst rupture, salpingitis
Neurological	Nerve root compression, herpes zoster
Metabolic	Diabetic ketoacidosis, Addisonian crisis, hypercalcaemia, acute intermittent porphyria
Miscellaneous	Sickle cell crisis, SLE, Henoch–Schönlein purpura, opiate withdrawal, familial Mediterranean fever

Peptic ulceration

Ulcers of the proximal alimentary tract caused by pepsin and gastric acid. Most develop in the duodenum, followed by the stomach and oesophagus. Rarely, they can arise within a Meckel's diverticulum due to the presence of gastric metaplasia. More than 80% are associated with *H. pylori* infection. Most of the remainder are caused by NSAIDs, with 10–30% of chronic users affected. Other risk factors predisposing to peptic ulcer disease include:
• Cigarette smoking.
• Alcohol.

- Medications: steroids (when provided with another risk/aetiological factor), bisphosphonates, COX-2 inhibitors, oral KCl, chemotherapy.

Clinical presentation

Although 'textbook' symptoms are said to arise from peptic ulcers, these are neither sensitive nor specific. Visualization of the GI tract is required to make or exclude the diagnosis. Classically, gastric ulceration causes postprandial epigastric pain (and thus associated with anorexia and weight loss), and duodenal ulceration causes pain when fasting (hence often nocturnal, waking patients from sleep) with relief after eating (and, therefore, associated with weight gain). The differential diagnosis of such pain includes malignancy, pancreatitis, cholecystitis, choledocholithiasis, gastro-oesophageal reflux disease, or cardiac or mesenteric angina. Related symptoms may include bloating, abdominal fullness, nausea, vomiting, heartburn, and waterbrash. Haematemesis or melaena indicate bleeding, mandating assessment in hospital.

Clinical examination may be normal or reveal epigastric tenderness. Peritonism should prompt immediate consideration of a perforation (obtain erect CXR ± CT) and exclusion of other causes of an acute abdomen.

Emergency presentations

The principal emergencies associated with peptic ulcers are haemorrhage and perforation. Rarely, patients present with consequences of peptic strictures (such as gastric outflow obstruction, see Chapter 4), or with fistulation (e.g. gastrocolic presenting with vomiting of faeces, choledochoduodenal manifesting with aerobilia).

Haemorrhage

Emergency bleeds present with haematemesis ± melaena (whereas subacute or chronic GI blood loss usually identified through investigation of IDA). The management of upper GI haemorrhage from peptic ulcers is detailed in Chapter 1. Note that posterior duodenal ulcers can invade the gastroduodenal artery, causing life-threatening bleeding; have a low threshold for surgical review in such patients.

Perforation

Presents with sudden onset epigastric or generalized abdominal pain. Examination may show fever, tachycardia, and abdominal tenderness with guarding and rebound. Be aware that elderly patients may not manifest these signs, and have a lower threshold for investigation.
- Obtain IV access, take bloods (FBC, U & E, LFT, clotting, amylase, and G & S), and provide IV fluids.
- Make NBM and inform the surgical team.
- Request an erect CXR to look for air under the diaphragm. Subsequently, obtain a CT if the patient is haemodynamically stable (proceed direct to surgery if not).
- Give broad-spectrum antibiotics IV (e.g. cefuroxime + metronidazole, or piperacillin-tazobactam) if perforation confirmed.
- Provide appropriate analgesia (e.g. morphine 5–10mg IV). Opioids *do not* mask signs of peritonism.

- For further details on the management of patients with generalized peritonitis, see 📖 p. 140. Definitive treatment is generally operative, although frail patients with high anaesthetic risk and a localized perforation may respond to being made NBM, IV fluid support and nutrition, and IV antibiotics.

Endoscopy

Urgent endoscopy is indicated for patients presenting with definite upper GI bleeding to make a diagnosis and achieve haemostasis (see Chapter 1). If a gastric ulcer is found, take a minimum of six biopsies to exclude malignancy (note that duodenal ulcers are rarely malignant). For patients found to have gastric or oesophageal ulcers, follow-up endoscopy should be performed after 8wk to confirm healing. Repeat endoscopy after 24–48h may be indicated with ulcers with high-risk stigmata for re-bleeding.

In the absence of overt haemorrhage or perforation, endoscopy for investigation of dyspepsia should be performed within 2wk for patients with:
- Progressive dysphagia.
- Unintentional weight loss.
- Epigastric mass.
- IDA.
- Persistent vomiting.
- Age >55y AND:
  - Persistent symptoms despite *H. pylori* testing/eradication and acid suppression therapy.
  - Previous gastric ulcer or surgery.
  - Continuing need for NSAIDs.
  - Increased risk of gastric cancer, or significant anxiety regarding the possibility of cancer.

Anti-secretory and antacid therapy

A number of therapeutic strategies are available.
- *Lifestyle measures.* Advise patients to stop smoking, and discontinue NSAIDs if possible. No special diet is required.
- *PPIs* (e.g. omeprazole 20mg od, lansoprazole 30mg od, pantoprazole 40mg od). First-line agents. Best taken immediately before meals. Prescribe for 8wk in uncomplicated ulcers, or 12wk if ulcer >2cm or complicated. Potentially need lifelong therapy in the elderly or those with significant co-morbidity. Limited suppression of fasting acid secretion therefore occasionally get nocturnal acid breakthrough. Healing rates 80–100% for duodenal and 70–85% for gastric ulcers. Side effects include diarrhoea, CYP450 inhibition, and 3-fold increased susceptibility to *C. difficile* in hospitalized patients.
- *Histamine receptor antagonists* (e.g. ranitidine 150mg bd or 300mg nocte, or cimetidine 400mg bd or 800mg nocte). Healing rates 70–80% for duodenal and 55–65% for gastric ulcers. Particularly effective for nocturnal acid secretion and may be synergistic with PPIs. Side effects include diarrhoea and deranged LFT. Cimetidine can cause gynaecomastia and CYP450 inhibition.

- *Misoprostol.* Synthetic prostaglandin analogue. Usual dose 400µg bd (with meals) for 4–8wk. Similar efficacy to PPIs for healing NSAID-induced ulcers but is little used due to side effects (diarrhoea, vaginal bleeding, miscarriage, and premature labour). Should not be given to women of childbearing potential unless effective contraceptive methods are employed. Marketed with diclofenac as Arthrotec®.
- *Antacids* (e.g. aluminium hydroxide 500–1000mg up to qds, or 10mL magnesium carbonate 3% up to tds). Effective for symptomatic relief. Aluminium may constipate, and magnesium is a laxative.
- *Sucralfate.* Combination of aluminium hydroxide and sulphated sucrose. Forms a barrier raft, protecting against acid and other irritants. Usual dose is 1g qds, separated from food by >1h. Avoid in renal failure. Rarely may cause gastric bezoars. Binds phenytoin and warfarin, reducing their absorption and efficacy. Little additional efficacy beyond PPIs.
- *Bismuth* (tripotassium dicitratobismuthate (De-Noltab®) 240mg bd). Side effects include darkening of the tongue, black faeces, and constipation. Can cause encephalopathy if absorbed, so maximum duration should be 12wk. Usually prescribed as part of *H. pylori* eradication.
- *Surgery.* Obsolete for uncomplicated peptic ulcers. Indications include bleeding unresponsive to endoscopic therapy, perforation, and gastric outlet obstruction not relieved by endoscopic dilatation. Operations include highly selective vagotomy or gastrojejunostomy. Subtotal gastrectomy with Roux-en-Y anastomosis may be required for refractory ulcers near the gastro-oesophageal junction.

H. pylori testing and eradication

All patients with peptic ulceration should be tested for *H. pylori*. Diagnosis may be achieved by urea breath test, stool antigen testing, or mucosal biopsy (followed by CLO™ test, histology, or culture). These methods have largely superseded serology which cannot distinguish past from current infection (although serology less susceptible than other methods to false negative results due to established PPI therapy).

Initial eradication therapy typically uses three agents (e.g. two from amoxicillin 1g bd, clarithromycin 500mg bd and metronidazole 500mg bd; and lansoprazole 30mg or omeprazole 20mg bd) for 7d (14d regime slightly superior). Resistance to amoxicillin is rare, ~15% for clarithromycin, and variable for metronidazole (but high in urban areas). This is curative in >85%.

Routine follow-up testing (e.g. by repeat urea breath test) is not generally required, although is used to confirm eradication in patients with 'complicated' ulcers, the elderly, or those with co-morbidities for whom repeat ulceration could be disastrous. Otherwise, failure of eradication is typically detected by symptom recurrence. Strategies for second-line therapy include addition of tetracycline 500mg qds, increasing length of treatment to 10–14d, and/or adding in a fourth agent (usually bismuth). Approximately 1% of patients are re-infected per annum.

What do I do if the ulcer fails to heal?

An ulcer is defined as refractory if it has not healed within 8wk of commencement of a PPI (12wk if ulcer was >2cm). Questions to ask before adding in second agents include:

• Was the patient compliant with treatment?
• Has *H. pylori* been eradicated?
• Is there ongoing (surreptitious) NSAID use or cigarette smoking?
• Is there evidence for a hypersecretory condition? Check serum gastrin (fasting, avoid acid secretory medication for 2wk before test).
• Is the ulcer peptic? Review histology. Other causes of upper GI ulceration (account for 5–10% of cases) include:
  • Adenocarcinoma.
  • Crohn's disease.
  • Gastrinoma (Zollinger–Ellison syndrome).
  • Carcinoid syndrome.
  • Sarcoidosis.
  • Sepsis.
  • Burns (Curling's ulcer).
  • Head injury (Cushing's ulcer).
  • Systemic mastocytosis, basophilic leukaemias (related to increased histamine release).
  • Diseases related to immunocompromise (see Chapter 12).

Gallstone disease

Gallstones are common (prevalence 10–15%), formed by aggregation of cholesterol, mucin, and calcium bilirubinate when their concentrations rise beyond supersaturation thresholds. Three major subtypes are seen (see Box 9.1). Most are discovered incidentally by US; 80% remain asymptomatic. The annual incidence of complications is 1%. Four acute syndromes are common: biliary colic, acute cholecystitis, acute cholangitis, and acute pancreatitis (see 📖 p. 134).

Box 9.1 Risk factors for gallstones

• Cholesterol stones (90%).
  • Age.
  • Female gender.
  • High parity.
  • Ethnicity (Native American, Hispanic).
  • Family history.
  • Diet: high calorie, high carbohydrate, high cholesterol, low fibre.
  • Dyslipidaemia (particularly type IV: high triglycerides, low HDL).
  • Oestrogens (OCP, HRT).
  • Rapid weight loss (although controlled weight loss protective).
• Brown pigment stones (5%)
  • Biliary infection (bacteria, helminths).
  • Abnormal biliary anatomy, Caroli's syndrome.
  • Post-cholecystectomy.

(Continued)

Box 9.1 *(Continued)*
- Black pigment stones (5%).
  - Haemolytic anaemia.
  - Hepatic cirrhosis.
  - Crohn's disease.
  - Cystic fibrosis.

① Biliary colic

Transient impaction of a stone, or possibly sludge, in the cystic duct. Presents with RUQ/epigastric pain, which may radiate to the right shoulder or scapula. This typically starts abruptly after eating (particularly fatty foods) due to gallbladder contraction, peaks within 1h, and resolves gradually within 5h as stones spontaneously de-obstruct. There may be associated nausea or vomiting. Episodes are recurrent.

① Acute cholecystitis

Persistent obstruction of the cystic duct leads to gallbladder inflammation. Although initially sterile, infection with bowel-derived organisms (particularly *Enterobacteriaceae*, enterococci, and anaerobes) then ensues.

Patients present with pain similar in nature to biliary colic but persistent. Vomiting and fever are usually present. Tenderness and guarding in the RUQ is characteristic. Murphy's sign is elicited by palpating at the level of the right ninth costal cartilage and asking the patient to take a deep breath in. It is positive if the patient arrests inspiration (corresponding to pressure on the inflamed gallbladder by the examining hand) but does not do so when a similar manoeuvre is attempted on the left side. A mass is palpable in 25% of patients after 24h of symptoms, although rare at initial presentation.

Infection may be severe enough to cause sepsis. Gangrene develops in 20% and perforation in 2%, with high mortality if the latter progresses from peri-cholecystic abscess to frank peritonitis. Emphysematous cholecystitis describes infection of the gallbladder wall with gas-forming organisms, which carries a more severe prognosis. Diagnose on imaging or, if palpable, crepitus in the RUQ.

⊙ Acute cholangitis

Obstruction of the biliary tree, resulting in ascending infection. Presents with RUQ pain (often constant but may be colicky), fever, and obstructive jaundice (Charcot's triad; all three features present in 50–75%). Reynold's pentad also includes confusion and hypotension, carrying a poor prognosis.

Obstruction is secondary to non-gallstone disease in 20%. Causes include extrinsic compression (head of pancreas mass lesions, adenopathy), benign or malignant biliary strictures, and intra-luminal parasitic infection (*Ascaris*, *Clonorchis*; see Chapter 17).

Investigation

Admit patients with 'complicated' gallstone disease:
- Pain not resolving within 5h.
- Severe vomiting or pyrexia.

- Localized abdominal tenderness.
- Blood tests showing raised WCC, CRP, LFT, or amylase.

Blood tests

In biliary colic, FBC, CRP, LFT, and amylase are normal. A lipid profile may be helpful in identifying modifiable risk factors for gallstone disease. Blood film and haemoglobinopathy screens are appropriate if an underlying haemolytic anaemia is suspected.

Acute cholecystitis and cholangitis are associated with raised WCC and CRP, and deranged LFT (particularly ALP, although transaminases can be higher). Visible jaundice is uncommon and, if present, should prompt consideration of an accompanying common bile duct (CBD) stone (choledocholithiasis) or Mirizzi syndrome (bile duct obstruction due to extrinsic compression by gallbladder or cystic duct stone). Take blood cultures if septic. Raised amylase suggests concomitant pancreatitis.

Imaging

- Abdominal US (following a 4h fast) is first-line for identifying gallstones (95% sensitive, although operator-dependent) and their complications. It is 98% sensitive for acute cholecystitis (gallbladder wall >5mm; ultrasonic Murphy's sign positive: inspiratory arrest as US probe presses on the gallbladder; and peri-cholecystic fluid). Can also provide functional dynamic information about postprandial gallbladder.
- Request MRCP if choledocholithiasis suspected despite a non-diagnostic US, to determine whether ERCP required prior to cholecystectomy.
- Plain AXR/CT of little value in uncomplicated gallstone disease or acute cholecystitis, as only 10% of gallstones are calcified.
- Scintigraphy (HIDA scan) rarely necessary; use generally limited to outpatient screening for sphincter of Oddi dysfunction.
- ERCP predominantly therapeutic rather than investigational in this context.
- Endoscopic US very accurate for imaging CBD. Largely redundant for investigating gallstone disease, except in patients with typical symptoms but normal basic investigations. It accurately predicts successful cholecystectomy in 90% of such patients by demonstrating biliary sludge and confirming presence of crystals within bile.

Management

The aims of treatment are to relieve symptoms, limit development or progression of gallstone-related complications, and prevent recurrence.

Asymptomatic gallstones

Prophylactic cholecystectomy is not recommended as the annual incidence of symptoms is only 1%. Seek specialist advice in those at higher risk of becoming symptomatic (congenital haemolytic anaemias, prior to bariatric surgery) or for developing cholangiocarcinoma (Caroli's disease, choledochal cyst, gallbladder adenoma, porcelain gallbladder).

Biliary colic

Definitive treatment is cholecystectomy, usually performed laparoscopically. This is not urgent if disease is uncomplicated. Recommend a low-fat diet and simple analgesia. Be aware that 20% patients who undergo surgery for presumed biliary pain remain symptomatic 2y later; more likely if symptoms are atypical, so a good history is paramount.

If patients refuse or are unfit for surgery, prescribe 10–15mg/kg ursodeoxycholic acid (UDCA) PO od if radiolucent cholesterol stones <5mm present, expecting ~1mm/month litholysis. Recurrence is ~50% within 5y. Extracorporeal shockwave lithotripsy, together with UDCA, can be attempted for larger stones if aggregate stone size is <30mm. Responses are poorer with radio-opaque and multiple stones.

Acute cholecystitis

Cholecystectomy is generally indicated, either performed within 7d of symptom onset or 2–3mo after inflammation has settled. During the acute episode, keep patients NBM, and provide IV fluids and analgesia. Antibiotic therapy with co-amoxiclav 1.2g IV tds, cefuroxime 750mg–1.5g IV tds, or ciprofloxacin 400mg IV or 500mg PO bd is appropriate; convert to oral preparations after 48h if improving.

In patients who are poor surgical candidates (ASA grade >3), conservative management can be tried. If this fails, percutaneous cholecystostomy under local anaesthesia and radiologic guidance can be attempted.

Ascending cholangitis

Keep patients NBM, and provide IV fluids and antibiotics as described in 'Acute cholecystitis' (see 📖 p. 133). Therapeutic ERCP is indicated within 72h for most patients. This should be accelerated to within 24h if there is suspected gallstone pancreatitis or severe sepsis.

ERCP can identify and remove or stent obstructing lesions. Sphincterotomy can prevent future gallstone obstruction but is associated with increased risk of procedural complications. Permanent metal stents are appropriate for patients with malignant strictures. Temporary pigtail stents are used to facilitate drainage in benign strictures or in patients with retained gallstones; these require removal/replacement every 3mo.

Patients too frail for ERCP, or in whom ERCP is technically impossible, should undergo external radiologically guided drainage. Thereafter, an internal stent(s) can be placed, either radiologically or as part of a combined procedure with an endoscopist. Open surgical exploration should be avoided where possible.

Once the emergency presentation has resolved, patients should be booked for elective cholecystectomy.

Complications of gallstones

- Acute cholecystitis.
- Gangrenous cholecystitis.
- Gallbladder empyema.
- Subphrenic abscess.
- Gallbladder perforation.
- Choledocholithiasis.

- Mirizzi's syndrome (extrinsic CBD obstruction by cystic duct stone or inflamed gallbladder).
- Ascending cholangitis.
- Cholangiocarcinoma.
- Pancreatitis.
- Gallstone ileus (consequent to a cholecystoenteric fistula, with subsequent stone impaction at the ileocaecal valve. AXR demonstrates a radio-opaque gallstone, small bowel obstruction, and aerobilia).

:O: Acute acalculous cholecystitis

Accounts for 5–10% of cases of cholecystitis. High morbidity and mortality as occurs in sick patients. Pathogenesis poorly understood. Three principal clinical subtypes are observed:

- Patients receiving TPN (usually for >3mo). It is possible that lack of gallbladder stimulation by absence of enteral feeding leads to biliary stasis and consequent irritation and inflammation of the gallbladder.
- Thromboembolic disease. Acute vascular compromise causes infarction of the gallbladder. This may also occur as part of the natural history of untreated acute calculous cholecystitis.
- Patients with HIV infection (see Chapter 12).

Manage with antibiotics as for 'Acute cholecystitis' (see 📖 p. 133), but have low threshold for cholecystectomy if condition continues to deteriorate, as higher risk of gallbladder perforation.

Intrahepatic gallstones

Rare in the Western world but more frequent in South East Asia. Intrahepatic stones can be formed *in situ* (almost always brown pigment stones related to parasitic infection) or migrate proximally from the gallbladder; distal biliary strictures predispose to the latter. Patients present with recurrent pyogenic cholangitis and are managed accordingly. Additional complications include liver abscess formation, secondary hepatic cirrhosis, and elevated risk of cholangiocarcinoma.

:O: Acute pancreatitis

Acute inflammation of the pancreas is associated with activation of proteases, leading to auto-digestion. Incidence 5–25/100,000, of whom 20% have severe disease and 2–4% of cases are fatal. Consider acute pancreatitis in patients with unexplained multiorgan failure or a SIRS.

Causes

Common

- Gallstones (30% of cases; affects 5% of patients with gallstones).
- Alcohol (30%; affects 10% of chronic alcohol misusers).
- Idiopathic (up to 20%).

Rare
- Infection:
  - Viral (mumps, coxsackievirus, HIV).
  - Bacterial (*Mycoplasma*, TB).
  - Parasitic (*Ascaris*, *Clonorchis*).
- Hypercalcaemia (± hyperparathyroidism).
- Hypertriglyceridaemia (>11mmol/L; causes 2–3% of cases).
- Hypothermia.
- Post-ERCP (in 2–9%, although 50% have raised amylase post-ERCP).
- Drugs (2%):
  - Steroids, azathioprine, sulfasalazine, mesalazine.
  - Oestrogens.
  - Furosemide.
  - NSAIDs.
  - Sodium valproate.
  - Anti-retrovirals (see Chapter 12).
- Autoimmune (associated with raised IgG4).
- Familial (genetic testing in young patients with 'idiopathic' disease).
- Anatomic:
  - Choledochal cyst.
  - Duodenal diverticula.
  - Possibly pancreas divisum.
- Pancreatic duct obstruction:
  - Ampullary and pancreatic tumours.
  - Sphincter of Oddi dysfunction.
  - Ductal stones and strictures.
- Trauma (rare, as pancreas is retroperitoneal).
- Ischaemia.
- Scorpion venom.

Diagnosis

Guidelines recommend that the diagnosis be established in all patients within 48h, with no more than 20% classified as idiopathic.

History
- Abdominal pain. Constant and severe, usually in left upper quadrant or epigastrium. Radiates to the back. Onset rapid (within 1h).
- Nausea and vomiting in 90%.
- Ask specifically about the conditions listed above.

Examination
- Upper abdominal tenderness ± peritonism.
- Ileus can occur secondary to local peritonitis.
- Bruising around the umbilicus (Cullen's sign) or flanks (Grey–Turner's sign) is due to intra-abdominal haemorrhage (occurs in 1%). Indicates severe disease.
- Fever is common.
- Assess volume status.
- Respiratory examination may reveal basal atelectasis or pleural effusions.

Blood tests
- Serum amylase:
  - Rise >3 times ULN in the absence of renal failure usually diagnostic of acute pancreatitis. Values do not correlate well with severity.
  - Lower levels are consistent but not diagnostic, as there are other causes of hyperamylasaemia (see Box 9.2).
  - Serum amylase may be normal in patients with acute-on-chronic pancreatitis, and falsely negative in patient with hypertriglyceridaemia.
  - If reason for raised amylase is unclear, measure amylase and lipase in blood, and amylase in urine. Serum lipase is disproportionately normal with extra-pancreatic amylase production, in which case request amylase isoenzymes to confirm a salivary source. Macroamylasaemia is suggested if urine amylase is disproportionately low compared to serum. Patients with HIV infection can have raised salivary amylase, which is of no consequence.
- Obtain FBC, U & E, LFT, CRP, calcium, glucose, bicarbonate, and ABG on admission and at 48h to detect complications and for prognostication (see 'Severity scores', 📖 p. 138).
- Serum triglycerides. Most accurate after normal oral intake has resumed. In patients with pancreatitis caused by hypertriglyceridaemia, it may not be possible to measure amylase in lipaemic serum. The diagnosis can instead be made on urinary amylase concentrations.

Imaging
- Plain AXR generally not helpful but may show a sentinel loop or ileus.
- CXR may show basal atelectasis or pleural effusion.
- Request urgent abdominal US to look for gallstone disease or biliary tree dilatation. Imaging of the pancreas is usually poor, as it is often obscured by overlying bowel gas. It is not accurate for identifying necrosis, or assessing severity of inflammation or fluid accumulation.
- CT performed with 500mL oral contrast and rapid bolus IV contrast is very helpful for confirming the diagnosis, but should be delayed beyond 72h (earlier scans may underestimate the extent of necrosis). It is not required if diagnosis robust and disease mild. Calcification of the pancreas suggests underlying chronic pancreatitis.
- MRI with gadolinium is as accurate as CT but more difficult to perform in critically ill patients. MRCP can define pancreatic duct involvement.

Box 9.2 Other causes of hyperamylasaemia
- Renal insufficiency.
- Macroamylasaemia (urine amylase will be low).
- Biliary tract disease.
- Intestinal obstruction, ischaemia, or perforation.
- Acute appendicitis.
- Ovarian cyst rupture, ectopic pregnancy.
- Parotitis or salivary gland disease.
- Diabetic ketoacidosis.
- Lung carcinoma.

Severity scores

CRP >150mg/L at 48h predicts severe disease. Numerous scoring systems have been constructed to help predict the severity of an episode of acute pancreatitis. The most commonly used are the Ranson or Glasgow criteria (see Tables 9.2 and 9.3), the APACHE-II score (not specific to pancreatitis) (see Box 9.3), and the CT severity index. Ranson and Glasgow are the most straightforward but require results from 48h post-admission. The CT severity index is a radiological grading system, calculated as the sum of the Balthazar CT score (5 grades running from A (score 0; normal) to E (score 4; defined by pancreatic enlargement, inflammation, and multiple fluid collections) and the percentage necrosis score (score 0 when necrosis absent, but 6 when >50%). A total score ≥5 predicts high morbidity and mortality.

Management

- Make patient NBM.
- Aggressive fluid resuscitation. Substantial third space fluid losses occur, and patients frequently require 1L/4h for the first 72h.
- Electrolyte replacement (particularly K^+) alongside fluids. Hypocalcaemia is common but usually due to hypoalbuminaemia. Supplementation not usually required unless ionized or corrected calcium is low, signs of neuromuscular instability are present (tetany, Chvostek's and Trousseau's signs), or the QT interval is prolonged on ECG. Mg^{++} is also often low.
- Provide supplemental O_2 to maintain SaO_2 >94%.
- Analgesia. Usually opioids (these do not exacerbate acute pancreatitis despite theoretical concerns about causing sphincter of Oddi spasm).
- Thromboprophylaxis with LMWH and graduated compression stockings.
- Prophylactic antibiotics are controversial, although recent evidence suggests these do not reduce mortality in the absence of sepsis or pancreatic necrosis.
- Catheterize in all but mild pancreatitis to guide fluid replacement. Insert CVP line if urine output remains low despite adequate fluid replacement (to prevent pulmonary oedema in the context of acute tubular necrosis).
- Early HDU/ITU involvement in severe disease. Mortality is 20% in these patients if this referral is delayed.

Box 9.3 APACHE-II score
- Calculated during the first 24h of ITU admission.
- Incorporates 12 physiological variables, including age, temperature, circulatory parameters, pH, electrolytes, renal function, FBC, ABG, and GCS.
- Scores >9 associated with 15% mortality.

Table 9.2 Ranson criteria

On admission	At 48h
Age >55 (>70)	Drop in Hct >10%
WCC >16 x 10⁹/L (>18)	Estimated fluid sequestration >6L (>4)
Glucose >11mmol/L (>12)	Calcium <2.0mmol/L
LDH >350IU/L (>400)	Urea increase >1.8mmol/L (>0.7)*
AST >250IU/L	Base deficit >4MEq/L (>6)
	PaO₂ <8kPa on air

* Following IV fluid resuscitation.

Originally devised and validated for alcoholic pancreatitis. Figures in brackets are adaptations for gallstone pancreatitis. Score ≥3 indicates severe disease. Mortality according to score: 0–2≈2%; 3–4≈15%; 5–6≈40%; 7–8≈100%. Reprinted with permission from the Journal of the American College of Surgeons, formerly Surgery Gynaecology & Obstetrics. 'Prognostic signs and the role of operative management in acute pancreatitis'. Randon JHC, Rifkind KM, Roses DF, et al., Surg Gynecol Obstet 1974;139:69–81.

Table 9.3 Modified Glasgow criteria

On admission	At 48h
Age >55	Calcium <2.0mmol/L
WCC >15 x 10⁹/L	Albumin <32g/L
Glucose >10mmol/L	LDH >600IU/L
Urea >16mmol/L	
PaO₂ <8kPa	

A score ≥3 indicates severe disease.

Reproduced from *Gut*, S.L. Blamey et al., 'Prognostic factors in acute pancreatitis', 25, 12, pp. 1340–1346, copyright 1984, with permission from BMJ Publishing Group Ltd.

Nutritional support
Should be provided to all patients likely to remain NBM for >7d and, in these patients, instituted within 72h. NJ feeding with a low-fat, high-protein diet is favoured to TPN in the absence of ileus, as it diminishes the incidence of bacterial translocation, avoids catheter sepsis, and reduces hospital stay. NG feeding may be suitable in less severe disease. Introduce oral fluids at ~24h in patients with mild disease, adding in a low-fat diet over the next 4d.

Gallstone pancreatitis
Urgent ERCP + sphincterotomy within 24h is indicated in patients with concomitant cholangitis. In the absence of sepsis, ERCP within 72h should

be performed if there is high suspicion of a retained CBD stone (based on MRCP or US) and bilirubin >70µmol/L (not settling at 48h). ERCP is not advised in all cases, as it may worsen pancreatitis and stones will pass spontaneously in 80%.

Patients with gallstone pancreatitis should undergo cholecystectomy following recovery but prior to hospital discharge, delayed by 2–3wk if severe necrotizing pancreatitis has occurred. Preoperative ERCP is required if LFT worsen or cholangitis develops; otherwise, intraoperative cholangiography will suffice to demonstrate a clear duct.

Pancreatic necrosis

Sterile necrosis does not usually require therapy. Antibiotic prophylaxis is controversial; at most, it should be restricted to patients with >30% gland necrosis by CT and continue for no more than 14d. Cefuroxime 1.5g + metronidazole 500mg IV tds, or meropenem 1g IV tds, are appropriate, as these display good penetration into pancreatic tissue.

Infected necrosis should be suspected in patients with known necrosis who deteriorate after 7d of illness. CT- or EUS-guided FNA should be performed, with Gram stain and culture of the aspirate to confirm infection (usually monomicrobial) and guide therapy. Probiotic use is associated with worse outcomes.

If patients continue to deteriorate, provide anti-fungal cover (fungal infection occurs in 10%, especially following antibiotic therapy) and consider endoscopic or radiological drainage of pus (although there is no definitive evidence this is helpful). Open surgical intervention is associated with high mortality, and thus conservative treatment is preferred.

Complications

Local

- Necrosis ± infection. Mortality 20%.
- Fluid collections and pseudocysts (walled-off collections lacking epithelial or endothelial cells). Require no therapy in the absence of infection or significant impingement on nearby organs (causing obstructive jaundice, gastric outflow obstruction, or intestinal obstruction). Symptomatic mature pseudocysts can be drained endoscopically, percutaneously, or surgically, depending on local expertise.
- Inflammatory masses.
- Pseudoaneurysm.
- Splenic and portal vein thrombosis.
- Chronic pancreatitis.

General

- Hypoxia:
  - Splinting of the diaphragm.
  - Atelectasis.
  - Intrapulmonary shunt.
  - Sympathetic pleural effusion.
  - Pancreatico-pleural fistula.
  - ARDS (20% of severe pancreatitis).

- Multiorgan failure.
- Electrolyte disturbances (particularly hypokalaemia, hypocalcaemia, and hypomagnesaemia).
- SIRS.
- DIC.

Prevention

Prevention of recurrence is achieved by treating the underlying cause. Patients with alcohol misuse should be referred for counselling. ERCP with sphincter of Oddi manometry is occasionally undertaken in patients with idiopathic disease despite complete investigation, although this itself causes pancreatitis in 25%.

:۞: **Peritonitis**

Inflammation of the peritoneum, which may be localized or generalized.

Causes

- Inflamed or perforated intra-abdominal viscera:
  - Peptic ulceration.
  - Cholecystitis.
  - Appendicitis.
  - Pancreatitis.
  - Diverticulitis.
  - Bowel infarction.
- Ectopic pregnancy.
- Spontaneous bacterial peritonitis (SBP; infection of ascites in patients with chronic liver disease).
- Trauma.
- Peritoneal dialysis with superinfection.
- Leakage of sterile body fluids (endometriosis, iatrogenic bile leak).
- TB.
- Peritoneal carcinomatosis.
- Rarer causes:
  - Connective tissue disease (SLE, rheumatoid arthritis).
  - Familial Mediterranean fever.
  - Acute intermittent porphyria.

Clinical presentation

Anorexia and nausea, shortly followed by acute abdominal pain. Pain is initially poorly localized (visceral peritoneal involvement). Development of focal signs implies involvement of somatically innervated parietal peritoneum. Examination reveals fever, tachycardia, abdominal guarding, and rebound tenderness. Ileus common, manifesting as abdominal distension, vomiting, constipation, and absent bowel sounds. Clinical signs may be suppressed in immunocompromised patients.

Investigation

- Blood tests. FBC (leukocytosis), U & E, LFT, calcium, amylase, CRP, coagulation screen, G & S, blood cultures. Blood gas to assess severity (lactate, pH, base excess).
- Urinalysis for haematuria or pyuria. Send urine for culture. Check β-HCG in all women of childbearing potential.
- Send stool for M, C, & S and *C. difficile* assay if diarrhoea.
- Peritoneal fluid if ascites. Send sample for cell count (SBP diagnosed if >250 polymorphs/mm^3), Gram stain and culture (using blood culture bottles inoculated at the bedside increases yield from 20% to >70%), amylase, and albumin.
- Imaging:
  - Erect CXR for air under diaphragm (indicates perforated viscus).
  - Plain AXR as screen for bowel obstruction.
  - Abdomino-pelvic CT is the most useful modality and should be requested urgently. Patients should be haemodynamically stabilized prior to imaging. If this cannot be achieved, proceed direct to surgery.
  - US if hepatic, biliary, renal, or gynaecological pathology suspected.
- Laparoscopy/laparotomy. Gold standard for diagnosis. Do not delay this in patients with severe sepsis due to likely underlying perforated viscus.

Management

Resuscitate the patient and treat the underlying disorder:
- *Aggressive* fluid and electrolyte replacement (e.g. 1L colloid stat, then 1L every 1–2h). CVP monitoring may be required for goal-directed therapy in transient or non-responders. Inform ITU of such patients early.
- Antibiotics. Typically a cephalosporin and metronidazole to cover Gram-negatives and anaerobes. Add staphylococcal cover (flucloxacillin) if penetrating abdominal trauma.
- Laparotomy indicated in most cases to determine and correct underlying abnormality; request urgent surgical review. Not indicated for SBP.
- Drain any collections radiologically if surgery delayed.

Complications

- Sequestration of fluid and electrolytes, resulting in shock and acute kidney injury.
- Sepsis, peritoneal abscess.
- Splinting of the diaphragm.
- Death. Mortality is <10% in otherwise healthy, young patients but rises to ~40% in the elderly or those with underlying chronic disease.

☼ Retroperitoneal haemorrhage

Although rare, this can cause significant morbidity and mortality and should be suspected in patients who appear to be bleeding without an obviously detectable source. Predisposing factors are:

- Leaking abdominal aneurysm.
- Haemorrhagic pancreatitis.
- Trauma.
- Cardiac catheterization using femoral access.
- Adrenal malignancy.
- Anticoagulation or bleeding diathesis (e.g. haemophilia, von Willebrand disease).

The patient may be shocked with abdominal or flank pain, although the signs of haemorrhage can initially be subtle. Peri-umbilical (Cullen's sign) or flank (Grey–Turner's sign) bruising may be present, although they occur late. If severe, abdominal compartment syndrome can develop, defined as intra-abdominal (usually measured as intravesical) pressure >20mmHg. This manifests with renal failure, reduced cardiac output, respiratory failure, and intestinal ischaemia.

Survival of the patient depends on rapid diagnosis, restoration of circulatory volume, and control of ongoing haemorrhage. CT is the investigation of choice and does not require IV contrast to establish the diagnosis. US is not useful. Treatments include transcatheter arterial embolization to stop ongoing bleeding, and surgical decompression of the haematoma if compartment syndrome is present.

Retroperitoneal fibrosis

Retroperitoneal fibrosis (RPF) is a rare disorder affecting 1/100,000 patients/year, with a 3:1 male predominance. Fibrosis encroaches on and engulfs the abdominal aorta, IVC, iliac vessels, and ureters. It has a protean presentation, most commonly with progressive abdominal, flank, and lower back pain of insidious onset. Colicky flank pain suggests ureteric obstruction. Constitutional symptoms (weight loss, malaise, anorexia, and low-grade pyrexia) are often present. Claudication, oedema, and macroscopic haematuria may develop.

Aetiology

- Idiopathic (up to 70%).
- Abdominal aortic aneurysm.
- Drugs (especially ergot derivatives such as methysergide).
- Abdomino-pelvic radiotherapy.
- Asbestosis.
- Retroperitoneal haemorrhage.
- IgG4-related systemic disease (may have coexisting pancreatitis).
- Mycobacterial infection.
- Carcinoid tumours.

Investigation

- Blood tests:
    - FBC. Anaemia of chronic disease and elevated WCC are common.
    - U & E. Renal failure mandates exclusion of ureteric obstruction. If present, arrange urgent imaging to assess for hydronephrosis.
    - Inflammatory markers. CRP and ESR usually elevated.
    - Serology. ANA positive in 60%. IgG4 elevated in ~50% of those with IgG4-related systemic disease (Stone et al., 2012).
- Imaging:
    - Arrange urgent US or CT KUB if abnormal renal function to exclude hydronephrosis.
    - CT appearances may be diagnostic, obviating need for biopsy.
    - CT-PET useful for monitoring disease activity and response to therapy (Jansen et al., 2010).
- Biopsy. Request if diagnosis uncertain to exclude neoplastic disease. Histology shows characteristic lymphoplasmocytic inflammation, storiform fibrosis, obliterative phlebitis, and eosinophilia. Specifically request IgG4 immunohistochemistry if immune-mediated RPF suspected.

Treatment

- Initiate prednisolone 1mg/kg/d PO for 4wk. Taper over 2mo to 10mg/d and continue for 6–18mo. Provide bone and gastric protection. Response in >80%, often within days of starting therapy.
- Long-term maintenance can be achieved with steroid-sparing agents (cyclophosphamide, methotrexate, azathioprine, mycophenolate mofetil, or rituximab).
- If hydronephrosis present, refer to urology, and arrange urgent nephrostomy and drainage. May subsequently require ureteric stenting. Monitor with fortnightly US.
- Secondary RPF often resolves if the underlying cause can be treated.

:O: Bowel ischaemia and infarction

Inadequate mesenteric perfusion leads to ischaemia and necrosis of the bowel wall. Compromise of the coeliac axis affects the foregut, liver, biliary system, and spleen; the superior mesenteric artery (SMA) the mid-duodenum to distal transverse colon; and the inferior mesenteric artery (IMA) the hindgut consisting of distal colon and rectum. Gastric ischaemia is very rare due to redundancy in its blood supply.

Acute mesenteric ischaemia describes severe interruption in blood flow, accounting for 60% of cases, with 60% mortality. Damage, mainly mediated by inflammatory mediators released on reperfusion, occurs after the primary hypoxic insult. Bowel ischaemia is initially reversible; oedema and cyanosis herald infarction, following which necrosis occurs (usually within 12h). This disrupts the mucosal barrier, allowing bacterial translocation and resulting in peritonitis and sepsis.

The SMA is most commonly affected, as it has the largest calibre and the shallowest angle of origin from the aorta. Embolic disease carries the worst prognosis, as patients with chronic arterial compromise may have developed significant collateral circulation. Emboli usually lodge 6–8cm from the SMA origin near the source of the middle colic artery; emboli at the SMA origin (15%) are often fatal. Multiple sites are affected in 20%.

Chronic mesenteric ischaemia ('intestinal angina') is less severe, episodic, and usually due to atherosclerosis.

Acute SMA ischaemia

- Embolic (50%, usually cardiac in origin):
  - AF.
  - Mural thrombus post-MI.
  - Infective endocarditis.
  - Mycotic aneurysm.
- Thrombosis (20%, usually occurs near vessel origin):
  - Atherosclerosis.
  - Vasospasm (vasopressors, cocaine, ergotamine).
  - Arterial dissection.
  - Arteritis.
- Superior mesenteric vein (SMV) thrombosis (5%):
  - Hypercoagulable states (intra-abdominal infection, sepsis, polycythaemia, OCP, inherited or acquired thrombophilias, previous DVT/PE).
  - Venous stasis (portal hypertension, compression by tumour mass).
  - Injury to vascular endothelium (trauma).
- Non-occlusive mesenteric ischaemia (NOMI) (25%, related to low-flow states/hypotension; co-morbidities predispose to mortality of 70%):
  - Septic shock.
  - Hypovolaemia/haemorrhage.
  - Cardiogenic shock.

Clinical presentation

Early diagnosis is challenging but crucial to prevent serious sequelae. Maintain high clinical suspicion in elderly patients with risk factors.

History

- Pain may be sudden onset (embolic) or over hours to days (thrombotic). It is usually central and of disproportionate severity compared to examination findings.
- Nausea, vomiting, and forceful bowel action follow; rectal bleeding is very unusual.
- A history of mesenteric angina (postprandial pain beginning soon after eating and lasting up to 3h, with associated weight loss, anticipatory anxiety of food, and early satiety) should be sought.
- Ask about risk factors for thromboembolic disease.

Examination

- Depend on degree of compromised blood flow.
- Peritonism develops over hours as transmural bowel infarction occurs, with abdominal distension, guarding, and rebound.

- Patients become pyrexial, tachycardic, tachypnoeic, hypotensive, and oliguric.
- Examine for a possible embolic source (AF, aneurysms) or evidence of arterial disease in other vascular territories (peripheral pulses, bruits).

Investigations

- Blood tests. Send FBC, U & E, LFT, calcium, amylase (often non-specific elevation), coagulation screen, and G & S.
- Take ABG. Patients with metabolic acidosis and abdominal pain have mesenteric infarction until proven otherwise. Raised lactate is 70–100% sensitive but <50% specific. It may only rise once infarction has occurred. However, do not discount the diagnosis if the clinical setting is compatible despite normal blood tests.
- ECG. Look for AF, evidence of recent MI (ST segment elevation or Q waves), or hypertensive heart disease (left ventricular hypertrophy).
- Imaging:
  - Erect CXR for air under the diaphragm.
  - Plain AXR for ileus or mural thickening (particularly in venous thrombosis).
  - CT angiography has sensitivity of 75% and specificity of 90%, revealing bowel wall oedema, mesenteric streaking, pneumatosis intestinalis, portal venous gas, and solid organ infarction.
  - Mesenteric angiography is the gold standard with sensitivity of 88%. Occlusive emboli have a sharp cut-off, whereas thrombi taper near the vessel origin. In non-occlusive disease, narrowing of multiple arterial branches is seen with regions of spasm and filling defects. The false negative rate for venous thrombosis is high, although features include the thrombus itself, reflux of contrast into the aorta, a prolonged arterial phase with contrast accumulation into the bowel wall or extravasation into the lumen, and an attenuated venous phase.
  - MRA has similar sensitivity and specificity but is usually impractical in the critically unwell patient.
  - Doppler US is operator-dependent and limited to assessing the origins of the major vessels.
  - Surgical exploration. In cases where the diagnosis is unclear, laparoscopy/laparotomy should not be delayed. It can identify and remove areas of necrotic bowel. Infusion of 1g fluorescein intraoperatively (visualized under Wood's lamp) demarcates potentially viable areas of bowel.

Management

- Patients should be NBM. Insert NGT.
- Provide supplemental oxygen and analgesia.
- Aggressive fluid and electrolyte correction.
- Invasive monitoring is indicated in those with haemodynamic instability, but vasopressors should be avoided as these tend to worsen ischaemia. Cardiac function should be optimized.
- Involve a vascular surgeon, interventional radiologist, and ITU early.

Occlusive arterial disease
- Percutaneous angioplasty may be effective.
- Thrombolyse within 8h of symptom onset in embolic disease. Administer alteplase 20mg by slow intra-arterial bolus (followed by a subsequent 20mg bolus 12h later). Contraindicated if bowel necrosis and peritonitis are present.
- Surgical revascularization is possible (endarterectomy for emboli, aorto-mesenteric bypass for thromboses), although the primary aim should be resection of necrotic bowel.

Non-occlusive arterial disease
Angiographically guided papaverine infusion at 30–60mg/h can be effective and should be continued for at least 24h, titrated to clinical response. In the event that the catheter slips out of the aorta, significant hypotension can occur. The drug is incompatible with heparin.

Veno-occlusive disease
- Administer unfractionated heparin. Provide an initial bolus of 80U/kg, then an infusion commencing at 18U/kg/h (to a maximum of 5,000U). Infusion rates should be adjusted according to the APTT.
- Afterwards, convert to warfarin.
- There is no role for surgical revascularization in venous disease.

Outcomes
Acute mesenteric ischaemia has an overall mortality of 70%. This rises to >90% in the presence of infarction but falls to 50% if recognized and treated early. Veno-occlusive disease has a better prognosis with 30d mortality of 15%.

⚙ Colonic ischaemia
More common than SMA occlusion but less severe (usually non-gangrenous ischaemia). Generally affects the elderly due to prevalence of cardiovascular risk factors. Any part of colon can be affected, but the splenic flexure and rectosigmoid are particularly susceptible, as blood supply derives from narrow terminal branches of the SMA and IMA, respectively, and these are watershed zones.

History
- Tissue hypoxia leads to bowel wall spasm, causing anorexia, nausea, vomiting, abdominal distension, and diarrhoea in 75%.
- Mucosal sloughing results in rectal bleeding, usually accompanied by mild lateral abdominal pain.

Examination
- Patients usually do not appear ill, although severity depends on degree of ischaemia/infarction.
- Patients with severe ischaemia may be pyrexial, tachycardic, tachypnoiec, hypotensive, and oliguric.
- Peritonitis presents with abdominal distension, severe generalized or focal peritonism, and absent bowel sounds.
- Examine for a possible embolic source (AF, bruits) or evidence of arterial disease in other vascular territories.

Investigations

- Baseline investigations are similar to SMA ischaemia, although profound metabolic acidosis is unusual.
- Send stool for culture and C. *difficile* assay. Send sample to parasitology if appropriate travel history.
- CT required in patients with severe symptoms/signs, although it may be normal acutely.
- Colonoscopy/flexible sigmoidoscopy should be performed early in patients presenting with rectal bleeding. Typically, segmental areas of submucosal haemorrhage are seen in the left or transverse colon, with characteristic histological features.
- Angiography is usually not indicated (occluding lesions are typically distal to major vessels and likely to have resolved by the time patients are hospitalized). May be required to exclude small bowel infarction.
- Laparoscopy required if gangrene suspected.
- ECG to look for cardiac dysrhythmia (elective 24h tape if normal), and transthoracic echocardiogram.

Management

- Provided analgesia, and correct fluid and electrolyte deficiencies.
- Blood transfusion rarely required.
- Keep NBM with NG drainage if ileus present.
- Avoid medications that compromise splanchnic blood flow (diuretics, β-blockers, NSAIDs).
- Provide antibiotics (e.g. cefuroxime + metronidazole) in moderate/severe disease.
- Surgical resection without prior bowel preparation if gangrene present.
- Treat venous thrombosis with heparin acutely, and warfarin long-term.
- Minimize risk of recurrence by addressing cardiovascular risk factors. Treat dysrhythmias, hyperlipidaemia, hypertension, and diabetes mellitus. Advise smoking cessation.

Outcomes

Colitis is non-gangrenous in 85%. Long-term sequelae are infrequent, and mortality is 6% (associated with patient co-morbidity). In 20%, segmental colitis or ischaemic strictures subsequently occur. Recurrence is rare if risk factors are treated. Peritonism or sepsis indicate gangrene, which is usually fatal; even with surgery, mortality remains high (50–75%).

☼ Volvulus

Twisting of the gut around its axis, causing luminal obstruction. Can progress to strangulation and infarction. Mortality high if untreated.

Colonic volvulus

Sigmoid and caecal volvuli account for the vast majority of cases. The former occurs in the elderly, the latter in middle age. Consider Hirschsprung's disease in young patients with sigmoid volvulus.

Clinical features

The history is one of acute obstruction with abdominal distension, absolute constipation, and pain with superimposed colic. Caecal volvulus presents with vomiting. Signs on examination are consistent with large (sigmoid volvulus) or small (caecal volvulus) bowel obstruction, showing abdominal distension, a tympanic abdomen, and tinkling or absent bowel sounds.

Investigation

- Blood tests. FBC, U & E, LFT, amylase, coagulation screen, G & S.
- ABG/VBG. Lactic acidosis implies significant ischaemia.
- Erect CXR to exclude perforation.
- Plain AXR. Shows 'coffee bean' sign with sigmoid volvulus.
- CT has the highest sensitivity and can exclude strangulation.

Management

- Make NBM and insert NGT.
- IV correction of volume and electrolytes deficiencies.
- Endoscopic decompression of sigmoid volvulus provides temporary relief, but recurrence in 50% (therefore, early elective surgery usually required). Recurrence of caecal volvulus even higher.
- Request surgical review:
  - Urgent laparoscopy/laparotomy required if infarction suspected (sepsis, peritonitis; occurs in 20%).
  - Caecal volvulus requires ileocaecostomy or caecopexy.
  - Sigmoid volvulus requires mesosigmoidopexy or Hartmann's procedure. Percutaneous endoscopic colostomy can be performed in those too frail for surgery who suffer recurrent volvulus.

Gastric volvulus

Rare. Most commonly presents in the fifth decade. In 60%, the stomach twists about its long axis (organo-axial), presenting acutely. In 40%, volvulus occurs about the short axis (mesentero-axial), more likely to be incomplete and to recur. Usually associated with diaphragmatic defect (para-oesophageal hernia, post-operative), laxity/absence of gastrosplenic or gastrocolic ligaments, or fixation due to adhesions.

Clinical features

- Acute obstruction in 70%. Presents with triad of epigastric or retrosternal pain, non-productive retching, and inability to pass NGT.
- Incomplete obstruction in remainder, with chronic symptoms of intermittent epigastric pain, early satiety, and dysphagia.

Investigation

- Blood tests as for colonic volvulus.
- Erect CXR and plain AXR often diagnostic during acute episode.

Management

- Make NBM. Insert NGT if possible.
- IV correction of volume and electrolytes.
- If no evidence of infarction, upper GI endoscopy to attempt detorsion.
- Surgery (open or laparoscopic) is indicated if infarction suspected, symptoms recur, or hiatus hernia repair required.

:✪: Bowel obstruction

Mechanical or functional bowel obstruction prevents normal transit of luminal contents. Obstruction can be partial or complete. Causes may be subdivided into intra-luminal, mural or extramural structural lesions, or functional amotility of an otherwise patent bowel. Bowel proximal to the level of obstruction dilates and accumulates secretions and swallowed air, resulting in significant fluid and electrolyte shifts. Progressive dilatation compromises blood flow, resulting in ischaemia and infarction.

Bowel strangulation is a surgical emergency, usually caused by oedematous bowel twisting around an adhesive band. It typically occurs with complete obstruction; when arising in patients with partial obstruction, it generally only occurs with a Richter's hernia (where part of the bowel circumference is trapped in the hernial orifice). If left uncorrected, it progresses to infarction and necrosis, intestinal perforation, peritonitis, and death. Mortality is 100% untreated, 8% if operated within 36h (compared to 1% in patients operated on for simple mechanical obstruction), and 25% with surgery thereafter.

Small bowel obstruction (SBO)

Causes
- Adhesions (60%). Can occur from 4wk post-operation; 3% patients undergoing diagnostic laparotomy subsequently develop SBO. Adhesions are rare following laparoscopy, although SBO can occur through a peritoneal defect caused by trochar placement.
- Incarcerated hernia.
- Neoplasia (particularly metastatic colonic and ovarian carcinoma).
- Stricturing Crohn's disease.
- TB.
- Intussuception.
- Volvulus.
- Ischaemic or radiation strictures.
- SMA syndrome.
- Foreign body (including bezoars).
- Gallstone ileus.

History
- Abdominal distension.
- Colicky central abdominal pain (constant focal pain is associated with strangulation).
- Vomiting.
- Constipation (after 12–24h).
- Ask about past medical history (including malignancy) and previous abdominal surgery.

Examination
Abdominal distension, tympanic percussion note, high-pitched tinkling, or absent bowel sounds. Check hernial orifices. Clinical signs of volume depletion (hypotension, reduced urine output, tachycardia) are common. Pyrexia, tachycardia, and peritonism occur late, with strangulation and perforation.

Large bowel obstruction (LBO)

Causes
- Neoplasia (60%). Left-sided lesions obstruct earlier.
- Adhesions.
- Hernias.
- Crohn's disease.
- Volvulus.
- Faecal impaction, severe constipation.
- Ischaemic or radiation strictures.

History
- Abdominal distension.
- Colicky lower abdominal pain.
- Absolute constipation (no passage of stool or flatus).
- Vomiting (late feature).
- Abrupt onset of symptoms makes an acute obstructive event, such as volvulus, more likely.
- Chronic constipation, straining, and change in stool consistency suggest carcinoma.

Signs
As for SBO. Be aware that the combination of a femoral hernia with LBO should prompt a search for a colonic tumour, as the hernia is frequently not the point of obstruction but has manifested as a result of a more distal lesion.

Investigation
- Blood tests:
  - FBC, U & E, Mg^{++}, clotting, G & S.
  - ABG if strangulation suspected. May reveal metabolic acidosis and raised lactate, although hypokalaemic alkalosis from vomiting may complicate interpretation.
- Imaging:
  - Plain AXR confirms obstruction in 75%. Signs include bowel distension (>3cm small bowel, >5cm large bowel) and air-fluid levels on erect film. Gas within rectum >24h after symptom onset unusual in complete SBO.
  - Erect CXR if perforation possible.
  - CT scanning is the investigation of choice if a mass lesion suspected or plain radiology equivocal. Oral contrast not required as intra-luminal fluid acts as a natural contrast agent. A serrated appearance at the point of obstruction suggests strangulation, as do bowel wall thickening, portal venous gas, and pneumatosis. Serial CT scans useful in patients managed conservatively.
  - Small bowel series or enema with water-soluble contrast (Gastrografin®, 100mL PO or PR) indicated if CT non-diagnostic. The appearance of contrast within the caecum at 24h following oral administration also predicts resolution, with sensitivity and specificity >95%; plain AXRs are required 6h, 12h, and 24h post-administration.
  - Consider requesting US/MRI of small bowel in patients with known or suspected Crohn's disease presenting with subacute obstruction.

- • Accurate for assessing mural inflammation and avoids cumulative radiation exposure in young patients.
- Endoscopy. Colonoscopy and small bowel endoscopy may be diagnostic and therapeutic if intra-luminal obstruction or volvulus suspected, but should not delay surgery if peritonitic.
- Laparoscopy/laparotomy. If imaging studies do not identify source of obstruction.

Management

- Request surgical review.
- Make patient NBM and insert NGT.
- Provide IV fluids and electrolytes (particularly K^+). Replace upper GI losses with 0.9% saline containing 20–40mmol/L KCl.
- Prescribe analgesia and anti-emetics as required.
- Octreotide is a useful palliative agent if anti-emetics insufficient.
- Gastrografin®. Adhesional bowel obstruction has been reported in some studies to respond to oral administration of Gastrografin®, as this is hypertonic and osmotically attracts water into the bowel lumen, decreasing mural oedema and stimulating motility. This has not been supported by a systematic review (Abbas et al., 2007).
- Endoscopy. Endoscopic removal of foreign bodies, decompression of volvulus, and stenting of neoplastic lesions can all be effective.
- Surgery. Laparotomy/laparoscopy ± intestinal resection is indicated for:
  - • Complete obstruction not resolving with 12–24h of conservative management.
  - • Incarcerated hernias.
  - • Volvulus not responsive to endoscopic therapy.
  - • Closed loop obstruction (obstruction at two sites, producing an isolated ischaemic segment, often with minimal signs).

'Virgin abdomens' (i.e. in patients who have not previously undergone surgery) usually progress to complete obstruction and, consequently, surgery. Emergency surgery is required if there is evidence of ischaemic bowel or perforation.

Outcomes

Up to 80% of partial obstructions respond to conservative management, although 50% recur within 10y. Improvement is evidenced by return of normal bowel sounds, passage of flatus, and reduction in NG aspirate volume (to <150mL/4h). Mortality is higher amongst patients managed surgically: this is largely associated with patients with malignant obstruction, who have 40% in-hospital mortality (thus, try to manage this group conservatively if possible).

① Acute colonic pseudo-obstruction (Ogilvie's syndrome)

Pseudo-obstruction (non-mechanical ileus) is common and refers to bowel amotility in the absence of any mechanical obstruction.

Causes

- Post-operative (not limited to GI operations).
- Peritonitis (any cause).
- Intra-abdominal sepsis.
- Severe pneumonia, cardiac disease, or other systemic illness.

- Electrolyte disturbance (particularly hypokalaemia, hypocalcaemia, or hypomagnesaemia).
- Trauma, especially spinal or retroperitoneal (affecting parasympathetic nerves).

Diagnosis is based on history and plain AXR. The latter shows globally dilated large ± small bowel. Check FBC, CRP, U & E, calcium, and Mg^{++}. Exclude underlying structural lesions (usually by abdominal CT) and toxic megacolon.

Management
- Conservative measures first. NBM, NG drainage if nausea/vomiting, IV fluid, and electrolyte correction. Regularly move patient to prone elevated hip position. Correct underlying cause if possible. Avoid certain medications (opiates, sedatives, anticholinergics). Monitor progress with daily AXR.
- Neostigmine (2mg IV over 1–3min) helpful in 75% when symptoms persist >24–48h and caecal diameter >8–10cm. Patients should be cardiac monitored, with atropine available in case of bradycardia. Can be repeated daily, up to three times.
- Endoscopic deflation using suction, with a flatus tube placed in the transverse colon, is indicated for progressive colonic dilatation to diameter >11 cm. Bowel preparation should not be given and CO_2 used for insufflation.
- Surgery only required in 10% in those who have signs of peritonitis or in whom conservative approaches fail.

Severe constipation

Constipation usually presents as a chronic symptom (see the *Oxford Handbook of Gastroenterology and Hepatology*, p. 44). It can, however, present acutely, particularly in the elderly, when it needs to be distinguished from an acute abdomen or intestinal ileus. Presence of an obstructing colonic lesion should be considered in all patients.

Clinical presentation
History
- Clarify normal bowel habit and duration of the problem. Recent changes require work-up for an organic cause. Complaints lasting several years are more likely to be functional in origin.
- Ask about stool consistency, and presence of blood or mucus.
- Concurrent nausea, vomiting, abdominal distension, and inability to pass flatus may indicate bowel obstruction, which may itself be secondary to chronic constipation.
- Alternating diarrhoea and constipation is common in irritable bowel syndrome.
- Ask about discomfort, excessive straining, and need to digitate rectally or vaginally (suggests rectocoele) to pass stool.
- Tenesmus suggests a rectal lesion.
- Pain during defaecation implies anorectal disease (e.g. anal fissure).

- Bloating is ubiquitous and does not differentiate functional from organic disease.
- Ask about weakness or sensory change in the lower limbs, and genitourinary symptoms, which may implicate a neurological cause (e.g. cauda equina syndrome).
- Past medical history may reveal conditions associated with dysmotility (diabetes, hypothyroidism, or primary neurological disease). Ask about immobility.
- Medication use should be carefully reviewed (opioids, anticholinergics, calcium channel blockers, iron, aluminium, laxatives).

Examination
- Abdominal distension or masses may be due to colonic stool, tumours, or bowel obstruction.
- Abdominal wall hernias can obstruct bowel or interfere with generation of sufficient pressures to allow defaecation.
- A complete anorectal examination is necessary in all patients to identify anal fissures or stenosis, rectal masses, and the quantity and nature of any stool within the rectum. Acute constipation with an empty rectum suggests LBO, which should be evaluated, as described in 'Large bowel obstruction' (see 📖 p. 150).
- Perform a neurological examination of the lower limbs (including a search for a sensory level), and look for saddle anaesthesia or diminished anal tone in patients with acute onset constipation.

Investigation
- Blood tests. FBC (+ haematinics if anaemic), U & E, calcium, and TFT.
- Imaging:
  - Plain AXR reveals faecal loading or megarectum.
  - CT scan if obstructing lesion, volvulus, or stricture suspected.
  - Barium contrast studies are not as useful as physiological tests.
- Endoscopy:
  - Flexible sigmoidoscopy valuable in patients who are acutely constipated if LBO suspected. It is virtually mandatory in patients with rectal bleeding, especially if they are >50y or have a significant family history of colorectal cancer.
  - Rectal biopsy can corroborate a history/suspicion of laxative abuse (melanosis coli); deep biopsies can reveal diagnoses such as Hirschsprung's disease (better diagnosed with anorectal manometry).
- Physiological studies:
  - Bowel diaries improve the accuracy of the history.
  - Anorectal manometry is useful in patients with probable chronic neurological disease.
  - Defaecography (barium or MRI) helps evaluate possible structural lesions.

Management
After acute illness and bowel obstruction have been excluded, medical care consists of a combination of enemas (e.g. phosphate enema 1–2 daily)

and laxatives. This should be preceded by manual disimpaction of stool if severe pain or absolute constipation present. Oral fluid intake should be encouraged and, conventionally, patients are advised to increase dietary fibre intake (although there is limited evidence of efficacy to support this). Consider referral to a gastroenterologist with an interest in bowel motility disorders for interventions such as biofeedback.

If severe symptoms persist >4–6wk, liaise with surgical and multi-disciplinary teams and patient regarding colectomy, correction of rectocoele (if present), or placement of a caecal irrigation device.

When to call the surgeon

Close liaison between medical and surgical teams, underpinned by good working relationships, always benefits patients with GI disease. However, always clarify the primary team responsible for care unless fully integrated care is well established (see Table 9.4). Medical (GI) nutritional advice should be sought in *all* patients who are anticipated to not eat for 5–7d.

Table 9.4 Conditions usually under medical (GI) care

Condition	When to call the surgeon
Peptic ulceration	Suspected perforation
	Gastric outlet obstruction despite 2wk high-dose acid suppression and unsuitable for endoscopic therapy
	Severe uncontrollable bleeding
Ascending cholangitis*	Post-ERCP awaiting elective cholecystectomy
Ogilvie's syndrome	Rapid or extensive (>10cm) dilatation
Severe constipation	Rarely if symptoms persist; rectocoele

Table 9.5 Conditions usually under surgical care

Condition	When to call the (GI) physician
Biliary colic	For ERCP prior to cholecystectomy if persistent choledocholithiasis
Cholecystitis	–
Acute pancreatitis*	For *urgent* ERCP if gallstone impacted at the ampulla of Vater
	To place NJ tube if required
	To endoscopically drain large, persistent pseudocysts
Peritonitis	–

(Continued)

Table 9.5 (Continued)

Condition	When to call the (GI) physician
Bowel ischaemia/infarction*	To manage long-term parenteral nutrition following small bowel infarction
	To optimize risk factors and manage sequelae following colon anoxia
Volvulus	For diagnostic/therapeutic endoscopy
Bowel obstruction	For therapeutic endoscopy (e.g. stenting colonic tumour)

* May be managed by alternative team, depending on local expertise.

Acute abdominal pain

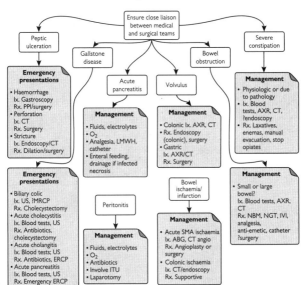

Further reading

Abbas S, Bissett IP, Parry BR (2007) Oral water soluble contrast for the management of adhesive small bowel obstruction. *Cochrane Database Syst Rev* **3**: CD004651.

Bloom S, Webster G, Marks D (2012) *Oxford Handbook of Gastroenterology and Hepatology, 2e.* Oxford University Press, Oxford.

Jansen I, Hendriksz TR, Han SH, et al. (2010) (18)F-fluorodeoxyglucose position emission tomography (FDG-PET) for monitoring disease activity and treatment response in idiopathic retroperitoneal fibrosis. *Eur J Intern Med* **21**: 216–21.

Stone JH, Zen Y, Deshpande V (2012) IgG4-related disease. *N Engl J Med* **366**: 539–51.

Malnutrition and chronic gastrointestinal disease

Anorexia and bulimia nervosa

Eating disorders arise from a severe preoccupation with food and body image, leading to disturbed eating habits and impaired physical and psychosocial functioning. For diagnostic criteria, see Box 10.1. Patients not fulfilling these criteria may be diagnosed with an 'eating disorder not otherwise specified' (EDNOS).

Anorexia nervosa is characterized by a set of adverse attitudes to body shape and weight, in which self-worth is largely determined by these parameters. It predominates in women between the ages of 16 and 25y. Body image is frequently distorted, with active maintenance of extreme low body weight (<85% ideal weight or BMI <17.5 kg/m^2). There may be associated bulimic behaviours.

Bulimia nervosa is a syndrome of episodic uncontrolled overeating (binges) followed by extreme, maladaptive weight control behaviours designed to correct for caloric intake. These include intense dieting, over-exercising, and purging with self-induced vomiting, or diuretic or laxative misuse (see 📖 p. 71). It affects 2–5% of adolescent females. Hallmark personality features include loss of control, low self-esteem, and guilt. Most bulimic individuals are of normal weight and perceive their behaviour as problematic, in contrast to anorexia nervosa.

Clinical features

Patients with severe anorexia nervosa may present with bradycardia, hypotension, yellow-orange cutaneous hue (from hypercarotenaemia), acrocyanosis, lanugo hair, and/or hypothermia (when very severe). Those with bulimia nervosa may develop parotid hypertrophy, dental enamel erosion, excoriations or calluses on the dominant hand (Russell's sign), and chronic pharyngitis; these result from digitally induced vomiting. Post-menarchal women may be amenorrhoeic.

Complications of both disorders include electrolyte disturbances (and consequent cardiac dysrhythmias and seizures), malabsorption syndromes, nutritional deficiencies, osteoporosis, growth retardation, subfertility, and predisposition to infection. GI complications include constipation, oesophagitis, Mallory–Weiss tears, peptic ulceration, melanosis coli, and deranged LFT/hepatic impairment. Pancreatitis should be considered if abdominal pain is present.

Ask about coexistent depression (up to 50%; several screening tools are available such as the Beck depression inventory scale) and suicide risk. Explore home and social circumstances.

Investigation

- Blood tests:
  - Electrolytes. Look for low K$^+$, Na$^+$ (from excessive water intake or purging), Mg^{++}, calcium, and PO$_4^{3-}$.
  - Endocrine. Low T$_3$, LH, FSH, oestradiol, and testosterone.
  - Serum transaminases and cholesterol may be elevated in starvation; albumin may be low.
  - Leukopaenia in severe disease.
  - Check amylase in all patients with abdominal pain.

- Exclude pregnancy as a cause of recurrent vomiting.
- ECG in patients with electrolyte disturbance. Look for prolonged QTc.

Box 10.1 DSM IV-TR diagnostic criteria for eating disorders

Anorexia nervosa*
- Refusal to maintain body weight at or above a minimally normal weight for age and height.
- Intense fear of gaining weight or becoming fat, even though underweight.
- Disturbance in the way body weight or shape are experienced, undue influence of body weight or shape on self-evaluation, or denial of the seriousness of current low body weight.
- Amenorrhoea (at least three consecutive cycles) in post-menarchal females.

Bulimia nervosa**
- Recurrent episodes of binge eating characterized by:
  - Eating (in a discrete time period) an amount that is larger than what most people would eat under similar circumstances.
  - A sense of lack of control over eating during the episode.
- Recurrent inappropriate compensatory behaviours to prevent weight gain. These may include self-induced vomiting, misuse of laxatives/diuretics/enemas/other medication, fasting, and excessive exercise.
- Binge eating and inappropriate compensatory behaviours both occur, on average, at least twice a week for 3mo.
- Self-evaluation is unduly influenced by body shape and weight.
- The disturbance does not occur exclusively during episodes of anorexia nervosa.

* May be subdivided into restricting types or binge eating/purging types. ** May be subdivided into purging and non-purging types.

Management

Treatment requires a multi-disciplinary approach (medical, dietician, and psychiatric teams need regular communication) to address the underlying psychosocial determinants, nutritional deficiencies, and other medical complications. It can be provided on an outpatient, day patient, or inpatient basis. Cognitive behavioural therapy forms the basis of psychological treatment. Antidepressant medication does not appear to be helpful in general but may have an adjunctive role in patients with depressive symptomatology or co-morbid obsessive-compulsive disorder (Aigner et al., 2011).

Be very aware that patients often try to divide teams. The therapeutic plan must be clear and understood by all caregivers and, ideally, only one person should make changes to this plan. Also be aware that patients can be particularly devious in their strategies to avoid being fed.

① Indications for admission

- Suicide risk.
- Adverse home circumstances.

- Failure of outpatient treatment.
- Severe low weight (BMI <13.5kg/m^2).
- Rapid weight loss, dehydration, hypoglycaemia, or oedema.
- Severe electrolyte disturbances.
- Cardiac abnormalities (bradycardia, hypotension, long QTc).
- Intercurrent infection.
- Failure to sit up from supine or squat without using their hands.

Admission can be to a general medical ward, or psychiatric unit with good access to general medical advice and assistance. Outcomes are better in units with staff experienced in the management of eating disorders. Inpatient interventions include IV or high-dose oral thiamine; calcium, vitamin D, and multivitamin/mineral supplements (e.g. Forceval®); daily measurement of plasma electrolytes (especially Mg^{++}, K$^+$, PO$_4^{3-}$) and correction of any abnormalities (see Table 10.1); cardiac monitoring and daily ECG. Specialized nurses should be in attendance. Patients are at high risk of developing re-feeding syndrome (for full details of its detection, management, and prevention, see Chapter 11). Conversely, it is important to increase calorie intake as soon as safe (re-judge daily).

Occasionally, patients need to be admitted and/or treated against their expressed wishes. The legal and ethical arguments to support this are complex and based on the following:
- Restriction of autonomy is justified only when a person is likely to do themselves considerable harm.
- Anorexia nervosa can cause considerable harm and lead to death.
- Being severely underweight produces cognitive distortion, providing a legal defence to administer non-consensual therapies.
- Thus, patients with severe anorexia can be detained for assessment for up to 72h (section 5(2) of the Mental Health Act), pending psychiatric and social worker review. Section 3 of the Act allows feeding against the patient's will. Common law allows for urgent life-saving treatment to be administered to very sick patients for whom psychiatric assessment has not yet occurred.
- If informed consent is not provided by the patient, forced (tube) feeding can be administered until the severe phase of anorexia has passed.
- See the MARSIPAN guideline, published in 2010, for more details on the medical and psychiatric management of patients with severe anorexia (see ℘ http://www.rcpsych.ac.uk/files/pdfversion/CR162.pdf).

Outcomes

Early mortality is 5%, but late mortality as high as 20% (largely attributable to suicide (Preti et al., 2011), cardiac dysrhythmias, and infection). Inpatients can be discharged once their physical state has normalized, which usually takes at least 1–2wk of observed feeding. Consider the need for endocrine supplementation therapies (including HRT) on discharge.

Table 10.1 Electrolyte replacement therapy

Electrolyte	Oral	IV (only if severe)
Hypokalaemia	Sando-K® 4–12/d	20–40mmol KCl in 1L 0.9% NaCl or 5% glucose over 4–6h
Hypophosphataemia	Phosphate-Sandoz® 4–6/d	Phosphate Polyfusor® 10mmol/12h
Hypomagnesaemia	Maalox® suspension 10–20mL/d	30mmol $MgSO_4$ in 500mL 5% glucose over 24h
Hypocalcaemia	Calcichew® 1–3/d	Calcium gluconate 10mL of 10%

From MARSIPAN guidelines, 2010. © The Royal College of Psychiatrists and The Royal College of Physicians. Full report available at ♒ http://www.rcpsych.ac.uk/files/pdfversion/CR162.pdf. Equivalents to the named proprietary preparations may be available and appropriate. Use oral route where possible.

⊙ Acute presentations of gastrointestinal malignancy

Although uncommon, GI malignancy can present acutely. Symptoms, often consciously ignored, usually predate the acute presentation and include:
- Change in bowel habit.
- Rectal bleeding.
- Abdominal pain.
- Weight loss.
- Anorexia, nausea.
- Abdominal distension.

Investigation is directed by the dominant symptom. Request standard blood tests (FBC, U & E, LFT, calcium, CRP, and glucose). Tumour markers should not be used to make a diagnosis, although CA-125, CEA, CA19-9, and α-fetoprotein are appropriate if there is a high index of suspicion for ovarian, colonic, pancreatic, or hepatocellular carcinoma, respectively. More specific tests include:
- Haematemesis. Gastroscopy.
- Vomiting. Plain AXR, followed by abdominal CT if suggestive of obstruction, or OGD if normal.
- Jaundice. Abdominal US and/or pancreatic-protocol abdominal CT. Proceed to MRCP if bile duct dilatation but urgent ERCP if the patient is septic or has gallstone pancreatitis.
- Weight loss and abdominal pain. CT abdomen and pelvis; if normal, request OGD and colonoscopy.
- IDA. Gastroscopy and colonoscopy. If normal, capsule endoscopy if alarm symptoms (see Chapter 3). Remember 1% caused by renal cell carcinoma.
- Change in bowel habit. Colonoscopy (CT pneumocolon if >80y).
- Abdominal distension. Abdominal US or CT, and pelvic US. Distension is non-specific and, therefore, generally only merits investigation if occurs in conjunction with other symptoms or signs. If possible, avoid radiation in those <60y.

Gastric tumours

Present with heartburn, dyspepsia, haematemesis, gastric outlet obstruction (vomiting), or anaemia. Emergency management may include gastroscopy to control bleeding (see Chapter 1), stenting, or (often with limited success) APC or laser to prevent chronic bleeding.

Small bowel tumours

Present with abdominal pain, haematochezia or melaena, anaemia, or bowel obstruction (vomiting followed by constipation). Emergency surgery is required if there is bowel dilatation proximal to obstruction, perforation (± peritonitis), or severe bleeding. If the patient is too frail for surgery, obstruction can be managed by NG decompression and IV fluid support, perforation with broad-spectrum antibiotics, and bleeding by angiographic embolization; mortality in these patients is high.

Colorectal tumours

Emergency presentations include bowel obstruction (absolute constipation, abdominal distension and, later, nausea and vomiting), haemorrhage, and perforation. The management of bowel obstruction is detailed in Chapter 9. Request colonic stenting, if available, within 24h if rapid colonic dilatation; the rate of change is more important than the absolute diameter. Stenting reduces operative mortality, in part, by allowing primary anastomosis. If stenting is not available, unsuccessful or perforation has occurred, emergency surgery is required. Haemorrhage usually predicates urgent surgery, although angiography with embolization or radiotherapy may be attempted if the patient is deemed too frail.

Lymphoma

GI symptoms correlate with the anatomical site of the tumour. B-symptoms (fever, night sweats, weight loss) and pruritus may be present. Emergency management may involve surgery and interventional radiology (as described in the above three sections on gastric, small bowel, and colorectal tumours), or oncological treatment (chemotherapy, radiotherapy, or biologics such as rituximab).

Hepatic, pancreatobiliary, and neuroendocrine tumours

Emergency presentations of hepatocellular carcinoma, pancreatic adenocarcinoma, cholangiocarcinoma, and GI neuroendocrine tumours are discussed in Chapter 21.

⊙ Short bowel syndrome

Defined as a combination of electrolyte ± calorie deficiencies, resulting from a diminished length of functional small bowel. Critical lengths of normal small intestine have been defined that guide likely mode of future food and fluid replacement (see Table 10.2). Optimal management often requires several weeks of inpatient care, with changes made every few days so as to tailor therapy to each patient. If staff are not experienced in treating such patients, it is appropriate to discuss care with a specialist centre.

Table 10.2 Small bowel length and likely nutrition and fluid supplementation requirements

	Small bowel length (cm)	Replacement
Jejunostomy	<75	HPN
	<100	HPE ± HPN
	<150	EN
	<200	Fluid restriction and ORS
Jejuno-colic anastomosis	<50	HPN
	<100	EN
	<150	Fluid restriction and ORS

HPN, home parenteral nutrition; HPE, home parenteral electrolytes; EN, enteral nutrition; ORS, oral rehydration solution.

Initial assessment

- Ensure accurate fluid balance recorded. Weigh patients daily.
- Measure baseline blood tests: FBC, U & E, LFT, bone, glucose, TFT, CRP, clotting, haematinics, coeliac screen, vitamin A, vitamin D, zinc, Mg^{++}, selenium.
- Request daily U & E, Mg^{++}; twice weekly FBC, bone profile, LFT.
- Measure urine Na^+ concentration weekly; <10mmol/L suggests dehydration.

Initial management

- Keep NBM for first 48h to assess basal stool output. High output, defined as >1L, is associated with development of dehydration and electrolyte abnormalities. Patients with <1L are less likely to require stringent management.
- Subsequently, restrict oral intake to 1,500mL/24h, at least 1L of which being ORS (e.g. St. Mark's solution: 2.5g $NaHCO_3$, 20g glucose, 3.5g NaCl in 1L water; or 1.5-strength Dioralyte®). Give cold, and add cordial if unpalatable). Replace excess fluid losses with IV 0.9% saline, ensuring urine output >800mL/d.
- Explain that hypotonic oral intake promotes Na^+ secretion in the proximal small bowel, leading to increased fluid output and dehydration in patients without functioning colon to resorb fluid. Patients, *and some doctors*, find this hard to comprehend, often leading to conflicting advice being given and to patients surreptitiously drinking water to quench increasing thirst. Prescribe loperamide 4mg PO qds, to be taken 30min before meals. Prescribe double-dose vitamins/minerals (e.g. Forceval® 1 tablet PO bd).
- Recommend six small meals/d, predominantly dry foods, avoiding fluids for 30min before and after eating. NG or IV nutrition may be necessary initially to supplement intake. Oral calorific intake needs to be 2–3 times likely energy expenditure if high output. Liquid feeds should contain >100mmol/L Na^+ with osmolarity >300mOsmol/kg.

- Highly osmotic fatty foods or sorbitol can exacerbate diarrhoea if the colon remains *in situ*. Recommend high carbohydrate intake (but see section on D-lactic acidosis under 'Long-term management' (see p. 165). Salt can be added as desired. Avoid foods containing excess oxalate (spinach, rhubarb, beetroot, nuts, chocolate, tea, wheat bran, strawberries) in patients with short small bowel and colon *in situ*, as calcium oxalate renal stones occur in 25%.
- The following can then be tried if diarrhoea remains problematic:
  - Prescribe codeine phosphate 30–60mg PO qds.
  - Increase each loperamide dose by 2mg, up to 16mg/24h.
  - If high-output jejunostomy, prescribe high-dose PPI to lower gastric secretion. Then consider octreotide 50–200µg SC tds (then depot octreotide IM if effective). If electrolyte imbalance present, try oral replacement with up to 24mmol magnesium glycerophosphate (although often poorly absorbed), 5–15 slow sodium tablets, 5–15 potassium tablets, and 1–9µg 1α-colecalciferol. Routine medication doses may also need to be increased due to malabsorption.
  - Consider colestyramine or colesevelam if >60cm of terminal ileum has been resected with small bowel anastomosed to colon, to prevent bile salt-associated diarrhoea. This can exacerbate steatorrhoea. Vitamin B12, fat, and fat-soluble vitamin malabsorption likely in longer term.
- Parenteral fluids will be required if, following treatment optimization, daily output is >1.5L. If 1–1.5L losses, then 1L 0.9% saline containing 4mmol magnesium sulphate can be provided SC overnight.
- Parenteral nutrition is indicated if >10% weight loss occurs despite optimal enteral nutrition, and should be anticipated if the amount of remaining small intestine is limited (see Table 10.2).
  - Infuse 25cal/kg ideal body weight, including 0.5–1g protein/kg/d (critically ill patients need up to double this amount), and 1g lipid/kg/d.
  - Excessive parenteral calories cause hyperglycaemia, associated with increased rates of infection.
  - Reduce protein content if significant renal or hepatic disease.

Long-term management

- Initially, measure FBC, U & E, LFT, Mg^{++}, calcium, PO_4^{3-}, and urinary Na^+ weekly. Reduce frequency when stable. Measure zinc, selenium, vitamin A, vitamin D, vitamin B12, red cell folate, and clotting 3–6-monthly, then annually when stable. Bone mineral density should be measured biennially.
- Weigh weekly. Consider overnight enteral, instead of parenteral, feeding if weight gain (possible in 20% of patients due to intestinal adaptation, enhancing absorption).
- Increased output can be caused by medication, excess drinking, sepsis, obstruction, or disease (e.g. coeliac, Crohn's disease). Consider bacterial overgrowth if colon *in situ*.
- Gallstones occur in up to 45% of patients with short bowel syndrome. UDCA, NSAIDs, or metronidazole can be tried to prevent recurrence.

- In addition to bile salt diarrhoea and calcium oxalate renal stones, patients with short functional small bowel anastomosed to colon can develop D-lactic acidosis. Glucose and starch are metabolized by colonic bacteria into D-lactic acid. This is absorbed but not broken down by L-lactate dehydrogenase.
  - Episodic metabolic acidosis develops after high carbohydrate intake.
  - Ataxia, slurred speech, and confusion occur (patients appear drunk).
  - Anion gap increased, acidosis present, but lactate levels normal (as laboratory assay only measures L-lactate).
  - Provide $NaHCO_3$ to correct acidosis and bowel sterilization with metronidazole or neomycin; avoid probiotics (as *Lactobacilli* produce D-lactate) and decrease carbohydrate intake.

① Protein-losing enteropathy

Rare syndrome characterized by loss of serum protein into the GI tract. GI symptoms themselves are frequently absent. Blood tests show profound hypoalbuminaemia, and there may be deficiencies of fat-soluble vitamins. Complications include peripheral oedema, ascites, and pleural and pericardial effusions. Causes include:

- IBD.
- Coeliac disease (see Colour plate 19).
- Tropical sprue.
- NSAID enteropathy.
- Whipple's disease.
- Ménétrier's disease (characterized by giant hypertrophic gastric folds, mainly involving the fundus).
- Intestinal lymphoma.
- Intestinal sarcoidosis.
- Amyloidosis.
- Mesenteric venous thrombosis.
- Intestinal lymphangiectasia.
- Sclerosing mesenteritis.
- Graft-versus-host disease.
- Severe right heart failure.
- Fontan procedure for a single cardiac ventricle (produces raised right heart pressures).

The initial step in evaluation is to exclude other aetiologies of protein loss, including malnutrition, chronic liver disease with impaired synthetic function, and nephrotic syndrome. If no other cause is identified, enteric protein losses can then be determined by measurement of α1-antitrypsin (A1AT) clearance from plasma. This is calculated based upon measurement of A1AT in a simultaneous blood sample and 24h stool collection. Normal clearance is <27mL/24h, although, in the context of diarrhoea (of any cause), this rises to <56mL/24h. As A1AT is degraded by a pH <3.5, it is recommended to perform the test whilst on acid suppression therapy if a gastric cause of protein loss is suspected.

There is no specific therapy for protein-losing enteropathy, and treatment is directed to the underlying cause. Careful monitoring of nutrition and correction of micronutrient deficiencies are required. A high-protein diet is generally recommended. There is anecdotal evidence to suggest that octreotide may usefully decrease protein exudation from the bowel. Long-term use of intermittent IV albumin infusions is generally unrewarding. Surgery may be required in refractory cases of severe protein loss. Treatment with cetuximab or gastrectomy should be considered in Ménétrier's disease. (Burdick et al., 2000)

Other causes of severe malnutrition

In-hospital malnutrition is multifactorial and very common. The most common cause is poor dietary intake, which may be iatrogenic. Frequent contributors are listed in Box 10.2; elderly patients are at particularly high risk. Actively try to identify and manage these by eliminating/reducing precipitants and encouraging changes to the hospital environment where relevant. Take a dietetic history, risk-assess (e.g. MUST score; see Fig. 10.1), and monitor nutritional replacement in patients staying in hospital >1wk.

> **Box 10.2 Common factors that impact on dietary intake in hospital**
> - Reduced mobility/inability to reach food.
> - Poor eyesight.
> - Difficulty feeding without assistance due to impaired motor skills.
> - Misplaced dentures.
> - Difficulty communicating hunger.
> - Unappetizing selection of food.
> - Non-catering for religious or personal preferences.
> - Reduced conscious level.
> - Dementia.
> - Being nil-by-mouth.
> - Nausea and vomiting.
> - Constipation.
> - Anorexia induced by medication.

Other causes of malnutrition/weight loss include:
- Cardiac cachexia.
- Malignancy.
- Severe COPD.
- Chronic renal failure.
- Infections (severe sepsis, TB, parasites, AIDS).
- Hyperthyroidism, Addison's disease.
- Alcohol or recreational drug misuse.
- Malabsorption:
  - Coeliac disease, tropical sprue.
  - Small bowel Crohn's disease.

- Pancreatic exocrine insufficiency.
- Whipple's disease.
- Small bowel bacterial overgrowth.
- Amyloidosis.

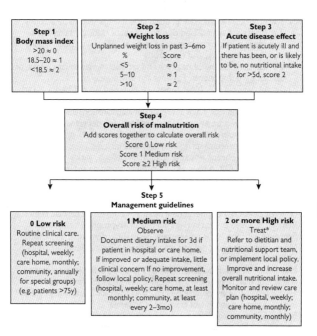

Fig. 10.1 Malnutrition Universal Screening Tool (MUST) score. The 'Malnutrition Universal Screening Tool' ('MUST') is reproduced here with the kind permission of BAPEN (British Association for Parenteral and Enteral Nutrition). For further information on 'MUST' see ℘ www.bapen.org.uk.

① Syndromes resulting from lack of essential nutrients

- Protein malnutrition. Principally seen in paediatric patients in developing countries. Syndromes include:
  - Kwashiorkor. Inadequate protein intake leads to muscle atrophy. Fat stores are maintained due to adequate caloric intake. Signs include reduced muscle mass, diarrhoea, irritability, poor quality hair, hepatomegaly, and dermatitis.
  - Marasmus. Wasting of muscles and fat due to inadequate intake of all dietary components. Patients are profoundly thin.
- Thiamine (vitamin B1). Most foods are enriched, so deficiency is rare, except in alcohol misuse (individuals often eat less as obtain calories from alcohol and may have associated malabsorption) and those on dialysis. However, be aware of the potential for deficiency in pregnant women with hyperemesis gravidarum (see Chapter 4), and patients with ongoing severe dysphagia. Syndromes include:
  - Wernicke's encephalopathy. Ophthalmoplegia, ataxia, and cognitive impairment. Often reversible if prompt thiamine replacement.
  - Korsakoff's psychosis. Retrograde and anterograde amnesia, compensated for by patient through confabulation. Irreversible.
  - Dry beriberi. Sensorimotor peripheral neuropathy.
  - Wet beriberi. Peripheral neuropathy + congestive cardiac failure.
- Pellagra. Caused by niacin (vitamin B3) or tryptophan deficiency. Presents with the '4 Ds': diarrhoea, dermatitis, dementia, and death. More common in alcohol misuse and those who eat large amounts of corn.
- Megaloblastic anaemia. Screen for B12 and red cell folate deficiency. Ask about diarrhoea, examine for glossitis, and look for evidence of associated autoimmune diseases (such as thyroiditis and vitiligo) that may support a diagnosis of pernicious anaemia.
- Scurvy (vitamin C deficiency). Signs include anaemia, ecchymoses, gingivitis and mucosal bleeding, pinpoint bleeding at base of hair follicles, and 'corkscrew' hairs.
- Osteomalacia (rickets in infancy/childhood). Caused by chronic deficiency of vitamin D and calcium. Consider in those with inadequate sun exposure (<10min/d), lactose-intolerant patients, and vegetarians. Presents with bony pain and proximal myopathy.

Malnutrition and chronic gastrointestinal disease

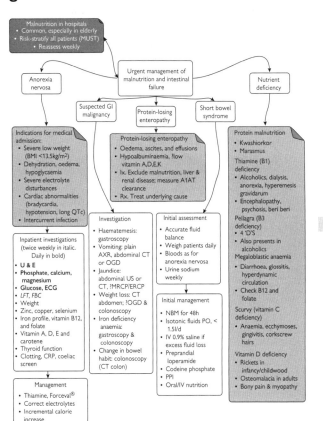

Malnutrition in hospitals
- Common, especially in elderly
- Risk-stratify all patients (MUST)
- Reassess weekly

Urgent management of malnutrition and intestinal failure

Anorexia nervosa

Suspected GI malignancy

Protein-losing enteropathy

Short bowel syndrome

Nutrient deficiency

Indications for medical admission:
- Severe low weight (BMI <13.5kg/m²)
- Dehydration, oedema, hypoglycaemia
- Severe electrolyte disturbances
- Cardiac abnormalities (bradycardia, hypotension, long QTc)
- Intercurrent infection

Protein-losing enteropathy
- Oedema, ascites, and effusions
- Hypoalbuminaemia, ?low vitamin A,D,E,K
- Ix. Exclude malnutrition, liver & renal disease; measure A1AT clearance
- Rx. Treat underlying cause

Protein malnutrition
- Kwashiorkor
- Marasmus

Thiamine (B1) deficiency
- Alcoholics, dialysis, anorexia, hyperemesis gravidarum
- Encephalopathy, psychosis, beri beri

Pellagra (B3 deficiency)
- 4 'D'S
- Also presents in alcoholics

Megaloblastic anaemia
- Diarrhoea, glossitis, hyperdynamic circulation
- Check B12 and folate

Scurvy (vitamin C deficiency)
- Anaemia, ecchymoses, gingivitis, corkscrew hairs

Vitamin D deficiency
- Rickets in infancy/childwood
- Osteomalacia in adults
- Bony pain & myopathy

Inpatient investigations (twice weekly in italic. Daily in bold)
- **U & E**
- **Phosphate, calcium, magnesium**
- **Glucose, ECG**
- *LFT, FBC*
- Weight
- Zinc, copper, selenium
- Iron profile, vitamin B12, and folate
- Vitamin A, D, E and carotene
- Thyroid function
- Clotting, CRP, coeliac screen

Investigation
- Haematemesis: gastroscopy
- Vomiting: plain AXR, abdominal CT or OGD
- Jaundice: abdominal US or CT, ?MRCP/ERCP
- Weight loss: CT abdomen; ?OGD & colonoscopy
- Iron deficiency anaemia: gastroscopy & colonoscopy
- Change in bowel habit: colonoscopy (CT colon)

Initial assessment
- Accurate fluid balance
- Weigh patients daily
- Bloods as for anorexia nervosa
- Urine sodium weekly

Initial management
- NBM for 48h
- Isotonic fluids PO, < 1.5l/d
- IV 0.9% saline if excess fluid loss
- Preprandial loperamide
- Codeine phosphate
- PPI
- Oral/IV nutrition

Management
- Thiamine, Forceval®
- Correct electrolytes
- Incremental calorie increase

Further reading

Aigner M, Treasure J, Kaye W, et al. (2011) World Federation of Societies of Biological Psychiatry (WFSBP) guidelines for the pharmacological treatment of eating disorders. *World J Biol Psychiatry* **12**: 400–43.

Burdick JS, Chung E, Tanner G, et al. (2000) Treatment of Ménétrier's disease with a monoclonal antibody against the epidermal growth factor receptor. *N Engl J Med* **343**: 1697–701.

Preti A, Rocchi MB, Sisti D, et al. (2011) A comprehensive meta-analysis of the risk of suicide in eating disorders. *Acta Psychiatr Scand* **124**: 6–17.

Stratton RJ, King CL, Stroud MA, et al. (2006) 'Malnutrition Universal Screening Tool' predicts mortality and length of hospital stay in acutely ill elderly. *Br J Nutr* **95**: 325–30.

Complications of nutritional support

☼ Venous catheter-related problems

Central or peripheral feeding?

- Above all else, 'if the gut works, use it'. Only consider IV feeding if patients are likely to be without enteral nutrition for >5d.
- Central venous catheter feeding (i.e. catheter tip in SVC, IVC, or right atrium) preferred to avoid thrombophlebitis from hyperosmolar feeds. Well-managed central catheters can be left *in situ* for a long time.
- Peripheral feeding with midline catheters (tip in proximal portion of arm) has a higher rate of catheter dysfunction than central catheters. Narrow gauge peripheral cannulae can be used but should be re-sited every 2d, and require low-calorie regimes (osmolality needs to be <900mOsm/L); therefore only useful in the short term (e.g. <1 wk) or supplemental to enteral intake.

Line sepsis

Line-related bloodstream infections are potentially lethal. Two-thirds are due to coagulase-negative staphylococci. The remainder are often caused by *S. aureus*, Gram-negative bacilli, *Candida* species, and *Pseudomonas*, and carry a worse prognosis. Line infection (significant growth from the line of >10^3cfu) should be differentiated from localized exit site cellulitis. One-third of patients with bacteraemia develop major complications, including septic shock, suppurative thrombophlebitis, metastatic infection, or endocarditis. Mortality is up to 10%.

Risk factors

- Site. Femoral >>> internal jugular > subclavian; leg >> arm.
- Technique and setting. Venous cut down > emergency > elective.
- Use. Parenteral nutrition (PN) > other uses.
- Number of hubs. Multi-lumen > single lumen.
- Duration of insertion >5d (although a well-managed, tunnelled central feeding catheter can be left *in situ* indefinitely).

Meticulous asepsis should be practised during insertion, using full barrier precautions and skin decontamination with 2% chlorhexidine. Lines should be routinely monitored and changed if infection confirmed or suspected in an unwell patient. Central feeding catheters should not be routinely changed, but peripheral (narrow gauge) feeding catheters exchanged every 2d. Use gauze dressings, and only change if contaminated. Administration sets should be changed at least every 3d. Antimicrobial-impregnated catheters associated with lower risk of infection.

Making the diagnosis

Bloodstream infection typically manifests with fevers and rigors, or complications. There may be associated exit site cellulitis. Take peripheral and central blood cultures (from every lumen) if temperature >38°C; label the origins clearly on the bottle. Definitive diagnosis requires identification of the micro-organism from both central and peripheral samples. Infections may be polymicrobial. All patients with *S. aureus* bacteraemia should have a transthoracic echocardiogram. Those with fungaemia require ophthalmological review.

When to remove the line

Clinical studies suggest that routine line removal results in loss of many that are sterile with no outcome benefits. They should not be exchanged over guidewires. Lines should only be withdrawn if:

- The patient has septic shock attributable to line infection.
- Non-tunnelled (temporary) central or peripheral catheter infection strongly suspected.
- Tunnelled central line infection recurs at least twice.
- Signs of venous thrombosis.
- New endocarditis.
- Significant purulence and erythema at the insertion site despite meticulous nursing care.

Management

Give empiric antibiotics if the patient is too ill to wait for definitive microbiology or a highly virulent organism is suspected. A glycopeptide (usually teicoplanin 400mg (6mg/kg if >85kg) IV bd for three doses, then 400mg (6mg/kg if >85kg) IV od for 5d) is appropriate, with a prolonged course of >4wk if there is deep-seated infection. In critically ill patients, it is appropriate to supplement with Gram-negative and pseudomonal cover (piperacillin-tazobactam 4.5g IV tds or meropenem 1g IV tds) ± fungal cover (liposomal amphotericin 3mg/kg IV od). Exit site abscesses may need surgical drainage or debridement.

Infection of tunnelled central feeding lines without severe cellulitis or severe sepsis is managed using central antibiotic administration (as per sensitivities) and cessation of feeding for 7d, with subsequent demonstration of sterile central cultures. Antibiotics are preferentially provided using catheter locks (Korbila et al., 2007).

Line occlusion

Central feeding lines can be flushed with urokinase. Aseptically, attach a three-way tap to the end of the catheter, with a 10mL syringe containing 5,000U urokinase in 2mL, and an empty 10mL syringe (with plunger depressed) to the vacant stopcocks. Pull on the empty syringe to create a vacuum in the catheter then, whilst maintaining suction, turn the three-way tap to allow the urokinase solution to be sucked into the catheter. Leave for 1h, then try and aspirate blood ± flush with 0.9% saline. This process may need to be repeated several times. Peripheral lines are usually removed if saline flushing ineffective.

ⓘ Venous thrombosis

The feeding catheter is removed and anticoagulation provided for 3–6mo. Vein patency is confirmed by Doppler US before further feeding catheters inserted in the same site. If these are intended for long-term use, they should be heparin-locked and anticoagulation continued.

Cannula insertion-related complications

Include pneumothoraces, malplacement and, rarely, cardiac tamponade. Pneumothoraces are treated by intercostal drain insertion and tamponade by pericardiocentesis under fluoroscopic guidance.

Other complications of parenteral nutrition

Liver disease

Clinically significant liver disease develops in ~5% adults on long-term PN, and up to 50% may have asymptomatic derangement of LFT. The clinical spectrum ranges from hepatic steatosis and cholestasis, through to hepatic fibrosis and cirrhosis (more common in infants). Predisposing factors include age, total caloric intake, duration on PN, and lipid or glucose overload. Soya-based lipid emulsions are particularly implicated. Note that liver dysfunction of onset <4wk after starting PN usually has another aetiology. LFT should be monitored weekly in the early phases of parenteral nutrition and 3-monthly in patients with established feeding.

Aberrant glycaemic control

Both hyper- and hypoglycaemia can occur with PN. Hyperglycaemia is associated with increased morbidity and mortality from cardiovascular events and sepsis (Cheung et al., 2005). These are readily managed/avoided by use of insulin.

Precipitous cessation of PN can provoke hypoglycaemia; slowly tapering the infusion rate over the last hour reduces the risk.

Psychological

Patients may experience acute grief or loss reactions due to bowel resection, lifestyle restrictions imposed by PN regimens, and altered body image. Depression is common (up to 80%), but deliberate self-harm rare (although must be considered in patients with recurrent central line infections).

Problems with enteral tubes

Complications directly related to the placement of percutaneous endoscopic gastrostomy (PEG) tubes include damage to surrounding structures (viscera and blood vessels), resulting in haemorrhage, perforation, or peritonitis. These occur more frequently in elderly patients and those with co-morbidity. The procedure has a directly attributable 30d mortality of ~1/150, serious morbidity of 1/30, and minor morbidity of 1/8.

Procedural risks are *much* higher in patients with advanced dementia, in whom PEG placement is relatively contraindicated (30d mortality >50%). Prior abdominal surgery does not preclude PEG but has a higher risk of colonic perforation. PEG is probably contraindicated in patients with ascites. Some complications can be easily prevented by correct traction (refer to PEG tube instructions). Correct Hb, platelets, and clotting as necessary before placement, and give peri-procedural IV antibiotics. The product instructions should be followed precisely. The external fixation device must be loosened 1cm at the skin surface 10d after insertion to avoid internal pressure necrosis and the tube rotated 360° every few days to avoid buried bumper syndrome.

☼ Immediate complications

Bleeding

Bleeding is uncommon but can be life-threatening if vascular injury at the time of PEG insertion. Localized vessel damage may respond to tamponade by tightening the intra-gastric flange against the skin (e.g. moving the marker at the skin surface from 4cm to 3cm). If persistent/life-threatening bleeding, consider interventional angiography or surgery.

Perforation

Usually involves the catheter passing through an anteriorly situated transverse colon. This can present with abdominal pain, peritonitis, or feed passing per rectum. Diagnosed by US. Emergency laparotomy is indicated if the patient is peritonitic. Otherwise, the PEG tube should not be used and the patient placed on broad-spectrum antibiotics for 4wk, at which time it can be removed endoscopically. The fistulous tract will gradually close, requiring only simple dressings.

Peritonitis

Peritonitis not due to colonic perforation should usually be treated conservatively with IV antibiotics. PEG feeding must not be given until resolved. Necrotizing fasciitis is a very rare, very serious infection that requires immediate surgical debridement.

Minor complications

Pneumoperitoneum is common after PEG placement and of no consequence in the absence of other worrying features. Surgical emphysema has also been described without any mishap having occurred.

Ileus may occur. Exclude perforation with a contrast study. Aspirate excess gastric air/fluid from the PEG. Resume feeding once resolves.

① Long-term PEG complications

Catheter occlusion

Common (up to 45%). May be re-opened by vigorous flushing with warm water (consider prior instillation of pancreatic enzymes in bicarbonate), or manually with a brush or balloon catheter. Wires should be avoided as may cause perforation. Tubes can be used immediately. To avoid recurrence, advise 4-hourly flushes with water (avoid saline as may crystallize) and ensure medication fully dissolved or in liquid formulation.

Dislodgement

Replace feeding catheter within 5d to maintain nutrition. If dislodged within 1m of original placement, relocate endoscopically to avoid peritoneal siting. By contrast, mature tracks are easily re-cannulated; maintain tract patency by placing a Foley catheter within 6–12h (may be successful up to 5d; if in doubt, perform under screening). Definitive tube replacement can then be performed under endoscopic or radiological guidance, or by placing a low-profile feeding device ('button'). If dislodgement is recurrent, review PEG care and consider using a larger catheter, larger balloon, or more durable silicone tube.

Leakage

Due to excessive tube motion or over-tight fixation of the PEG to the skin surface causing pressure necrosis. Exclude partial obstruction. Treat malnutrition and skin infection, ensure good glycaemic control if diabetic and avoid over-tight external fixation devices. Larger catheters usually ineffective (tissue growth and healing more important), Removal of PEG tube for 2–48h to allow partial tract closure has been reported to be successful when established tracts leak, but often a new puncture site will be required.

Cellulitis

Peri-stomal cellulitis is common and usually presents with localized erythema and tenderness; systemic upset is rare. Infections are mostly due to S. aureus and/or β-haemolytic streptococci. Candida super-infection may occur. Treatment involves stoma care, culture, and oral antibiotics (co-amoxiclav 625mg tds, or clindamycin 300–450mg qds if penicillin-allergic). The PEG may need to be removed and infection treated before a new tube is sited. MRSA colonized patients should have topical suppression therapy (e.g. chlorhexidine body wash daily for 5d, chlorhexidine shampoo 3 times/wk for 1wk, and mupirocin nasal ointment tds for 5d) prior to PEG (re)placement.

Bleeding

Late occurring bleeds most frequently due to oesophagitis or gastric ulcers; these should be visualized and treated endoscopically, together with PPI.

Obstruction

Gastric outlet obstruction occurs if the internal flange lodges in the pylorus or duodenum, most frequently after replacement. Presents as proximal small bowel obstruction, with reflux of stomach contents through the PEG. Diagnose with contrast studies. Management involves withdrawing the tube and fixing it at the skin surface. Often 'partial obstruction' represents gastroparesis (see 📖 p. 54).

Diarrhoea

The usual cause is intolerance of the feed preparation. Try feeds with reduced osmolarity or lower fibre content. Small doses of loperamide may be beneficial.

The rare complication to exclude is gastrocolic fistula. Patients may be asymptomatic for months, and the PEG may function normally. Often presents when a PEG tube is inadvertently replaced into the bowel lumen. The characteristic symptom is transient diarrhoea, occurring within minutes of feed, associated with passage of undigested feed per rectum or faecal material through the PEG. Most cases can be managed by removal and re-siting of the PEG; the residual track closes within days. Tubes may require laparoscopic replacement, following which any residual fistula can be excised. (see 'Perforation', 📖 p. 175).

Buried bumper syndrome

Rare but under-recognized complication in which gastric mucosa overgrows and seals the internal tube lumen. Thought to arise due to excessive tension between the inner and outer bolsters. Presents as mechanical failure to deliver feed and associated with abdominal pain during feeding.

Endoscopic examination confirms blockage and may allow the bumper to be released (techniques include snare cautery, laser, simple traction, and the 'push/pull technique'). All symptomatic patients should have their tubes replaced. Prevented by rotating the tube every few days following placement and releasing tube traction at 10d once the tract has formed.

Reflux and aspiration

Reflux and aspiration is common with long-term PEG feeding, particularly in patients with gastroparesis (e.g. Parkinson's disease, diabetes mellitus). Pulmonary aspiration is likely if feed aspirated from the mouth (can be clarified by injecting blue ink through the PEG) or if chest infections recur. If suspected, avoid opiates and agents that predispose to constipation, correct electrolytes (K^+, Na^+, Mg^{++}), reduce rate of feed, avoid feeding when patient supine, and prescribe prokinetics (e.g. domperidone linctus). Endoscopic jejunal extension tubes (JETs) can be used but often kink. Radiological JETs are of wider gauge and may be more effective.

PEG use in pregnancy

PEG feeding has been successfully conducted in pregnancy, and the associated complications are similar to those outlined in the sections under 'Immediate complications' and 'Long-term PEG complications' (📖 pp. 175–6). Intractable hyperemesis gravidarum may require conversion to a (radiological) JET.

⊙ Re-feeding syndrome

Re-feeding syndrome is characterized by severe fluid and electrolyte shifts in severely malnourished individuals in whom nutritional support has been commenced. Occurs following the introduction of both enteral and parenteral nutrition. Risk factors are shown in Table 11.1.

The principal pathogenetic mechanism involves the insulin response to re-introduction of carbohydrates. This stimulates glycogen, lipid, and protein synthesis (processes that deplete PO_4^{3-}, Mg^{++}, and thiamine), and drives potassium intracellularly. Fluid shifts occur due to osmotic gradients.

Clinical features

- Fluid shifts.
- Disordered Na^+ balance.
- Hypokalaemia.
- Hypomagnesaemia.
- Hypophosphataemia. Serum inorganic PO_4^{3-} <0.5mmol/L predisposes to rhabdomyolysis, immunosuppression, cardiorespiratory failure, hypotension, muscle weakness, cardiac arrhythmia, and seizures.
- Hypocalcaemia.
- Wernicke's encephalopathy. Presents with confusion, ocular signs, and ataxia. May lead to Korsakoff's psychosis.

NICE guidelines recommend starting re-feeding at no more than 50% of energy requirements (25% if very high risk). This does not need to wait for correction of fluid and electrolyte imbalances, which can be done concurrently. Parenteral vitamin supplementation should be commenced immediately and continued for the first 3–5d of re-feeding. Electrolytes and ECG should be monitored daily for 1wk, then three times the following week. Examine daily for oedema, heart failure, and confusion.

Management
- Identify at-risk patients (e.g. chronic alcohol misuse, anorexia, neglect).
- Check K^+, Mg^{++}, PO_4^{3-}, and calcium.
- Prior to feeding, administer IV thiamine (Pabrinex® 1 + 2), continued tds for 3–5d; oral thiamine 200–300mg bd is an alternative. Long-term supplementation with vitamin B co-strong 1–2 tablets PO od, thiamine 100mg PO od, and multivitamin/mineral supplements, e.g. Forceval® 1 tablet PO od, are recommended.
- Start feeding at 10kcal/kg/d (5kcal/kg/d in high-risk patients) on d1–3. Increase to 20kcal/kg/d thereafter (Ormerod et al., 2010). Then increase further to allow weight gain once metabolically stable (usually within first week).
- Rehydrate cautiously; supplement and correct K^+, PO_4^{3-} (see Table 11.2), Mg^{++} (see Table 11.3), and calcium as required.

Table 11.1 Predicting risk of re-feeding syndrome

≥1 of	or ≥2 of
BMI <16kg/m²	BMI <18.5kg/m²
>15% weight loss in 3–6mo	>10% weight loss in 36mo
Minimal nutritional intake for ≥10d	Minimal nutritional intake for ≥5d
Pre-existing electrolyte disturbance	Alcohol or drug misuse, use of antacids or diuretics

Table 11.2 Phosphate replacement

Severity	Serum level	Replacement
Maintenance	>0.85mmol/L	0.3–0.6mmol/kg/d PO
Mild	0.6–0.85mmol/L	0.3–0.6mmol/kg/d PO
Moderate	0.3–0.6mmol/L	9mmol IV over 12h
Severe	<0.3mmol/L	18mmol IV over 12h

Table 11.3 Magnesium replacement

Severity	Serum level	Replacement
Maintenance	>0.7mmol/L	0.2mmol/kg/d IV or 0.4mmol/kg/d PO
Mild-to-moderate	0.5–0.7mmol/L	0.5mmol/kg IV over 24h, then 0.25mmol/kg/day IV for 5d
Severe	<0.5mmol/L	24mmol IV over 6h, then as for mild-to-moderate

Complications of nutritional support

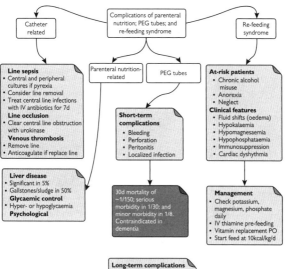

Catheter related

Line sepsis
• Central and peripheral cultures if pyrexia
• Consider line removal
• Treat central line infections with IV antibiotics for 7d
Line occlusion
• Clear central line obstruction with urokinase
Venous thrombosis
• Remove line
• Anticoagulate if replace line

Liver disease
• Significant in 5%
• Gallstones/sludge in 50%
Glycaemic control
• Hyper- or hypoglycaemia
Psychological

Complications of parenteral nutrition; PEG tubes; and re-feeding syndrome

Parenteral nutrition-related

PEG tubes

Short-term complications
• Bleeding
• Perforation
• Peritonitis
• Localized infection

30d mortality of ~1/150; serious morbidity in 1/30; and minor morbidity in 1/8. Contraindicated in dementia

Long-term complications
• Catheter occlusion
• Dislodgement
• Leakage
• Cellulitis
• Bleeding
• Obstruction
• Diarrhoea
• Buried bumper
• Reflux/aspiration

Re-feeding syndrome

At-risk patients
• Chronic alcohol misuse
• Anorexia
• Neglect
Clinical features
• Fluid shifts (oedema)
• Hypokalaemia
• Hypomagnesaemia
• Hypophosphataemia
• Immunosuppression
• Cardiac dyshythmia

Management
• Check potassium, magnesium, phosphate daily
• IV thiamine pre-feeding
• Vitamin replacement PO
• Start feed at 10kcal/kg/d

Further reading

Cheung NW, Napier B, Zaccaria C, *et al.* (2005) Hyperglycaemia is associated with adverse out-comes in patients receiving total parenteral nutrition. *Diabetes Care* **28**: 2367–71.

Korbila IP, Bliziotis IA, Lawrence KR, *et al.* (2007) Antibiotic-lock therapy for long-term catheter-related bacteremia: a review of the current evidence. *Expert Rev Anti Infect Ther* **5**: 639–52.

Ormerod C, Farrer K, Harper L, *et al.* (2010) Refeeding syndrome: a clinical review. *Br J Hosp Med (Lond)* **71**: 686–90.

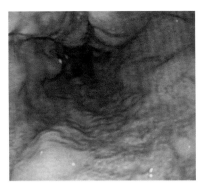

Colour plate 1 Oesophageal varices. Reproduced with kind permission from the Chelsea and Westminster Hospital.

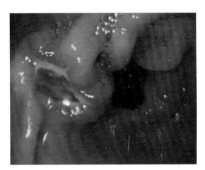

Colour plate 2 Benign pre-pyloric ulcer. Reproduced with kind permission from the Chelsea and Westminster Hospital.

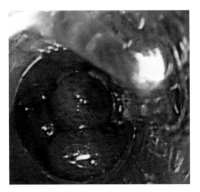

Colour plate 3 Oesophageal varices post-banding. Reproduced with kind permission from the Chelsea and Westminster Hospital.

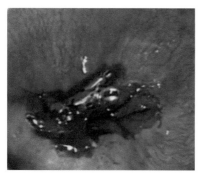

Colour plate 4 Clipped bleeding in Mallory–Weiss tear. Reproduced with kind permission from the Chelsea and Westminster Hospital.

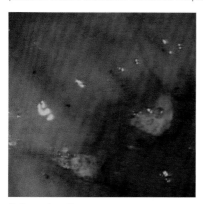

Colour plate 5 Linear antral gastritis. Reproduced with kind permission from the Chelsea and Westminster Hospital.

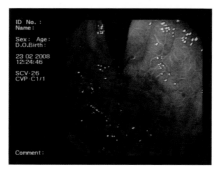

Colour plate 6 Portal hypertensive gastropathy. Reproduced with kind permission from the Chelsea and Westminster Hospital.

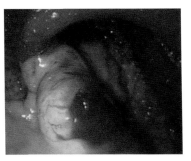

Colour plate 7 Bleeding gastric varix. Reproduced with kind permission from the Chelsea and Westminster Hospital.

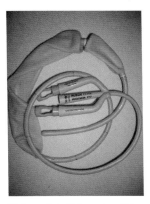

Colour plate 8 Sengstaken–Blakemore tube. Reproduced with kind permission from the Chelsea and Westminster Hospital.

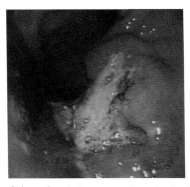

Colour plate 9 Gastric cancer. Reproduced with kind permission from the Chelsea and Westminster Hospital.

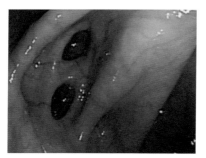

Colour plate 10 Colonic diverticulosis. Reproduced with kind permission from the Chelsea and Westminster Hospital.

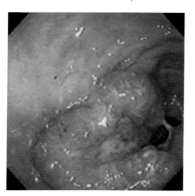

Colour plate 11 Colon cancer. Reproduced with kind permission from the Chelsea and Westminster Hospital.

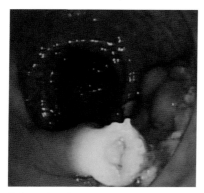

Colour plate 12 Snare cautery of pedunculated colonic polyp. Reproduced with kind permission from the Chelsea and Westminster Hospital.

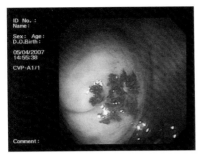

Colour plate 13 Angiodysplasia on the ileocaecal valve. Reproduced with kind permission from the Chelsea and Westminster Hospital.

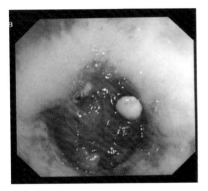

Colour plate 14 Haemorrhoids. Reproduced with kind permission from the Chelsea and Westminster Hospital.

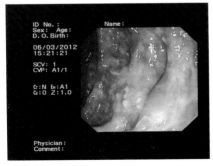

Colour plate 15 Pseudomembranous colitis. Reproduced with kind permission from the Chelsea and Westminster Hospital.

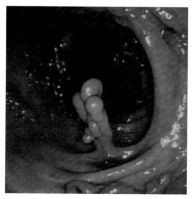

Colour plate 16 Pseudopolyps in a patient with quiescent ulcerative colitis. Reproduced with kind permission from the Chelsea and Westminster Hospital.

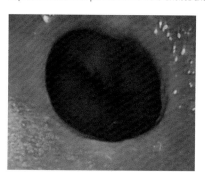

Colour plate 17 Oesophageal Schatzki ring. Reproduced with kind permission from the Chelsea and Westminster Hospital.

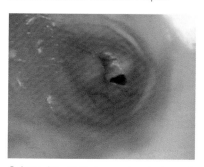

Colour plate 18 Benign oesophageal stricture. Reproduced with kind permission from the Chelsea and Westminster Hospital.

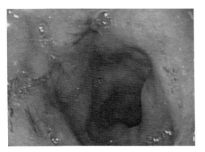

Colour plate 19 Duodenal coeliac disease. Reproduced with kind permission from the Chelsea and Westminster Hospital.

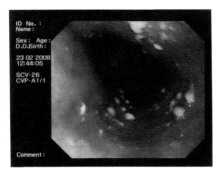

Colour plate 20 Oesophageal candidiasis. Reproduced with kind permission from the Chelsea and Westminster Hospital.

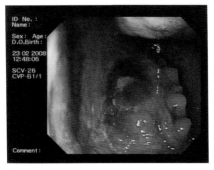

Colour plate 21 Oral Kaposi sarcoma. Reproduced with kind permission from the Chelsea and Westminster Hospital.

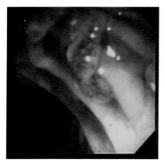

Colour plate 22 Liver fluke following ERCP extraction from the common bile duct. Reproduced with kind permission from the Chelsea and Westminster Hospital.

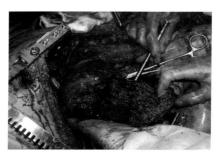

Colour plate 23 Hepatic trauma following blunt injury. Reproduced with kind permission from David Nott OBE.

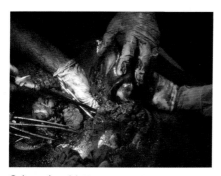

Colour plate 24 Hepatic trauma following shrapnel injury. Reproduced with kind permission from David Nott OBE.

HIV disease and the gastrointestinal tract

General principles

HIV-infected patients with low CD4 counts frequently develop acute GI and hepatobiliary disease. Whilst susceptible to the same disorders as immunocompetent patients, the differential diagnosis is broader. The aim is to identify treatable disorders. Clinical presentations are rarely specific, and patients usually require investigation rather than empiric treatment.

Opportunistic infections are unusual with CD4 >200/mm³ and, therefore, the degree of immunosuppression guides the differential diagnosis, investigation, and management (Nelson et al., 2011). Indeed, many of the infections described here are now rare, given the widespread use of highly active anti-retroviral therapy (HAART). Microbiologists and histopathologists should be alerted to HIV status, CD4 count, and viral load. Complications also vary according to mode of HIV acquisition, with differences between heterosexual and vertical infection, IV drug use (IVDU), and men who have sex with men (MSM). Co-infection with HIV and hepatitis B and/or C virus is common, as is non-pathogenic colonization of the GI tract (so direct demonstration of microbial tissue invasion remains the gold standard). Involve the HIV team early. Successful anti-retroviral therapy is often sufficient to induce remission and prevent relapse.

① Luminal disease

Upper GI disease

Presentations include nausea, vomiting, chest pain, fever, weight loss, dysphagia, odynophagia, and haematemesis. Approximately 10% of patients develop oesophagitis (not too dissimilar to population rates). Heartburn and regurgitation are usually due to gastro-oesophageal reflux disease. Endoscopy is required for diagnosis, with thorough mucosal examination and multiple biopsies of any lesion. Management of upper GI haemorrhage is similar to immunocompetent patients, except that CMV-negative blood should be used for resuscitation in seronegative immunosuppressed individuals.

Candida

Most patients with dysphagia or odynophagia have mucocutaneous candidiasis if CD4 <200/mm³. Oropharyngeal disease is characterized by painless, white mucosal plaques, easily removed by scraping with a tongue depressor. Erythematous patches and angular chelosis can also be seen. Oesophageal candida presents with retrosternal burning pain or odynophagia. The absence of oropharyngeal candida does not rule out oesophageal involvement. Endoscopy reveals thickened mucosal folds and confluent exudative white plaques, which may ulcerate (see Colour plate 20). Cytology or culture demonstrate yeast infection.

Empirical therapy is often appropriate for patients with odynophagia and oral thrush; request gastroscopy if no improvement in oesophageal symptoms within 72h:

- Treat mild oral disease with fluconazole 50mg PO od for 7–14d.
- Moderate or severe disease requires fluconazole 100mg PO od for 7–14d (21d if oesophageal involvement).

- Severe oesophageal disease refractory to 1wk of fluconazole requires caspofungin IV (70mg loading dose followed by 50mg od) or liposomal amphotericin 3mg/kg IV od for 14d. Caspofungin possesses the more favourable side effect profile.
- Initiation of HAART often hastens recovery and prevents recurrence.
- Prophylaxis with fluconazole 50–100mg PO od recommended when CD4 <100/mm³.

Herpes simplex virus (HSV)

Causes oesophagitis when CD4 <200/mm³. Characteristic endoscopic findings are 1–3mm vesicles, usually in the distal oesophagus, the centres of which slough to form volcano lesions. Diagnosis is confirmed by viral culture or PCR. Complications include haemorrhage and stricturing, mucosal necrosis, oesophageal perforation, tracheo-oesophageal fistulation, and HSV pneumonia.

Treatment is aciclovir 5–10mg/kg IV tds (whilst unable to take medication orally), followed by 400mg PO five times/d for a total of 14d. Reduce frequency of administration in renal failure. Alternative is valaciclovir 1g PO bd. Resistant viruses may respond to foscarnet 90mg/kg IV bd.

Cytomegalovirus (CMV)

Causes oesophagitis when CD4 <100/mm³. Presents with fever, nausea, and odynophagia. Demonstration of mucosal ulceration with characteristic intracytoplasmic and intranuclear inclusion bodies on biopsy is required for diagnosis, supported by detection of CMV antigen by PCR or immunohistochemistry. Viral cultures take >2wk and are prone to contamination in patients with CMV viraemia. Request ophthalmology review to identify coexistent retinitis.

Treatment is ganciclovir 5mg/kg IV bd, switching to valganciclovir 900mg PO bd once oral therapy tolerated for at least 14d or until no evidence of ongoing CMV viraemia. Foscarnet 60mg/kg IV tds is used for resistant disease. Side effects include renal failure with all agents, pancytopaenia with ganciclovir, and hypocalcaemia and hypomagnesaemia with foscarnet. Maintenance therapy indicated if multiple relapses.

Neoplasia

Both Kaposi's sarcoma (see Colour plate 21) and non-Hodgkin's lymphoma can involve the upper GI tract. Potential treatment options include observation, surgical resection, immunomodulatory agents (such as interferon), chemotherapy, and radiotherapy. Initiation of anti-retrovirals improves prognosis, and full staging (imaging and bone marrow examination) is mandatory. Involve oncologists early.

Idiopathic ulceration

If infection excluded, ulcers may respond to a 3wk course of prednisolone 40mg PO od in combination with a PPI. Thalidomide 200mg PO od has been reported as effective.

Diarrhoea

Also see Chapter 5. Risk greatest with low CD4 counts, and MSM.
- Large-volume, watery stools associated with peri-umbilical pain imply small bowel disease.

- Frequent, small-volume stools with or without blood, associated with faecal urgency, tenesmus, or lower abdominal cramping, indicate colorectal involvement.
- Fever suggests mucosal invasion or bacteraemia.

A minimal, stepwise diagnostic work-up is appropriate, as intensive screening does not detect significantly more treatable disorders and non-specific treatment is often effective:

- Stool samples for routine M, C, & S and *C. difficile* toxin × 2. Peripheral blood cultures if febrile. If CD4 <200/mm³, blood cultures for mycobacteria, and stool samples for modified acid-fast stain or immunofluorescence (cryptosporidia) and modified trichrome stain (microsporidia).
- If above negative, non-bloody diarrhoea, normal inflammatory markers, and CD4 >200/mm³, empiric antidiarrhoeal (loperamide 2–4mg, up to qds). Octreotide 50–200µg SC tds only rarely required. Empiric tinidazole 2g stat PO, and repeated after 1wk, often provided to combat parasitic infection, especially in MSM.
- Otherwise, flexible sigmoidoscopy to examine for CMV colitis (histology) and mycobacteria (histology and culture). Save additional sample in glutaraldehyde for electron microscopy if microsporidia suspected.
- If above non-diagnostic and CD4 <200/mm³, request OGD and colonoscopy. Take biopsies as outlined for flexible sigmoidoscopy.

Specific aetiologies include:

Drug side effect
Common with anti-retrovirals, particularly nelfinavir and ritonavir. May affect up to 50% of patients on HAART. Usually a diagnosis of exclusion.

Bacterial infection
Salmonella, *Shigella*, and *Campylobacter* are more common, even if CD4 count is normal. *C. difficile* is now a common cause of diarrhoea (Sanchez et al., 2005). See Chapter 6.

Giardiasis
Risk of acquisition and re-acquisition increased with oro-anal intercourse (see ⚏ p. 86).

Small bowel bacterial overgrowth
Presents with generalized malabsorption of carbohydrates, fat, protein, fat-soluble vitamins, and vitamin B12. Definitive diagnosis by duodenal aspiration and culture of >10⁵ colonies/mL rarely performed, as breath tests are less invasive (but only 70% sensitive). Efficacy of broad-spectrum antibiotics is not clinically proven, although they are often used empirically. Common choices are tetracycline 250mg qds, co-amoxiclav 625mg tds, co-trimoxazole 960mg bd, or ciprofloxacin 500mg bd for 7–10d. Value of probiotics unproven.

CMV
Occurs in up to 10% of patients with AIDS, with CD4 count usually <100/mm³. Virus sexually transmitted in MSM, of whom 90% are seropositive.

Ileocolitis presents with pain, diarrhoea, and bleeding; perforation has been reported. Diagnosis and management are as for CMV oesophagitis (see 📖 p. 183) commence or optimize HAART. Relapse common (approximately 40%) and therefore maintenance therapy may be indicated.

HSV

Causes severe, relapsing proctocolitis. Treatment for 7–14d with aciclovir 400mg PO five times/d (5mg/kg IV tds if severe) or valaciclovir 1g PO bd.

Mycobacterium tuberculosis

HIV infection significantly increases risk of re-activation of latent TB. Can present at any stage of HIV disease, although is more common as immunodeficiency progresses. Most frequently involves the ileocaecal region, although all parts of the gut can be affected. Diagnosis usually requires colonoscopy or laparoscopy. Immunosuppression reduces sensitivity of interferon-γ release assay (e.g. QuantiFERON TB Gold®) and tuberculin skin testing. Management follows standard BHIVA guidelines (Pozniak et al., 2011).

Mycobacterium avium intracellulare

Rare following widespread use of anti-retrovirals. Generally presents when CD4 <100/mm^3 as a systemic disseminated illness with fever and severe anaemia; night sweats and weight loss are less common. GI tract involved in up to 80% and may manifest with diarrhoea, malabsorption, and/or abdominal pain.

Endoscopy most frequently demonstrates duodenal involvement, followed by ileocaecal and colorectal disease. Characteristic 1–3mm white nodules are seen; microscopically, there is chronic inflammation, typically without granulomas. Diagnosed by demonstrating organism in tissue samples, bacteraemia (rapid culture results in 5–12d, single culture usually adequate), or bone marrow involvement. Stool culture unhelpful as does not differentiate colonization from tissue invasion.

Treatment requires at least two agents, usually a macrolide with amikacin, rifabutin, or ethambutol. Isoniazid and pyrazinamide are ineffective. Adverse drug reactions are common, occurring in up to 45%. Prophylaxis with azithromycin or clarithromycin.

Cryptosporidium

Protozoal infection acquired from ingesting contaminated water. Susceptible when CD4 <50/mm^3, although infection can occur in immunocompetent individuals. Incubation period 7d. Predominantly infects small bowel mucosa. Presents with high-volume (often >2L/d), liquid, non-bloody stools and nausea, vomiting, and abdominal cramps. Four clinical patterns: chronic (60%), transient with spontaneous resolution within 2mo (30%), fulminant (5%), and asymptomatic (5%). Send stool microscopy for ova and parasites using modified acid-fast stain or immunofluorescence. If negative, consider duodenal and/or colonic biopsies. Treatment is primarily supportive, with correction of dehydration and electrolytes. The mainstay of treatment is HAART, and there is often spontaneous resolution if anti-retrovirals restore CD4 counts to within normal limits. In recalcitrant disease, nitazoxanide 500mg PO bd for 3d is effective in immunocompetent individuals but not shown to be better than placebo in patients with immunocompromise (Fox and Saravolatz, 2005). Paromomycin 500mg PO qds (or 1g PO bd) for up to 12wk can also be tried, although there is limited clinical experience with this approach.

To prevent recurrent infection, counsel patients about the importance of hand washing, to drink bottled or boiled water, and to avoid raw shellfish and oro-anal contact.

Microsporidia

Presentation and management similar to cryptosporidium. Mucosal biopsy with Giemsa or modified trichrome stain and electron microscopy can demonstrate parasites. Treatment is largely supportive with optimization of HAART. If no response, albendazole 400mg PO bd for 21d may be required (particularly effective against *Encephalitozoon intestinalis*). Thalidomide 100mg PO nocte for 1mo also reported to be effective for symptom control in small series.

Cyclospora

Coccidian parasite of the small bowel. Widespread in the tropics and responsible for food-borne illnesses in the USA. Causes prolonged bouts of watery diarrhoea. Diagnosis established on stool microscopy for oocysts or PCR. Treatment is with co-trimoxazole 960mg PO bd for 7d.

Isospora belli

Implicated in 10–20% of cases of chronic HIV-related diarrhoea in tropics. Presentation similar to *Cyclospora*. The best management strategy is to initiate or optimize HAART. If this does not control infection, may respond to co-trimoxazole 960mg PO qds for 10d (although 960mg PO bd also appears effective).

Histoplasmosis

Fungal infection that causes diffuse patchy colitis, presenting with diarrhoea, fever, abdominal pain, and weight loss. Diagnosis established by blood or urine antigen tests, or demonstration of the organism in biopsies. Treat with itraconazole 200mg PO tds for 3d, then bd for 2wk. Use liposomal amphotericin 3mg/kg IV od if severe.

HIV enteropathy

Chronic IBD apparently not attributable to infection; a diagnosis of exclusion. Histopathology shows non-specific chronic inflammatory cells in small and large bowel, with a preponderance of CD8 T cells. Duodenal biopsies reveal villous flattening. Reduced absorption of D-xylose may be demonstrable. Small case series suggest therapeutic responses to standard IBD immunosuppressants and, possibly, to institution of HAART.

Inflammatory bowel disease

Preliminary data suggest that ulcerative colitis (but not Crohn's disease) is more common in patients with HIV infection. Long-term follow-up data from patients with both HIV and IBD demonstrate lower relapse rates as CD4 counts fall (Viazis et al., 2010).

Neoplasia

Diarrhoea may be the presenting symptom of both lymphoma and Kaposi's sarcoma. Investigation and management as for oesophageal disease.

Anorectal disease

Most commonly present in MSM. Diagnoses includes viral warts (condylomata acuminata), squamous cell carcinoma (related to human papilloma virus infection; annual incidence 37:100,000 (20-fold relative risk) in MSM but twice that in HIV-infected MSM), chlamydial infection (*C. trachomatis* and lymphogranuloma venereum; the latter diagnosis should be considered in any HIV-infected MSM presenting with acute ± bloody colitis), and *N. gonorrhoeae*.

① **Pancreatitis**

Causes specific to HIV-infected patients include:
- Drug-induced:
  - Anti-retrovirals (didanosine, stavudine). These drugs are now rarely encountered in the UK but often used in Eastern Europe and sub-Saharan African settings, and thus need to be considered in patients recently arriving from these locations.
  - Antimicrobials (pentamidine, co-trimoxazole).
- Infectious: CMV, mycobacteria (*M. tuberculosis* and *M. avium*), cryptococcus, HSV, toxoplasma, cryptosporidium (in prolonged infection).
- Neoplastic: lymphoma, Kaposi's sarcoma.

Request CT with pancreatic protocol. Radiologically guided FNA of inflamed pancreas can obtain cells for cytology to diagnose neoplastic lesions. CMV inclusions may be demonstrable in ductal epithelial or acinar cells.

① **Hepatobiliary disease**

Deranged LFT are common in advanced HIV disease, often with no identifiable hepatobiliary cause. Jaundice is usually not related to HIV infection per se (unless due to disseminated opportunistic infections) but more commonly caused by decompensated liver disease from another aetiology. An approach to investigating patients with deranged LFT is as follows:
- Elevated serum transaminases >2× ULN should be investigated by serology for hepatotropic viruses (HAV, HBV, HCV, HDV if HBV-positive, EBV, and CMV) and consideration of drug causes (see Chapter 18). Send PCR for HCV RNA, as negative serology does not exclude infection. Remember to ask about over-the-counter medicines and herbal remedies. Also screen for autoimmune liver disease (immunoglobulins, AMA, ANA, anti-smooth muscle antibody, anti-LKM1), Wilson's disease if <40y (caeruloplasmin and serum copper in the first instance), and hepatocellular carcinoma (α-fetoprotein). Request US.
- Elevated serum ALP may indicate infiltrative disease or cholangiopathy. If biliary dilatation present on US, request MRCP (possibly followed by ERCP, which allows tissue sampling and sphincterotomy if required). CT indicated if mass lesions or adenopathy suspected (e.g. patients with systemic symptoms and hepatomegaly).

- Liver biopsy should only be performed if US and CT are non-diagnostic. It rarely identifies lesions not previously demonstrated in other tissues. Transjugular biopsy mandated in patients with coagulopathy.
- If an infectious cause is considered (i.e. CD4 <200/mm^3), send blood for mycobacterial and fungal cultures and CMV antigen/PCR.
- Measure lactate if US shows steatosis, as mitochondrial dysfunction due to HAART may be the cause. Older anti-retroviral drugs (e.g. didanosine, stavudine) were associated with mitochondrial dysfunction and hyperlactataemia (although acidosis unusual); these are now rarely seen.

Hepatic disease
CD4 count guides differential diagnosis. If >500/mm^3, suspect a drug reaction, neoplasia, or co-infection with hepatotropic viruses. If <200/mm^3, opportunistic infections are more common.

Drug-induced hepatitis
See Chapter 18. Common side effect of anti-retrovirals (indinavir, saquinovir, ritonavir, stavudine, nevirapine (10% get severe toxicitiy), didanosine, zidovudine) and antimicrobials (co-trimoxazole, pentamidine, ketoconazole, rifampicin, isoniazid, pyrazinamide). Presents with raised serum transaminase levels, fever, rash, leukocytosis and, occasionally, eosinophilia. Anti-retrovirals can cause fulminant hepatic failure with hepatomegaly, steatosis, and lactic acidosis through mitochondrial toxicity; this is reversible if diagnosed early and the offending agent withdrawn. It is appropriate to discontinue drugs if transaminases rise >5× ULN.

Hepatotropic viruses
Infection with HBV, HCV, and HDV is more common in HIV-infected patients due to shared routes of transmission. HBV frequently re-activates in advanced HIV disease (even if previously thought to be immune) and, in patients with advanced HIV disease, vaccination is ineffective at generating long-lasting immunity. IVDUs typically develop more severe disease than MSM. Progression of liver disease is more rapid in HIV-infected compared to non-infected patients.

Management is similar to HIV-uninfected patients (see Chapter 14), and often anti-viral drugs are chosen with activity against both infections. Be aware that immune reconstitution with early introduction of anti-retrovirals may elicit fulminant liver failure.

Mycobacterium avium intracellulare
Associated with late-stage disseminated infection, although liver disease usually clinically silent. Patients typically have CD4 <100/mm^3. Liver biopsy is sensitive for diagnosis and shows acid-fast mycobacteria; granulomata are either absent or poorly formed.

Mycobacterium tuberculosis
Can present at any stage of HIV infection, although is more common as immunodeficiency progresses. Typically arises as re-activation of latent disease rather than re-acquisition. Most prevalent in IVDU.

Bacillary peliosis hepatitis

Extremely rare systemic infection caused by *Bartonella* species. Presents with fever, lymphadenopathy, hepatosplenomegaly, and cutaneous lesions. May be diagnosed by serology although, if negative, liver biopsy shows dilated vascular lakes within the hepatic parenchyma. Bacilli can be visualized on silver stain. Treat with co-trimoxazole 960mg PO bd for 14d.

Fungi

Typically occur in late-stage HIV disease as part of a systemic disseminated infection. Histoplasmosis most common in endemic areas (e.g. the USA). Patients frequently have hepatomegaly. Organisms usually identified in bone marrow, pulmonary specimens, or peripheral blood smears. Capsular antigen assay is available, although mostly the diagnosis is obtained on culture. Liver biopsy rarely required although, if taken, shows fungi within granulomata. Cryptococcosis, coccidiomycosis, and blastomycosis also reported. Treatment is with liposomal amphotericin 3mg/kg IV od for 14d.

Pneumocystis jirovecii

Dissemination seen rarely, principally in patients receiving nebulized pentamidine prophylaxis. Treat with co-trimoxazole 120mg/kg IV in 2–4 daily divided doses for 14d.

Neoplasia

Non-Hodgkin's lymphoma is the most common clinically manifesting neoplasm (usually Burkitt's lymphoma). Approximately 10% hepatic. Fever is an inconsistent feature.

Kaposi's sarcoma is common (up to 50%) in post-mortem specimens, particularly in MSM, although it is rarely clinically apparent. Diagnosis is through CT and biopsy. Management as for oesophageal disease.

Biliary disease

Biliary tree obstruction can occur as part of an infective process or through extra-luminal compression by lymph nodes. Two complications are more specific to HIV infection.

HIV cholangiopathy

Presents with RUQ pain and elevated ALP due to infections, e.g. *Cryptosporidium* (therefore, diarrhoea often present). Occurs with CD4 <100/mm^3. Jaundice unusual, as complete obstruction is rare. Most common in MSM. ERCP reveals three clinical patterns: distal biliary stricturing with papillitis (most common), diffuse biliary strictures similar to PSC, or a mixed picture. Treat infectious agent if possible. Endoscopic sphincterotomy indicated if CBD dilated, and often successful at relieving pain.

Acalculous cholecystitis

Late-stage complication, often occurring in association with opportunistic infection elsewhere (e.g. CMV, histoplasma). Presents with RUQ pain, nausea and vomiting, elevated WCC and CRP, and deranged LFT. Occasionally, severe enough to constitute a surgical emergency. US shows thickened gallbladder wall in the absence of gallstones. Radionuclide scans can demonstrate obstruction of the cystic duct. Cholecystectomy is curative.

HIV disease and the gastrointestinal tract

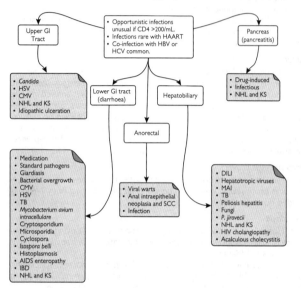

Upper GI Tract

- *Candida*
- HSV
- CMV
- NHL and KS
- Idiopathic ulceration

- Opportunistic infections unusual if CD4 >200/mL.
- Infections rare with HAART
- Co-infection with HBV or HCV common

Pancreas (pancreatitis)

- Drug-induced
- Infectious
- NHL and KS

Lower GI tract (diarrhoea)

Hepatobiliary

Anorectal

- Medication
- Standard pathogens
- Giardiasis
- Bacterial overgrowth
- CMV
- HSV
- TB
- *Mycobacterium avium intracellulare*
- Cryptosporidium
- Microsporidia
- Cyclospora
- *Isospora belli*
- Histoplasmosis
- AIDS enteropathy
- IBD
- NHL and KS

- Viral warts
- Anal intraepithelial neoplasia and SCC
- Infection

- DILI
- Hepatotropic viruses
- MAI
- TB
- Peliosis hepatitis
- Fungi
- *P. jirovecii*
- NHL and KS
- HIV cholangiopathy
- Acalculous cholecystitis

Further reading

Fox LM, Saravolatz LD (2005) Nitazoxanide: a new thiazolide antiparasitic agent. *Clin Infect Dis* **40**: 1173–80.

Nelson M, Dockrell D, Edwards S, *et al.* (2011) British HIV Association and British Infection Association guidelines for the treatment of opportunistic infection in HIV-seropositive individuals 2011. *HIV Med* **12** Suppl 2: 1–140.

Pozniak AL, Coyne KM, Miller RF, *et al.* (2011) British HIV Association guidelines for the treatment of TB/HIV coinfection 2011. *HIV Med* **12**: 517–24.

Sanchez TH, Brooks JT, Sullivan PS, *et al.* (2005) Bacterial diarrhea in persons with HIV infection, United States, 1992–2002. *Clin Infect Dis* **41**: 1621–7.

Viazis N, Vlachogiannakos J, Georgiou O, *et al.* (2010) Course of inflammatory bowel disease in patients infected with human immunodeficiency virus. *Inflamm Bowel Dis* **16**: 507–11.

Assessment of liver function

Interpretation of liver function tests

Liver function tests (LFT) can be divided into markers of hepatocyte or biliary epithelial cell integrity (ALT, AST, ALP, γGT), and those indicative of synthetic/metabolic function (albumin, INR/PTT, bilirubin, ammonia). In addition, hypoglycaemia, lactic acidosis, and elevated lactate dehydrogenase (LDH) can be non-specific markers of severe hepatic dysfunction.

Deranged LFT need to be correlated with the clinical picture. The patient may have overt jaundice (see Chapter 14) or be apparently well. No single test is sensitive or specific. Abnormal results, therefore, require validation with other markers (to exclude an extrahepatic source) ± imaging or liver biopsy. Deranged LFT are not infrequently found in patients without liver disease or other significant pathology. However, as some conditions can present in this way during their asymptomatic phase (e.g. primary biliary cirrhosis (PBC), see 🔲 p. 227), with an opportunity for early introduction of disease-modifying therapies, serial testing ± further investigation is strongly recommended.

Bilirubin

- Normal range: ~3–17μmol/L.
- Breakdown product of heme. Bilirubin is transported into hepatocytes, where it is conjugated to make it water-soluble prior to excretion into bile.
- Elevated levels may reflect:
  - Increased production (haemolysis). Predominantly unconjugated hyperbilirubinaemia.
  - Impaired uptake/conjugation (hepatocyte dysfunction).
  - Impaired biliary excretion (usually secondary to obstruction).
- The causes of very high bilirubin concentrations, but otherwise near normal LFT, are massive haemolysis, Weil's disease, and intra-abdominal sepsis.
- For the emergency evaluation and management of the jaundiced patient, see Chapter 14.

Serum aminotransaminases

Serum alanine (ALT) and aspartate (AST) transaminase both rise following hepatocyte injury. If these dominate the LFT derangement, it is termed a 'hepatitic' picture and suggestive of parenchymal injury due to aetiologies such as viral infection, alcohol, drugs, ischaemia, autoimmune hepatitis, and non-alcoholic fatty liver disease (NAFLD).

- ALT:
  - Normal range: ~5–50IU/L.
  - More specific than AST.
  - Also present in muscle, so myositis, rhabdomyolysis, and MI can cause false positive elevation. Measurement of creatine kinase (CK) can clarify.
- AST:
  - Normal range: ~5–45IU/L.
  - Other sources (and hence false positive results) include erythrocytes, cardiac and skeletal muscle, kidney, and brain.

- ALT:AST ratio sometimes correlates with the aetiology of hepatitis:
  - ALT > AST suggests viral hepatitis or NAFLD.
  - AST > ALT suggests alcoholic liver disease. Serum concentrations are rarely >200IU/L and never >400IU/L (in which case look for another cause).
- Transaminases >1,000IU/L almost always imply acute hepatocyte injury due to drugs, viruses, ischaemia, or autoimmune hepatitis.
- The only causes of massive serum transaminases >10,000IU/L are paracetamol overdose, herpes simplex hepatitis, and severe ischaemic hepatitis.
- In the well patient with elevated serum transaminases and no clear cause following a routine screen (see 📖 p. 210–11), advise weight loss, abstinence from alcohol, and cessation of all medications where possible, then re-test after 2mo.

Alkaline phosphatase (ALP)
- Normal range: ~40–165IU/L.
- Derived from biliary epithelium. Rise implies bile duct obstruction, extra- or intrahepatic cholestasis, or diffuse infiltration of the liver.
- Also present in bone, kidney, intestine, and placenta. Causes of non-hepatobiliary elevation include:
  - Fractures.
  - Paget's disease of the bone.
  - Skeletal tumours (primary or metastatic).
  - Renal osteodystrophy.
  - Pregnancy.
  - Growth spurts in childhood.
- Organ-specific isoenzymes can be measured to clarify the source, but this is rarely necessary as concomitant elevation in γGT supports biliary origin.
- US mandated to exclude biliary tree dilatation and hepatic tumours.

Gamma glutamyltransferase (γGT)
- Normal range: ~10–60IU/L.
- More specific for cholestasis than ALP, and principal clinical use is to clarify source of the latter.
- Disproportionate elevation of γGT in comparison to other LFT (including ALP) suggests alcohol misuse or alcoholic liver disease.
- Isolated asymptomatic elevations in γGT are common:
  - May occur due to enzyme induction by alcohol or drugs (steroids, anticonvulsants, statins, NSAIDs, St. John's wort).
  - Also seen in NAFLD.
  - Extensive investigations rarely yield significant pathology (although persistently raised γGT is associated with increased all-cause mortality).
  - Such patients should have blood tests repeated after 3–6mo, and only be investigated further if additional biochemical abnormalities emerge, there has been a further significant rise in γGT, or symptoms have developed.

Albumin

- Normal range: ~35–50g/L.
- Since it is synthesized specifically by the liver, hypoalbuminaemia is an indicator of impaired synthetic function. However, it is not specific, with other causes of low albumin, including:
  - Malnutrition/malabsorption.
  - Active inflammation (including hepatitis). Albumin synthesis is down-regulated during acute phase responses.
  - Severe sepsis (serum levels can fall precipitously, as albumin redistributes to the extracellular space).
  - Nephrotic syndrome.
  - Protein-losing enteropathies (see Chapter 10, 📖 p. 165).
- In the absence of a confounding cause, hypoalbuminaemia reflects disease severity and is one of the prognostic factors in chronic liver disease (see 'Child–Pugh score', 📖 p. 256).

International normalized ratio (INR)/prothrombin time (PTT)

- Normal ranges:
  - INR: 0.8–1.2.
  - PTT: varies between laboratories but ~10–13s.
- Measure of the extrinsic coagulation pathway. Since PTT measurements vary between laboratories, the INR is derived to standardize measurements, and defined as the PTT of the patient divided by the PTT of a healthy control.
- Best guide to liver synthetic function (specifically the vitamin K-dependent clotting factors II, VII, IX, and X), in the absence of vitamin K deficiency. The latter can be excluded, if necessary, by giving vitamin K 10mg PO/IV for 3d.
- Strong prognostic indicator of poor outcome in acute hepatitis and decompensated chronic liver disease, and need for liver transplantation (see Chapter 15).

Ammonia

- Normal range: ~10–80µg/dL.
- Predominantly produced by catabolism of protein. Most of this is derived from the GI tract and reaches the liver via the portal venous system, where it is metabolized to urea. Impaired hepatocyte function can lead to hyperammonaemia, thought to be important in the pathogenesis of hepatic encephalopathy (see 📖 p. 245).
- To obtain an accurate measurement, blood must be sampled from an artery or vein *without* use of a tourniquet. It should be transported immediately on ice to the laboratory (phone ahead to warn them the sample is on its way).

- Although elevated blood ammonia level supports a diagnosis of hepatic encephalopathy, it is neither sensitive nor specific, and rarely adds to the clinical impression in patients with known chronic liver disease. In particular:
  - Normal serum ammonia does not exclude hepatic encephalopathy.
  - There is generally no role for serial ammonia measurements in patients with encephalopathy, as other clinical indicators are superior.
  - Hyperammonaemia may also result from a high protein load (upper GI haemorrhage, TPN), bypass of hepatic metabolism (TIPS), drugs (particularly sodium valproate), or congenital urea cycle disorders.
  - Be wary of ascribing altered GCS in a chronic liver disease patient to encephalopathy solely on the basis of elevated ammonia levels. Up to 70% of patients with chronic liver disease have ammonia concentrations higher than the ULN with no evidence of encephalopathy (Ong et al., 2003). Search for alternative explanations (e.g. intracranial haemorrhage, sepsis).
- Hyperammonaemia is a poor prognostic factor in acute liver failure (Kumar et al., 2012).

α-fetoprotein (α-FP)

- Normal range: ~1–10ng/mL.
- Glycoprotein, elevated in 60–80% of patients with hepatocellular carcinoma (HCC; higher in African and Far East Asian populations). Concentrations >400ng/mL strongly suggestive of HCC.
- Raised levels also seen in:
  - Germ cell tumours of testis/ovary.
  - Gastric, biliary tract, or pancreatic carcinoma (usually in context of liver metastases).
  - Active hepatitis or cirrhosis.
  - Ataxia-telangiectasia.
  - Pregnant women carrying a foetus with a neural tube defect or Down's syndrome.
- Not used in isolation for screening for HCC as negative in up to 40%, hence combine with another modality (US or double contrast CT) in at-risk patients. Conversely, α-FP concentrations >100ng/mL mandate exclusion of HCC.
- Difficult to interpret during episodes of active hepatitis or flares of chronic liver disease, although trend is helpful. If explained by active liver disease, subsequent serum levels will fall towards normal, as opposed to rising, if there is an underlying HCC.

Imaging

Persistently deranged LFT without a clear extrahepatic source mandate imaging of the liver. This should be performed within 24h for patients with new-onset jaundice, acute liver failure, decompensated chronic liver disease, or cholangitis; and within 1wk for patients with an obstructive/cholestatic pattern of their LFT. Isolated elevations in serum transaminases <5× ULN in an otherwise well patient can be monitored by serial blood tests in the first instance but investigated further should they persist or the clinical picture evolve.

Ultrasound scan (US)

US is the initial imaging modality of choice in almost all patients presenting with deranged LFT. It is useful for detecting most focal and diffuse hepatobiliary abnormalities and, where necessary, guides choice of second-line investigation. Its strengths are that it displays soft tissue and vascular flow in real time and does not involve ionizing radiation, and it can be performed at the bedside. Weaknesses include operator dependence, reduced image quality with greater distances from the skin or in obese patients, and windows can be obstructed by bowel gas or bone. Its roles are as follows:
- Hepatitic picture:
  - Excludes mass lesions (most sensitive modality). US detects 85–90% of HCCs (false negatives usually occur with tumours <2cm). CT does not outperform and is reserved for cases of diagnostic doubt.
  - Sensitive for diffuse heterogeneous steatosis seen in NAFLD and venous dilatation consistent with congestive hepatopathy (secondary to right heart failure).
  - Doppler analysis characterizes flow in the portal and hepatic veins and can identify thrombosis (Budd–Chiari syndrome). Proceed to CT or MRA if equivocal.
  - Proceed to CT if further imaging of liver parenchyma required.
- Cholestatic picture:
  - Excludes large duct obstruction and obstructive hepatic neoplasia.
  - US is ideal for evaluation of gallbladder lesions, with >90% sensitivity and specificity for gallbladder stones (but only 50% sensitivity for stones in the CBD).
  - If biliary tree dilatation is seen on US, an obstructive lesion is likely (possible diagnoses include choledocholithiasis, carcinoma of the head of pancreas, cholangiocarcinoma, hilar adenopathy, biliary strictures, and papillary stenosis). Note biliary dilatation can be normal in the elderly and following cholecystectomy. Evaluate further with MRCP (CT if contraindications). If the patient has cholangitis with very high suspicion of a large CBD stone, proceed directly to ERCP.
  - If US is normal, possible diagnoses are PBC, primary sclerosing cholangitis (PSC), a drug reaction, or hepatic granulomas. Request serum AMA and ANA; if positive, proceed down the management pathway for PBC (see 📖 p. 227). Also review medication history; discontinue any likely causal agents (see Chapter 18) and observe.

If neither of these steps yields a diagnosis, request an MRCP to exclude PSC. If normal, liver biopsy is indicated.

- If US demonstrates a focal hepatic lesion, diagnoses include HCC, liver metastases, abscesses (see Chapter 17), hepatic adenoma, focal nodular hyperplasia, or haemangioma. Doppler analysis is helpful for assessing vascularity of larger lesions. Measure serum α-FP, and request a double or triple phase contrast CT. Liver biopsy may subsequently be required for tissue diagnosis.

- Intervention. Liver biopsy and intralesional therapies have higher success rates and fewer complications when performed under US guidance.

- Imaging of other abdominal viscera. US is also used to identify other intra-abdominal abnormalities, particularly the presence of ascites, splenomegaly (coexistent disease involvement or secondary to portal hypertension), and renal tract disease (polycystic disease, exclusion of urinary tract obstruction in patients with possible hepatorenal syndrome).

- For full guidance on investigation and management of cholestatic liver disorders, see EASL Clinical Practice Guidelines (2009).

Computed tomography (CT)

CT is typically the second-line imaging modality for assessing the liver parenchyma. Spiral CT can now obtain images within a single breath hold. Detection of lesions is enhanced with use of iodinated IV contrast.

- Compared to MRI, CT is more widely available with better spatial resolution (but worse tissue contrast). Other advantages include greater capacity to image other areas of the body and detect distant lesions, and relative ease of access for ITU patients (less accessible in an MRI scanner, and requires compatible equipment).

- Discuss the clinical questions and possible diagnoses with the radiologist in advance to ensure most appropriate imaging protocol performed. Biphasic images (arterial and portal dominant phases) are particularly sensitive for diagnosis of hypervascular lesions (e.g. HCC), which enhance during the arterial phase. Arteriography is also helpful when planning surgical resection, intra-arterial chemotherapy, or embolization (see Chapter 21).

- CT contrast angiography (including triple phase: arterial, portal, and venous) can be performed to look for vascular occlusions, although is less sensitive than MRI.

- CT is less sensitive than US for focal liver lesions, with accuracy for detecting hepatic metastases of 60–80%.

- Diffuse liver lesions are similarly neither reliably detected nor characterized (hence need to consider biopsy following a non-diagnostic scan). Exceptions include the strikingly low attenuation observed in hepatic steatosis and high attenuation in haemochromatosis, heavy metal toxicity (but not copper in Wilson's disease, due to insufficient quantities deposited), or iodine-mediated hepatitis (secondary to amiodarone).

- Biphasic contrast CT also has high sensitivity for pancreatic mass lesions in patients with obstructive cholestasis.

- Contraindications. There are no absolute contraindications. Relative contraindications include:
  - Radiation dose. A single abdominal CT exposures the patient to ~10mSv (≈500 CXRs) ionizing radiation. This extrapolates to an estimated risk of cancer death of 1/2,000–4,000 per scan (highest in young, female and/or obese patients). Consider other modalities (usually MRI) in young or pregnant (particularly during first trimester) patients but, if risks of not performing CT outweigh small risk from radiation, then proceed to scan.
  - IV contrast. Do not administer in patients with previous allergy or anaphylaxis to iodine-based contrast media. Use with caution in patients with renal impairment, as risk of contrast nephropathy if eGFR <45mL/min/1.73m². In such patients, ensure adequate pre- and post-hydration with 0.9% saline or 1.26% sodium bicarbonate; discontinue any nephrotoxic drugs (and metformin due to risk of precipitating lactic acidosis), and monitor U & E after 48h and 72h. There is no evidence to support prophylactic use of N-acetylcysteine (Stacul et al., 2011).

Magnetic resonance imaging (MRI)

MRCP provides detailed imaging of the biliary and pancreatic ductal systems without the risks of invasive ERCP.

- MRCP outperforms US for the detection of bile duct stones, for which it is 92% sensitive and 97% specific. False negatives can occur for stones <3mm diameter, and false positives with air bubbles.
- It is the imaging modality of choice for investigation of biliary strictures, and of hepatic parenchyma when US and CT are equivocal. Sensitivity for focal lesions slightly superior to CT but inferior to US. Infiltrative processes involving metals (e.g. haemochromatosis) demonstrate low T_2-weighted signal. MRCP before and after secretin injection useful in evaluation of possible sphincter of Oddi dysfunction in patients with chronic pancreatitis, but rarely indicated.
- MR is superior to US and CT for evaluation of the hepatic vasculature.
- Other advantages of MRI over CT include avoidance of ionizing radiation and better tissue contrast resolution (although spatial resolution is inferior).
- Disadvantages include lower availability of scanners, greater expense, longer scans (typically 30–45min, compared to 15min for CT), and more difficult access for ITU patients.
- Contraindications:
  - Ferromagnetic implants (certain cardiac pacemakers, intracranial aneurysm clips, intraocular metal).
  - Severe claustrophobia.
  - Renal failure. Avoid gadolinium-based IV contrast in patients with eGFR <30mL/min/1.73m² due to risk of nephrogenic systemic fibrosis (which is, nonetheless, much rarer than adverse events with iodinated contrast).

Endoscopic retrograde cholangiopancreatography (ERCP)
See Chapter 14 (📖 p. 229).

Nuclear medicine studies
Scintigraphic studies are of limited use in investigating hepatobiliary disease, having been largely superseded by other modalities. The following still have applications:
* Positron emission tomography (PET):
    * Usually employs ^{18}F-fluorodeoxyglucose (FDG) as the radioisotope, and combined with CT for better anatomic resolution.
    * Useful in cancer staging and as part of the evaluation of masses >1cm of unknown aetiology (non-avid lesions unlikely to be malignant).
    * Less sensitive for neuroendocrine tumours due to their lower metabolic rates.
    * False positives with active inflammation and granulomatous disease.
* Octreotide scan. Used in the diagnosis and monitoring of neuroendocrine tumours (see Chapter 21).
* Hepatobiliary iminodiacetic acid (HIDA) scan:
    * Measures excretion of radionuclide tracer from the liver into bile.
    * Previously used for investigation of suspected cholecystitis, including cystic duct patency.
    * Still occasionally used for investigation of possible biliary pain and sphincter of Oddi dysfunction, although now largely superseded by MRCP and ERCP.

Liver biopsy

Liver biopsy should be considered if no cause is found for deranged LFT despite initial investigations and if these remain >2× ULN for >6–12mo. It may also be required to define the degree of liver injury where a cause has been identified, including histological grade (inflammatory activity) and stage (fibrosis and cirrhosis). Advances in imaging techniques (e.g. FibroScan® US) and blood markers of fibrosis (e.g. FibroTest®, ELF®) may obviate the need for invasive biopsy in the future.
* The results of liver biopsy only alter management in ~30% of cases.
* Where possible, biopsy should be perfomed under US guidance (increases sensitivity, reduces complications).
* Transjugular biopsy should be performed in patients with significant or uncorrectable coagulopathy, or those with ascites.
* Indications for liver biopsy include:
    * Unexplained hepatitis or abnormal LFT where non-invasive investigations have not been diagnostic.
    * Chronic HBV/HCV. Staging and grading may impact upon need and timing of anti-viral therapy (see Chapter 14). Biopsy rarely needed in acute viral hepatitis.
    * Alcoholic hepatitis. For confirmation of diagnosis, as clinical diagnosis incorrect in 20%.
    * Genetic haemochromatosis. To stage.

- Autoimmune hepatitis. During initial work-up and probably in assessing treatment response.
- NAFLD. Biopsy is the only means of differentiating simple steatosis from non-alcoholic steatohepatitis (which can progress). Selection of those patients who require biopsy is not yet clearly defined and, at present, based largely on expert opinion rather than evidence-based guidelines. Most only biopsy those with persistent LFT >2× ULN.
- Focal liver masses. To achieve tissue diagnosis. Can be avoided in patients where imaging definitive (also avoids tumour seeding needle track).
- Routine use in PBC, PSC, and Wilson's disease not required where the diagnosis established by other means.
- Contraindications include:
  - Coagulopathy (INR >1.3). Perform under FFP cover or via transjugular approach. Percutaneous plugged biopsy can be attempted in patients with moderate coagulopathy (INR 1.4–1.6), in which gelatin is injected down the biopsy track after removing the needle, although this technique may be challenging and is associated with higher risk of liver laceration.
  - Thrombocytopaenia (platelets <60 × 10⁹/L) or dysfunctional platelets. Perform with platelet transfusion cover.
  - Agitated patient (sudden movement can cause liver laceration).
  - Significant ascites. Drain first or use transjugular approach.
  - Biliary obstruction.
  - Amyloidosis. Increased risk of intraperitoneal haemorrhage.
  - Cystic lesions. Risk of biliary leak if communicate with biliary tree; anaphylaxis if inadvertently biopsy hydatid cyst; and cutaneous tracking and amoeboma formation with amoebic liver abscess.
- Technique. See Box 13.1.
- ⚙: Complications of liver biopsy (significant morbidity in 1%):
  - Subcapsular haematoma. Seen in >20% on US. Rarely symptomatic.
  - Intraperitoneal haemorrhage.
  - Peritonitis.
  - Gallbladder perforation.
  - Pneumothorax.
  - Injury to colon or kidney.
  - Overall 7d mortality is 0.2%, but this occurs principally in those being investigated for malignancy. The figure falls to 0.01% when investigating for non-malignant indications (West and Card, 2010).

Box 13.1 Technique for percutaneous liver biopsy

- Obtain informed consent.
- Check platelet count and INR, and correct as described in the 'Coagulopathy' bullet point under the 'Contraindications' bullet point (see p. 202), if needed. Antiplatelet agents should be stopped at least 1wk prior to procedure (discuss first with cardiologist if patient on clopidogrel for coronary artery stent).
- Lie patient supine, with right hand behind head.
- Perform under US guidance if possible (otherwise, identify liver by percussion).
- Usual approach is in the mid-axillary line between the lower ribs.
- Use aseptic technique. Clean skin with chlorhexidine.
- Infiltrate 4–6mL 1–2% lidocaine into the skin, then down to the liver capsule, aiming just above the upper border of the lower rib to avoid the neurovascular bundle.
- Make a 5mm scalpel incision into the skin.
- Biopsy performed, using either cutting (Tru-Cut) or suction (Menghini) needle. Ask patient to take full expiration (elevates diaphragm, minimizing risk of pneumothorax) and hold breath (minimizes traumatic injury) before needle insertion.
- Post-procedure, instruct patient to lie in the right lateral position for 1h (helps tamponade liver capsule), then supine for 2h.
- Monitor in hospital for 6h post-procedure. Request observations every 15min for 2h, then every 30min for 2h, then hourly. Most complications occur within the first 10h and >60% within 2h.

The patient with persistently deranged liver function tests but normal investigations

If all the above diagnostic investigations are unrewarding and significant LFT derangement persists, consider and test specifically for diagnoses of:

- Undeclared alcohol misuse.
- α1-antitrypsin (A1AT) deficiency.
- Coeliac disease.
- Glycogen storage disease.
- Addison's disease.

These explanations should ideally be screened for prior to proceeding to liver biopsy, but may also be suggested by the histological appearances.

Assessment of liver function

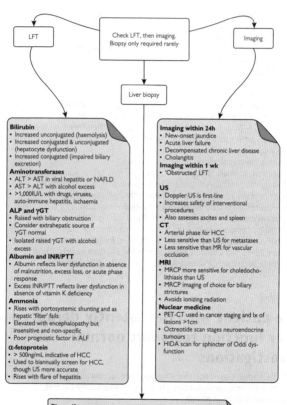

Check LFT, then imaging.
Biopsy only required rarely

LFT

Imaging

Liver biopsy

Bilirubin
- Increased unconjugated (haemolysis)
- Increased conjugated & unconjugated (hepatocyte dysfunction)
- Increased conjugated (impaired biliary excretion)

Aminotransferases
- ALT > AST in viral hepatitis or NAFLD
- AST > ALT with alcohol excess
- >1,000IU/L with drugs, viruses, auto-immune hepatitis, ischaemia

ALP and γGT
- Raised with biliary obstruction
- Consider extrahepatic source if γGT normal
- Isolated raised γGT with alcohol excess

Albumin and INR/PTT
- Albumin reflects liver dysfunction in absence of malnutrition, excess loss, or acute phase response
- Excess INR/PTT reflects liver dysfunction in absence of vitamin K deficiency

Ammonia
- Rises with portosystemic shunting and as hepatic 'filter' fails
- Elevated with encephalopathy but insensitive and non-specific
- Poor prognostic factor in ALF

α-fetoprotein
- > 500ng/mL indicative of HCC
- Used to biannually screen for HCC, though US more accurate
- Rises with flare of hepatitis

Imaging within 24h
- New-onset jaundice
- Acute liver failure
- Decompensated chronic liver disease
- Cholangitis

Imaging within 1 wk
- 'Obstructed' LFT

US
- Doppler US is first-line
- Increases safety of interventional procedures
- Also assesses ascites and spleen

CT
- Arterial phase for HCC
- Less sensitive than US for metastases
- Less sensitive than MR for vascular occlusion

MRI
- MRCP more sensitive for choledocho-lithiasis than US
- MRCP imaging of choice for biliary strictures
- Avoids ionizing radiation

Nuclear medicine
- PET-CT used in cancer staging and Ix of lesions >1cm
- Octreotide scan stages neuroendocrine tumours
- HIDA scan for sphincter of Oddi dysfunction

Biopsy if
- LFT >2x ULN for >6mo not otherwise explained
- Assess degree of fibrosis and inflammation in chronic liver disease
- Unknown focal liver lesion

Causes significant morbidity in 1%. Changes managment in <50%

Further reading

European Association for the Study of the Liver (2009) EASL Clinical Practice Guidelines: management of cholestatic liver diseases. *J Hepatol* **51**: 237–67.

Kumar R, Shalimar, Sharma H, et al. (2012) Prospective derivation and validation of early dynamic model for predicting outcome in patients with acute liver failure. *Gut* **61**: 1068–75.

Ong JP, Aggarwal A, Krieger D, et al. (2003) Correlation between ammonia levels and the severity of hepatic encephalopathy. *Am J Med* **114**: 188–93.

Stacul F, van der Molen AJ, Reimer P, et al. (2011) Contrast induced nephropathy: updated ESUR Contrast Media Safety Committee guidelines. *Eur Radiol* **21**: 2527–41.

West J, Card TR (2010) Reduced mortality rates following elective percutaneous liver biopsies. *Gastroenterology* **139**: 1230–7.

Jaundice

Assessment and causes of jaundice

Jaundice refers to yellow pigmentation of the skin and sclera caused by elevated bilirubin levels. It is usually clinically detectable when serum bilirubin concentrations rise above 60µmol/L. Jaundice usually requires urgent investigation and diagnosis, as it may herald the onset of severe hepatitis or acute liver failure, or indicate biliary obstruction (which can be complicated by cholangitis and septicaemia). Drug-induced liver injury (DILI) leading to jaundice is associated with 10% mortality, and any potential causative agents should be stopped immediately. In one study, pancreatic and biliary carcinoma (20%), gallstone disease (13%), and alcoholic liver cirrhosis (10%) were the most frequent diagnoses. Gilbert's disease (5% of the population) causes unconjugated hyperbilirubinaemia, although serum bilirubin is usually <80µmol/L; other LFT are typically normal unless there is coexisting fatty liver disease (common) or other liver pathology. In the assessment of the jaundiced patient, the aims are to establish:

- Type of jaundice (pre-hepatic, hepatic, or obstructive).
- Aetiology.
- Presence of underlying liver disease.
- Evidence of liver failure.

History

- Non-specific symptoms include anorexia, pruritus, malaise, lethargy, drowsiness, or confusion.
- Dark urine and pale stools may be features of either obstructive jaundice or hepatitis.
- Colicky RUQ pain, previous biliary colic, or known gallstones suggest gallstone disease. Fever, rigors, abdominal pain, and fluctuating jaundice should raise suspicion of cholangitis. Painless jaundice and weight loss suggest pancreatic or bile duct malignancy.
- Take a detailed drug history, including homeopathic or proprietary preparations, especially Chinese herbal preparations. Ask specifically about use of paracetamol and alcohol. Be aware of inadvertent paracetamol overdose in chronic alcoholics.
- Risk factors for viral hepatitis include IV drug use, unprotected sex, and foreign travel. There is an increased risk of viral hepatitis from blood transfusion, unprotected anal intercourse, ingestion of shellfish, tattooing, and in patients from Eastern Europe or Asia.
- Ask about past medical history and family history, particularly of known liver disease, autoimmune disorders, and haemolytic anaemias.
- Take an alcohol history (see 📖 p. 221).

Examination

- Note the degree of jaundice, and look for stigmata of chronic liver disease (clubbing, leukonychia, palmar erythema, Dupuytren's contractures, xanthelasma, Kayser–Fleischer rings, parotitis, spider naevi, telangiectasia, gynaecomastia, loss of secondary sexual hair, testicular atrophy). Lymphadenopathy may reflect malignancy.
- Look for needle marks, tattoos, and stigmata of deliberate self-harm.
- Hepatic encephalopathy results in falling conscious level and liver flap (asterixis). It usually signifies chronic liver disease (see Chapter 16).

- Note BP. MAP falls with liver failure, leading to oliguria or shock.
- Examine for pleural effusions (may occur concurrent with ascites).
- Examine for ascites, hepatomegaly, splenomegaly (portal hypertension or intravascular haemolysis), and abdominal masses.
- Test the urine for bilirubin. Absent bilirubin suggests Gilbert's disease or other conjugation defects, or haemolysis.

Tips on diagnosis
- See Table 14.1 for causes.
- The urine is dark in both hepatic and cholestatic jaundice.
- Itching suggests either extrahepatic (e.g. gallstones or pancreatic mass) or intrahepatic cholestasis (e.g. PBC or PSC).
- Severe haemolysis, sepsis with DIC, or rhabdomyolysis can mimic acute severe hepatitis.
- Ischaemic hepatitis occurs when there is (often unrecognized) hypotension in hypoxic patients with a raised JVP and congested liver.
- The only causes of a very high transaminase level (>10,000U/L) are paracetamol overdose, herpes simplex hepatitis, and severe hepatic ischaemia.
- Causes of very high bilirubin with other LFT being nearly normal include massive haemolysis (usually sickle cell disease), Weil's disease, or intra-abdominal sepsis.
- Severe alcoholic hepatitis may have a normal ALT, although clotting is often deranged.
- The transaminases are never >400U/L in alcoholic hepatitis (and rarely >200U/L), with AST > ALT.
- Jaundice in middle-aged women with high transaminases (>1,000U/L): think autoimmune or infectious hepatitis.
- Acute hepatitis A can cause high fever (40°C).
- Muscle injury or excessive exercise can increase both AST and ALT (and CK).

The most frequent diagnoses are:
- Biliary obstruction (stones, tumour; 35%).
- Alcoholic hepatitis (15%).
- Decompensated cirrhosis (15%).
- Viral hepatitis (8%).
- Autoimmune hepatitis (5%).
- Drug-induced hepatitis (3%).
- Haemolytic anaemia (3%).
- Sepsis (2%).
- Ischaemic hepatitis (1%).
- Other (13%).

Table 14.1 Causes of jaundice

Acholuric	Hepatitis	Obstructive
Haemolysis	Viral hepatitis (HAV–HEV, EBV, CMV, HSV)	Choledocholithiasis
Defective conjugation (Gilbert's disease, Crigler–Najjar)	Alcohol	Malignant (adenocarcinoma of pancreatic head, cholangiocarcinoma, metastases)
Impaired bilirubin excretion (Dubin–Johnson, Rotor syndrome)	Drug-induced (including paracetamol)	PSC
	Ischaemic	Benign biliary strictures (ischaemic, traumatic)
	Metabolic (haemochromatosis, Wilson's disease, A1AT deficiency)	Extrinsic compression (aneurysms, hilar adenopathy)
	PBC	HIV cholangiopathy (see Chapter 12)
	Non-alcoholic steatohepatitis	Parasitic (clonorchiasis, ascariasis, amoebiasis; see Chapter 17)
	Autoimmune hepatitis	
	Veno-occlusive disease (Budd–Chiari syndrome)	
	Granulomatous hepatitis (including sarcoidosis)	
	Pregnancy-related liver disease (see Chapter 19)	
	Bacterial infection (sepsis, Weil's disease; see Chapter 17)	
	Malignant infiltration	

Urgent investigations

- FBC. Decreased Hb in haemolysis (blood film may show abnormal RBC morphology, schistocytes ± reticulocytosis). Leukocytosis in sepsis and alcoholic hepatitis. Thrombocytopaenia in chronic liver disease with hypersplenism, alcoholism, paracetamol overdose, and malaria (request thick and thin blood film if appropriate travel history).
- U & E. Exclude renal failure (hepatorenal syndrome).
- LFT. If abnormal, determine whether pattern is hepatitic or cholestatic (see Chapter 13). Ascertain level of hyperbilirubinaemia and whether predominantly conjugated or unconjugated. Low serum albumin may reflect impaired hepatic synthesis or an acute phase response.
- PTT/INR. Elevated in acute liver failure, DIC, or malnutrition.

- Glucose. Diabetes is common in haemochromatosis and pancreatic carcinoma. Hypoglycaemia occurs in acute liver failure.
- Paracetamol levels. If overdose suspected or possible. Can cause very high transaminases (>10,000U/L).
- Haemolysis screen (LDH, haptoglobin, Coombs test).
- Urinalysis. Absence of bilirubinuria in a jaundiced patient suggests haemolysis, Gilbert's disease, or a conjugation defect.
- CXR. To look for associated pleural effusions, tumours, or metastases.
- US. If the patient is unwell or septic, exclude biliary obstruction that may require urgent decompression (91% sensitive, 95% specific). Note spleen size (portal hypertension) and any masses in the liver. Request Doppler imaging to rule out portal or hepatic vein thrombosis.
- CT performs comparably to US, but IV contrast may be contraindicated if there is associated kidney injury.

These investigations will delineate between a hepatitic cause of jaundice and cholestasis. Haemolysis is a rare cause of jaundice without being obvious. Imaging will determine whether there is biliary obstruction, portal hypertension, or a pancreatic mass.

Semi-urgent investigations

- Viral serology. Anti-HAV IgM, HBsAg and anti-HBc, anti-HCV, anti-HEV, and anti-EBV/CMV/HSV IgM and IgG.
- Immunology. ANA, anti-SM, AMA, anti-LKM1, and immunoglobulins.
- Ferritin and iron studies. Note that ferritin increases in any acute inflammatory disease (e.g. alcoholic hepatitis).
- α-FP. Elevated in HCC (low sensitivity), germ cell tumour metastases.
- Other investigations (copper studies, parasitology, microbiology for leptospirosis) according to clinical picture.
- MRCP is used for further investigation of proven biliary obstruction. Consider ERCP if large duct obstruction demonstrated.

Liver biopsy

Rarely required but has a role in diagnosis and management when:
- No cause is found for parenchymal injury.
- Where grading (degree of inflammation) and staging (degree of fibrosis) will guide treatment (e.g. viral hepatitis pre-treatment).
- Perform transjugular biopsy if INR >1.3 or platelets <80 × 10⁹/L.

Viral hepatitis

Hepatitis A virus (HAV), hepatitis B virus (HBV), or delta co-infection of HBV carriers can lead to acute hepatitis with jaundice. Acute hepatitis C can present with jaundice, although this is unusual (<25%). EBV infection frequently causes abnormal LFT, including mild or moderate jaundice, associated with splenomegaly during the acute phase. Be aware that subacute liver failure often carries poor prognosis, requiring liver transplantation to survive. Although a patient may be conventional virus-negative, disease could potentially be caused by an as yet unidentified infective agent. Patients should be asked about IV drug use, recent tattoos, sexual contacts, and any family or contact history of jaundice or hepatitis.

- Illness is characterized by a 'flu-like' prodrome with very high serum transaminases (up to 4,000U/L), and a small increase in ALP activity.
- If there is no coagulopathy, encephalopathy, or renal failure, send the patient home and await virology results. Advise the patient to avoid alcohol and sexual intercourse until LFT normal. Arrange repeat LFT and clotting at 2–3d intervals, and review the results (but not necessarily the patient). See the patient within 1wk. Instruct to return if increasingly unwell or drowsy.

Hepatitis A

- Causes 50% of reported acute viral hepatitis in the UK.
- Transmission faeco-oral through infected water or uncooked shellfish.
- High risk in travellers to endemic areas, although vaccine-preventable. Incubation ~30d, with jaundice within first week of symptoms.
- May be associated with high fever (40°C).
- ALT and AST often >1,000U/L during icteric phase.
- Diagnosis confirmed by serum HAV IgM antibodies, present at symptom onset.

Patients with acute hepatitis A require no specific treatment, but all household and school contacts should be immunized with HAV vaccine. This replaces previous guidelines that state that contacts should receive normal human immunoglobulins. Patients with acute hepatitis A rarely develop acute liver failure (<0.1%), although the prognosis is relatively good (>80% survival) with conservative management. Prolonged cholestasis occurs in 5%.

Hepatitis B

HBV is extremely common worldwide and endemic in South East Asia (up to 20% prevalence in some areas). The most frequent mode of infection is peri-natal, although blood inoculation and sexual transmission are also important.

Investigation

- For interpretation of HBV serology, see Table 14.2.
- HBsAg appears in serum 1–10wk after HBV exposure, and prior to symptom onset (jaundice, malaise, RUQ pain) or increased ALT. Most HBV infections are silent, with <50% presenting with jaundice.

- As HBsAg disappears, HBsAb titres rise (although there may be a window period when both are negative), so check anti-HBc IgM.
- Detection of anti-HBc IgM is usually regarded as an indication of acute HBV infection, but it may remain detectable for up to 2y or reappear during exacerbations of chronic HBV.
- Isolated presence of anti-HBc IgM indicates the period between HBsAg to anti-HBs seroconversion. Isolated anti-HBc IgG is found many years following recovery from acute HBV (by which time anti-HBs is no longer detectable) or after many years of chronic HBV infection (when HBsAg may have become undetectable). The latter cohort is susceptible to HBV flares following introduction of immunosuppression, including chemotherapy.
- In patients who subsequently recover, HBsAg usually becomes undetectable after 4–6mo; persistence beyond 6mo is arbitrarily defined as chronic infection. Progression from acute to chronic HBV occurs in <5% of adult-acquired infections (but >90% following vertical infection).
- HBeAg implies high infectivity (even if ALT is normal).
- Measure HBV DNA 6-monthly for 18mo in HBsAg-positive/ HBeAg-negative patients to assess whether ongoing viral replication, and measure in HBeAg-positive patients to determine risk of progression (and so stratify treatment). Viral replication is associated with HBV DNA >2,000IU/mL and usually raised ALT.
- HBV genotyping is available but does not (yet) influence treatment.
- Test for co-infection with HCV, HDV and (in all patients) HIV, and immunity to HAV. Monotherapy with lamivudine is only used to prevent re-activation in the context of immune suppression, but it should be avoided in HIV-infected patients to avoid anti-retroviral monotherapy.
- Liver biopsy is rarely needed in the acute phase but is helpful for chronic HBV if active therapy considered. Non-invasive markers of liver fibrosis are increasingly being validated in clinical practice.

Table 14.2 Interpretation of HBV serology

Result	Interpretation
HBsAg⁺	Ongoing active infection*
αHBs	Resolved infection or vaccinated (other serology normal)
αHBc IgM	Acute infection or exacerbation
αHBc IgG	Previous resolved or chronic infection
HBeAg⁺	High viral replication and infectivity
αHBe	Low infectivity (reciprocal of HBeAg⁺)

* May rarely be negative at presentation, especially in fulminant disease.

① *Complications*

- Cirrhosis. Usually develops 30–40y post-infection but highly variable.
- HCC. 100-fold risk compared to general population, and 2–6% annual risk if cirrhotic (0.5%/y otherwise). Screen every 6mo using serum α-FP and liver US.
- Membranous glomerulonephropathy.
- Polyarteritis nodosa.

The highest rate of complications arises in highly replicating chronic hepatitis (HBeAg-positive or αHBe-negative).

Treatment

Patients with acute HBV do not generally require anti-viral treatment. Over 95% of patients clear virus spontaneously during the acute phase, as do a further 1%/y of presumed chronically infected individuals.

- Acute HBV. Consider treating patients with:
  - Severe hepatitis (e.g. those who develop coagulopathy).
  - Acute liver failure. Occurs in <2%. Treatment reduces likelihood of re-infection post-liver transplant.
  - Protracted course (persistent symptoms/jaundice for >4wk).
  - Immunocompromise (including old age).
  - Concomitant HCV or delta virus infection.
  - Pre-existing liver disease.
- Chronic HBV (see Fig. 14.1). European guidelines (EASL Clinical Practice Guidelines, 2012) suggest considering anti-viral therapy in all patients with liver inflammation and HBV DNA >2,000IU/mL. Note that ALT is a poor surrogate for liver inflammation and fibrosis, and hence liver biopsy or (in the future) non-invasive markers of fibrosis are required.
- Health care workers should be considered for anti-viral therapy even if they do not fulfill typical criteria. Those who are HBsAg-positive with HBV ≥2,000IU/mL should receive a potent anti-viral with low resistance (e.g. entecavir or tenofovir). HBV DNA should be ≤2,000IU/mL (and ideally undetectable) before resuming exposure-prone procedures.

The goal of therapy is to suppress HBV replication, maintain HBsAg loss (this is infrequent, although may become more common as newer agents are used more regularly), induce HBeAg-positive seroconversion to HBeAg-negative/anti-HBe-positive, and minimize liver injury. Treatment is a fast-moving field but, at the time of writing (2013), anti-viral agents include:

- Pegylated interferon-α:
  - Induces HBeAg seroconversion in 30% and HBsAg loss in 10% at 1y.
  - Limited treatment course required (48wk). No risk of anti-viral resistance.
  - Disadvantages include SC administration and side effects (flu-like syndrome, autoimmune reactions, myelosuppression, depression).
  - Contraindicated in decompensated liver disease.
  - Predictors of good response: low pre-treatment HBV DNA level, ALT >3× ULN, high inflammatory score on biopsy, HBV genotype A or B.

- Treatment failure defined as absence of a log decrease in HBV DNA level at 12wk, or HBV DNA >2,000IU/mL at 24wk, in which case switch to an oral anti-viral agent.
- Lamivudine:
  - Oral nucleoside analogue.
  - Side effects minimal.
  - HBeAg seroconversion in 25% at 1y and 50% at 3y.
  - Treatment-resistant YMDD mutations in >40% after 3y, hence only used to prevent re-activation in those likely to become immunosuppressed (e.g. with concomitant chemotherapy).
- Tenofovir:
  - Oral nucleotide analogue. Recently approved for use in HBV.
  - Low rates of resistance, with high rates of viral control.
  - Avoid if severe renal disease.
  - Appropriate for first-line monotherapy (as of 2013).
- Entecavir:
  - Oral nucleoside analogue.
  - Potent anti-viral but higher risk of treatment resistance than with tenofovir, particularly if pre-existing lamivudine resistance.
  - Appropriate for first-line monotherapy (as of 2013).
- Adefovir:
  - Oral nucleotide analogue reverse transcriptase inhibitor.
  - Used to treat lamivudine-resistant HBV.
  - Less efficacious and more expensive than tenofovir, thus rarely used.
- Emtricitabine is currently under evaluation. As of 2013, only used for HIV therapy (as Truvada®, combined with tenofovir), although it is active against HBV.
- Telbivudine is licensed for HBV treatment but has less potency than tenofovir or entecavir, so rarely used.
- If HBeAg seroconversion is achieved, continue anti-viral therapy for at least an additional 6–12mo (and consider long-term treatment).
- Be aware that the nucleoside and nucleotide analogues also have activity against HIV, and it is important to avoid anti-retroviral monotherapy.

The 5y survival in chronically infected patients is ~80%; this falls to 35% after an episode of hepatic decompensation.

For HBsAg-positive patients, first-degree relatives and sexual partners should be tested for HBsAg, HBsAb, and anti-HBc IgM, and vaccinated against HBV (see also 🔲 p. 220). Prophylactic specific hepatitis B immunoglobulin (HBIg 500U IM) is protective if given within 10d of exposure. However, only use for persons with clear exposure to HBsAg-contaminated material (needlestick or sexual contacts who are HBsAb-negative). Follow-up for at least 6mo to ensure either no infection or that the virus is cleared in those who do develop acute HBV (i.e. HBsAg-negative, HBsAb-positive). Vaccinate against HAV if non-immune.

Offer vaccination to travellers to areas of endemicity, IVDU, MSM, health care workers, and patients with haemophilia or chronic liver disease. A 1mL vaccination, repeated at 6 and 12mo, provides 95% protection at 5y.

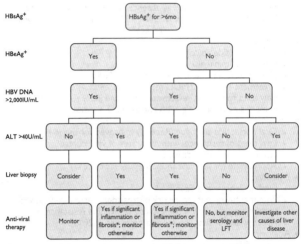

* High relapse rate

Fig. 14.1 Decision-making algorithm for HBV investigation and treatment. Adapted from Stuart Bloom, George Webster, and Daniel Marks, *Oxford Handbook of Gastroenterology and Hepatology*, second edition, 2012, Fig. 3.10, p. 345, with permission from Oxford University Press.

Hepatitis C

Acute hepatitis C is said to account for up to 20% of cases of acute viral hepatitis in the USA, although the figure is much lower (<5–10%) in the UK. HCV is transmitted predominantly through blood exposure; sexual or peri-natal transmission is rare (<5% risk). Most cases are asymptomatic; <25% develop discernible jaundice and serum ALT is usually <1,000U/L. About 70% develop chronic HCV (infection >6mo), although a significant number subsequently clear the virus. It is now recognized that polymorphisms near the IL-28 gene stratify for self-limiting (C/C allele, 50% clearance, found in Europeans) or chronic (T/T allele, 20% clearance, found in Africans) infection (Thomas et al., 2009).

• The presence of HCV RNA in serum confirms ongoing infection and is detectable within days to 2mo following exposure.
• Anti-HCV ELISA tests become positive from 8wk after exposure (but may take many months). These confirm exposure to, but not persistence of, disease; 50% of patients presenting with acute hepatitis C have antibodies at presentation.
• Determine viral genotype (affects treatment regimen and response).
• Liver biopsy allows staging and grading, although non-invasive markers are being increasingly used.

- Also test for HBV and HIV co-infection (as shared routes of exposure, and liver disease is more severe), and for associated autoimmune hepatitis and thyroid disease.

Complications
- HCC. Guidance as for HBV.
- Cryoglobulinaemia:
  - Detectable in 36–54%. Mostly asymptomatic.
  - Arthralgia and pruritus in 18%.
  - Neuropathy and glomerulonephritis in 2%.
- Mesangiocapillary and membranous glomerulonephritis.
- Lichen planus.
- Autoimmune disease:
  - Autoimmune hepatitis.
  - Sjögren's syndrome.
  - Thyroiditis.
- Polyarteritis nodosa.
- Porphyria cutanea tarda.

Treatment
All patients diagnosed with HCV should be followed up and treated once it is established they have chronic disease (i.e. anti-HCV+, HCV RNA+, elevated serum transaminases, and moderate/severe hepatitis or well-compensated cirrhosis on liver biopsy); for current European guidelines, see EASL Clinical Practice Guidelines (2011).
- Treat acute genotype 2 or 3 HCV with pegylated interferon-α and ribavirin for 24wk. This provides sustained virological response (undetectable HCV RNA) in 80% (Kamal *et al.*, 2004) at 6mo (genotypes 1 and 4 ~50% less responsive; therefore, alternative agents now used).
- As of 2012, standard of care for genotype 1 patients is triple therapy with pegylated interferon, ribavirin, and a protease inhibitor (e.g. telaprevir or boceprevir).
- Pegylated interferon-α monotherapy reserved for ribavirin intolerance.
- Ribavirin is contraindicated in pregnancy (advise effective contraception). Haemolysis common (fall in Hb by 2g/dL usual) and should be avoided in those with pre-existing haemolytic anaemias.
- Treatment algorithms provided here may not be applicable beyond 2013, as rapid drug development is occurring.
- Cessation of alcohol slows progression of liver disease. Vaccinate against HAV and HBV. Advise not to donate blood, or to share razors or toothbrushes. Advise use of barrier contraception.
- There is no established re-treatment algorithm in the event of treatment failure. Seek specialist advice.
- End-stage liver failure requires transplantation.

For anti-HCV+ patients, try and determine the source. Check LFT and HCV RNA in contacts, and follow them up since the majority of untreated patients will need treatment.

Hepatitis D (delta virus)

RNA virus that requires HBV for complete virion assembly; 5% HBV carriers are co-infected. Runs a more severe course, although has lower risk of HCC. Presence of HBsAg is necessary for a diagnosis of hepatitis D. Treatment is with interferon alone, although response rate is lower.

Hepatitis E

RNA virus endemic in the Indian subcontinent, South East Asia, and Middle East. Outbreaks have been reported in the UK (with pigs as the presumed reservoir).
- Transmission faeco-oral, incubation period 15–65d.
- Usually causes acute icteric hepatitis although occasionally a cholestatic picture is seen.
- Diagnosis by detection of anti-HEV IgM.
- Treatment supportive, as infection usually settles within 6wk.
  However, mortality high in pregnant women (>20% in third trimester).
- Acute liver failure/fulminant hepatitis may require transplantation.

① Needlestick injuries

The major blood-borne pathogens of concern associated with needlestick injuries are HBV, HCV, and HIV. There is also potential for transmission after mucocutaneous exposure to infected body fluids, although this is of lower magnitude. Significant stress and psychological trauma can result from needlestick injuries (even when no infection is ultimately acquired) due to long periods of uncertainty regarding the outcome, working restrictions, and side effects from post-exposure prophylaxis (PEP). Although the greatest fear tends to be of HIV infection, HCV and HBV are more common and more transmissible (the risk of HIV transmission from a needle of unknown origin is <1/30,000). The following are associated with higher risk of transmission:
- Injury from a device exposed to donor artery or vein.
- Blood exposure (as opposed to bloodstained fluid).
- Injury from hollow bore (as opposed to solid) needle.
- Deep injury.
- Visible blood on needle.
- No use of personal protective equipment (e.g. gloves).

Needlestick injury (no known risk factors)
- Initiate first aid treatment. If skin punctured, free bleeding should be gently encouraged and the wound washed with soap or chlorhexidine and water (but not scrubbed or sucked). If the mouth or eyes are involved, they should be washed thoroughly with water.
- Send serum from recipient to virology lab. This will usually not be tested at this stage (too early to demonstrate virus acquisition) but can subsequently be used in the event of seroconversion to confirm occupational acquisition.
- Clarify recipient's HBV vaccination status, including number of doses previously received, date of last booster, and most recent HBsAb titre.
- Counsel the recipient regarding:
  - Seroconversion risks (general and situation-specific, see sections on needlestick injury, 📖 pp. 219–20).

- Steps to reduce risk of blood-borne virus transmission.
- Follow-up procedure and rationale for this.
- Concept of a 'window period'.
- Infection control precautions during follow-up period: safe sex, no blood donation, and any work restrictions (none if low-risk exposure).
- Allow time to discuss anxieties and concerns.
- Test donor if they provide consent. The pre-test discussion should be carried out sensitively and not by the exposed member of staff (who has a conflict of interest):
  - Explain what has happened and the policy for requesting consent for blood-borne virus testing.
  - Keep details of recipient confidential.
  - Discuss practical implications of testing (positive and negative), including personal relationships, employment, medical follow-up, and life insurance (companies should only ask about *positive* test results).
  - Describe the procedure for having blood taken and arrangements for communicating results to the donor.
  - If consent provided, test for HBsAg, anti-HCV, and HIV antibodies. Write 'donor patient in needlestick incident' on the request form.
  - Donor testing cannot be undertaken without express consent (this cannot be provided by a third party).
- Report exposure to Occupational Health.
- If the recipient tests positive for a blood-borne virus, refer on to appropriate specialty.

Needlestick injury (known HBV carrier)

- Risk of seroconversion up to 30% (highest if donor HBeAg-positive with high HBV DNA).
- Basic management as outlined under 'Needlestick injury (no known risk factors), (see 📖 p. 218).
- If the recipient is not HBV-immune, check HBsAg status urgently. Vaccinate and test for HBsAg at 6wk, 3mo, and 6mo.
- PEP protocols as shown in Table 14.3 (see 📖 p. 220).
- Report exposure to Occupational Health.

Needlestick injury (known HCV carrier)

- Risk of seroconversion 0.5–1.8% for needlestick exposure to blood with detectable HCV RNA (transmission unlikely if undetectable).
- Basic management as outlined under 'Needlestick injury (no known risk factors)', (see 📖 p. 218). There is no PEP available for HCV.
- Report exposure to Occupational Health.
- Request follow-up blood tests for HCV RNA at 4wk, and HCV antibodies and ALT at 3 and 6mo.

Needlestick injury (known HIV carrier)

- Risk of seroconversion 0.3% (needlestick) and 0.1% (mucocutaneous). Correlates with viral load.
- Basic management as outlined under 'Needlestick injury (no known risk factors)', (see 📖 p. 218).

Table 14.3 HBV PEP if significant risk exposure

HBV status of recipient	HBV status of donor		
	HBsAg⁺	Unknown	HBsAg⁻
<2 doses HBV vaccine pre-exposure	Accelerated course of HBV vaccination + HBIg	Accelerated course of HBV vaccination	Initiate HBV vaccination course
≈ 2 doses HBV vaccine pre-exposure (αHBs not known)	1 dose HBV vaccine + second dose 1mo later	1 dose HBV vaccine	Finish HBV vaccination course
Known HBV vaccine responder (αHBs >10mIU/mL)	Consider HBV vaccine booster	Consider HBV vaccine booster	Consider HBV vaccine booster
Known HBV vaccine non-responder (αHBs <10mIU/mL 2–4mo post-immunization)	HBIg + consider HBV vaccine booster. Give second HBIg dose at 1mo	HBIg + consider HBV vaccine booster. Give second HBIg dose at 1mo	Consider HBV vaccine booster

An accelerated course of vaccine consists of doses spaced at 0, 1, and 2mo. Reproduced with permission from the Health Protection Agency, 'Exposure to hepatitis B virus: guidance on post-exposure prophylaxis', PHLS Hepatitis Subcommittee, *Communicable Disease Report Review*, 2, 9, August 1992. (see https://www.wp.dh.gov.uk/immunisation/files/2012/10/GreenBook-updated-251012.pdf).

- In cases of definite exposure to blood or other high-risk body fluids, PEP should be offered as soon as possible (preferably within 1h but up to 72h after exposure).
- If risk of exposure uncertain, it is reasonable to initiate PEP whilst clarification obtained.
- The current recommended regimen for PEP is Truvada® (tenofovir 245mg/emtricitabine 200mg) 1 tablet bd + Kaletra® (lopinavir 200mg/ritonavir 50mg) 2 tablets bd for 28d. The regimen may need modification if the donor is infected with a resistant virus (discuss with their HIV physician).
- Side effects include nausea, vomiting, abdominal pain, fatigue, diarrhoea, myelosuppression, rash, deranged LFT, pancreatitis, and peripheral neuropathy. Monitor FBC, U & E, LFT, and amylase, and co-prescribe an anti-emetic and loperamide.
- Report exposure to Occupational Health.

① Alcoholic hepatitis

Taking an alcohol history

There is a tendency to diagnose alcoholic liver disease when all other causes have seemingly been excluded despite the fact that an alcohol drinking history may be absent. Some patients drink a lot of alcohol but are not dependent on alcohol, and these are the patients most amenable to treatment. Patients generally need to drink 80U/wk for at least 10y to get alcoholic liver disease (a bit less in women and a bit more in men). If a patient denies alcohol abuse and their partner confirms this, believe them and look for other causes. Ask:

- What alcohol they drink.
- If they drink beer, what beer and what % alcohol it contains.
- Whether they drink every day.
- CAGE questionnaire: comprises discriminating questions where two affirmative questions strongly predicts alcoholism (see *Oxford Handbook of Gastroenterology and Hepatology*, p. 207).
- Whether their drinking ever affects their work.
- Be wary of the patient who boldly states the number of units they drink each week. Most people don't know how to calculate this and don't care.

Presentation and diagnosis

Acute alcoholic hepatitis may be asymptomatic, or present with jaundice on a background of anorexia, nausea, vomiting and, rarely, RUQ pain. Fever may reflect severe liver damage, but infection needs to be excluded. Acute alcohol withdrawal is unusual since most patients have stopped drinking alcohol before presentation; an undefined trigger initiates severe inflammation and hepatic neutrophil infiltration. Most patients with alcoholic hepatitis have cirrhosis at presentation.

On examination, patients are usually malnourished, with clinically evident jaundice and stigmata of chronic liver disease, including multiple spider naevi, palmar erythema, and a hyperdynamic circulation. The liver is usually enlarged and may be grossly so (if the liver is impalpable, then consider whether the patient is developing end-stage liver failure). It is unusual to be able to palpate the spleen. Cirrhotic patients often have ascites, with thin skin and visible superficial veins over the abdomen. The presence of xanthelasma suggests PBC. Approximately 15% have hepatic encephalopathy at presentation, with confusion, somnolence, and asterixis.

Investigations

- The term 'alcoholic hepatitis' is a misnomer since transaminases rarely exceed 200U/L (and are always <400U/L). The AST is always higher than the ALT.
- Serum γGT is often grossly elevated and, in those who stop drinking, it takes ~1mo for levels to halve.
- Bilirubin may be up to 1,000µmol/L.
- Albumin is often decreased.
- A prolonged INR usually signifies underlying cirrhosis.

- The FBC often shows macrocytosis, with leukocytosis ± left shift (even without infection), anaemia, and thrombocytopaenia. Thrombocytopaenia suggests cirrhosis but may be a direct result of alcohol abuse.
- Renal failure (hepatorenal syndrome) occurs in 20–40% of patients with severe alcoholic hepatitis (GAHS >9).
- Screen for bacterial and fungal infections: blood and urine and, if present, ascitic fluid microscopy and culture; and CXR.
- Liver biopsy confirms the diagnosis (neutrophil infiltration, hepatocyte ballooning/necrosis, Mallory bodies) and the presence of cirrhosis.

Assessing the severity of alcoholic hepatitis

Glasgow alcoholic hepatitis score (GAHS)
Considered to be the best scoring system for alcoholic hepatitis (see Table 14.4). Each variable is given a score, and then a combined score of 5–12 is obtained. A score >9 is associated with poor prognosis.

Table 14.4 The Glasgow alcoholic hepatitis score

Score given	1	2	3
Age (y)	<50	≥50	–
WCC (× 10⁹/L)	<15	≥15	–
Urea (mmol/L)	<5	≥5	–
INR	<1.5	1.5–2.0	>2.0
Bilirubin (μmol/L)	<125	125–250	>250

Reproduced from *Gut*, Forrest EH et al., 'Analysis of factors predictive of mortality in alcoholic hepatitis and derivation and validation of the Glasgow alcoholic hepatitis score', 54, 8, pp. 1174–1179, copyright 2005, with permission from BMJ Publishing Group Ltd.

Maddrey discriminant index (DI)
The classic way to calculate severity of alcoholic hepatitis is:

$$DI = serum\ bilirubin/17 + (prolongation\ of\ PTT \times 4.6)$$

A DI >31 is associated with >35% 4wk mortality.

Treatment

- Since alcoholic hepatitis can be associated with high short-term mortality, it is best to admit patients to hospital unless mild (bilirubin <50μmol and normal INR) and the patient lives in an abstinent environment.
- Institute general supportive measures (supplemental oxygen, IV fluids) as necessary. Insert CVP line (correct coagulopathy first) if shocked, bleeding, or renal failure.
- Many patients with alcoholic hepatitis are malnourished and some are deficient in thiamine. Give Pabrinex® IV and oral thiamine (200mg/d), and folic acid and multivitamins.
- Monitor and correct K^+, Mg^{++}, PO_4^{3-}, and glucose.
- Start high-calorie, high-protein (>1.2g/kg/d) diet.

- Provide vitamin K 10mg IV for 3d.
- Consider enteral feeding overnight for those with severe malnutrition. Moderate initial intake to avoid re-feeding syndrome.
- If infection clinically suspected, start broad-spectrum antibiotics (e.g. cefotaxime 1–2g IV od). Give fluconazole 100mg IV/PO od as prophylaxis against fungal infections. Note that many patients with alcoholic hepatitis have fever or leukocytosis that does not respond to these agents.
- Patients with severe alcoholic hepatitis (GAHS >9 or DI >32) should be treated with prednisolone 40mg PO od for 4wk. The only practical contraindication is untreated sepsis; if in doubt, give broad-spectrum antibiotics for 24–48h prior to steroids.
- An alternative treatment is pentoxifylline 400mg PO tds for 4wk. This is suggested to improve survival and decrease occurrence of hepatorenal syndrome, although its benefit is not yet proven (Whitfield et al., 2009). There is no evidence for combination therapy with steroids.

☼ Wernicke's encephalopathy

If a patient is confused and somnolent at times but with no features of hepatic encephalopathy, consider Wernicke's encephalopathy or Korsakoff's psychosis.

- Wernicke's encephalopathy is characterized by disorientation, indifference, inattentiveness, and impaired memory. Patients may have impaired oculomotor function (nystagmus, lateral rectus or gaze palsies) and gait ataxia. Less than 10% have a depressed level of consciousness although, if untreated, they will progress to stupor, coma, and death.
- Wernicke's encephalopathy may be precipitated by high carbohydrate loads, including IV glucose (hence administer thiamine beforehand if any clinical suspicion of deficiency).
- Treatment is with high-dose thiamine (Pabrinex® IV tds for 5d followed by long-term thiamine 200mg/d PO).
- Check serum Mg^{++} and correct if low, as thiamine may be ineffective if hypomagnesaemic.
- Korsakoff's psychosis is characterized by marked irreversible deficits in short-term memory and apathy, with an intact sensory system and relative preservation of long-term memory and other cognitive functions.
- The diagnosis is supported by low serum vitamin B1 (thiamine) or red cell transketolase, measured on a pre-treatment sample.

☼ Delirium tremens

- Delirium tremens does not seem to be a major problem in patients presenting with alcoholic hepatitis, since many have stopped drinking by the time they present to hospital.
- If symptomatic, manage with oral clomethiazole or low-dose diazepam. In recent years, clomethiazole has been avoided since the IV preparation was used inappropriately in some patients; however, the oral preparation may be safer than chlordiazepoxide. The latter accumulates in patients with cirrhosis (half-life up to 150h) and is not easily cleared if the patient becomes drowsy.
- Treat seizures according to standard protocols.

Zieve's syndrome

Acute metabolic disturbance that can occur following an alcohol binge or during withdrawal from protracted alcohol use. It is caused by depletion of hepatic lipid and characterized by jaundice, upper abdominal pain, haemolytic anaemia, and hyperlipoproteinaemia. Typically resolves within 3wk of abstinence.

⊙ Drug-induced hepatitis

Drug-induced jaundice is always severe (see Chapter 18). Patients with drug-induced jaundice should be monitored 3 times/wk and, ideally, admitted for observation, as many are serious and may not resolve. Hepatitic drug reactions are far more serious (10% mortality) than cholestatic reactions. Paracetamol-induced liver injury is a different case and discussed separately (see 🕮 p. 243 and p. 296). Withdraw the suspected drug and observe. Look for rash and eosinophilia and exclude other causes of liver injury. Some of the more common drugs causing jaundice are listed in Table 14.5; drugs causing a rise in serum transaminases, but rarely jaundice, are not listed. In the UK, all drug-induced causes of jaundice should be reported to the CSM (yellow pages at the back of the BNF).

Table 14.5 Common drugs that may cause jaundice

Hepatitic	Cholestatic	Mixed
Paracetamol	Chlorpromazine	Sulfonamides
Rifampicin	Flucloxacillin	Sulfasalazine
Allopurinol	Azathioprine	Carbamazepine
NSAIDs	Captopril	Dapsone
Halothane	Co-amoxiclav	Ranitidine
Methyldopa	Penicillamine	Amitriptyline
Hydralazine	Erythromycin	Nitrofurantoin
Isoniazid	Anabolic steroids	Co-amoxiclav
Phenytoin	Oral contraceptive	

⊙ **Autoimmune hepatitis**

Autoimmune hepatitis arises in 5–10/100,000 of the population, with a 4:1 female predominance. It is strongly associated with HLA-DR3 and HLA-DR4 haplotypes, the former predicting younger onset and more severe disease course. Most patients present with gradual onset disease, although acute hepatitis develops in up to 40%; acute liver failure remains rare. It is associated with other autoimmune conditions in 50% (thyroiditis, arthritis, vitiligo, ulcerative colitis, diabetes mellitus, pernicious anaemia), hepatitis C and, rarely, minocycline use (see Chapter 18). Overlap syndromes with PBC and sclerosing cholangitis are seen.

Investigations

- Serum transaminases are elevated, usually <2,000U/L.
- Polyclonal elevation in IgG. If total globulins (total protein minus albumin) is >45g/L, this is often due to autoimmune hepatitis.
- Serology facilitates diagnosis (titre >1:80) and division into subtypes:
  - Type 1 (~80%). ANA and anti-smooth muscle antibody positive. Good response to immunosuppression in 80%, although 25% have cirrhosis at presentation.
  - Type 2 (~20% in Europe but rare in the USA). LKM1 and LC-1 antibody positive but ANA and anti-smooth muscle antibody negative. Usually diagnosed in children. Rapidly progressive, with a poor response to immunosuppression.
  - Type 3. Presents with a similar clinical picture to type 1, but ANA, anti-smooth muscle, and LKM1 antibodies are undetectable. Associated with antibodies against soluble liver antigen.
  - Elevated anti-LKM1 titres are detectable in 2–5% of HCV-positive patients.
- Liver biopsy. Demonstrates periportal/lobular hepatitis but no pathognomonic features. Grade and stage predict prognosis.

Treatment

Indications for treatment include a serum transaminase level >1.5× ULN, serum IgG >2× ULN, or moderate or severe hepatitis on liver biopsy (patients can benefit from immunosuppression even if cirrhotic). Give prednisolone 30–40mg PO od for 2wk, then taper by 5mg every 10d to maintain at 5–15mg daily. Prednisolone is protein-bound, so reduce dose in patients with serum albumin <20g/L. Budesonide (3mg PO tds) for 6–12mo is at least as effective as prednisolone but has fewer side effects (Manns *et al.*, 2010). Start azathioprine simultaneously at 1–1.5mg/kg/d. This can subsequently be up-titrated to 2–2.5mg/kg/d according to response and tolerance, and used as monotherapy once remission is established. Case reports and series also support efficacy of ciclosporin, tacrolimus, and mycophenolate mofetil as steroid-sparing agents.

Immunosuppression induces sustained remission in 80% of patients at 4y (untreated, 5y mortality is 50%, compared to 90% survival at 10y with active therapy). Drug withdrawal should not be attempted within 2y of initiation and only then as guided by histology (100% of patients relapse if there has been progression to cirrhosis whilst on treatment, compared to only 20% with histological resolution).

Up to 10% of patients progress despite steroid therapy (in patients <30y, consider whether a diagnosis of Wilson's disease has been missed). Liver transplantation is required in these individuals, particularly if progression occurs within 4y of diagnosis or there is early hepatic decompensation. Autoimmune hepatitis may recur in the graft but rarely leads to its loss. Overall, post-transplant survival is 90% at 5y and 75% at 10y.

⊙ Haemochromatosis

Iron overload may be primary (genetic) or secondary (termed haemosiderosis, most commonly due to repeated blood transfusions). Normal body iron content is 3–4g; in haemochromatosis, this rises to >20g. Genetic haemochromatosis is caused by the autosomal recessive C282Y polymorphism in the *HFE* gene in 90% of cases. Up to 10% of Northern Europeans are heterozygous for this substitution, and 0.25% homozygous. Disease frequency, however, is lower as it has limited penetrance (~13%), partly explained by menstrual iron losses in pre-menopausal women. For full current guidelines on diagnosis and management, see EASL Clinical Practice Guidelines (2010).

Clinical features
- Hepatomegaly.
- Cirrhosis.
- HCC (15% of untreated cases).
- Cardiomyopathy (most commonly dilated but occasionally restrictive).
- Diabetes mellitus.
- Hypogonadotrophic hypogonadism.
- Skin pigmentation ('bronze diabetes').
- Porphyria cutanea tarda.
- Arthralgia/arthritis (chondrocalcinosis, pseudogout).

Investigations
- Blood tests:
  - Iron studies. Serum ferritin >1,000µg/L and iron-binding saturation >60% are strongly suggestive of haemochromatosis.
  - *HFE* gene analysis for C282Y and H63D polymorphisms is useful but still requires supportive biochemical studies to confirm the diagnosis, given their incomplete penetrance and existence of other mutations.
  - LFT. Typically hepatitic picture but often normal or only minimally deranged.
  - Screen for HCC with α-FP (and US) in those with cirrhosis.
  - Check glucose and HbA1c to screen for diabetes mellitus; LH, FSH, and testosterone in males for hypogonadism (response to gonadotrophin also impaired); and TFT, prolactin, and IGF-1 for evidence of panhypopituitarism.
- Imaging:
  - MRI is 84–91% sensitive and 80–100% specific for significant hepatic iron overload.

- US to screen for HCC in patients with cirrhosis.
- DEXA scan to screen for osteoporosis.
- Joint X-ray for chondrocalcinosis or arthritis.
- Liver biopsy is the gold standard for diagnosis as well as allowing assessment of severity and measurement of hepatic iron index. It is not required to determine extent of fibrosis in those who do not drink excess alcohol, in whom serum ferritin is <1,000μg/L and who have normal transaminases.
- Cardiac investigations. ECG (abnormalities found in a one-third of patients), echocardiogram, and 24h tape if cardiac symptoms. Cardiac MRI can quantify iron accumulation and assess function.

Treatment

- Venesect 1U blood (450mL) every 1–3wk. Measure ferritin and Hb after every three venesections. Aim for Hb at lower end of the normal range and ferritin <50–100μg/L (may take 2y to achieve).
- Iron chelation with desferrioxamine 2g IV three times/wk is used when venesection not tolerated, but is less effective.
- Advise alcohol cessation.
- Treatment of diabetes mellitus follows standard protocols. Refer to endocrinologist for management of hypogonadism.
- Arthralgia and arthritis are managed with simple analgesia or anti-inflammatory agents. The response to venesection is usually poor.
- Screen relatives for genetic haemochromatosis:
  - If the index case is C282Y or H63D homozygote or compound heterozygote, screen using genetic studies and serum iron studies.
  - If the index case does not carry these polymorphisms, screen biochemically.

Wilson's disease

See Chapter 15.

Primary biliary cirrhosis

Typically presents insidiously, with progressive fatigue and pruritus; jaundice occurs late (see the Oxford Handbook of Gastroenterology and Hepatology, p. 456). On examination, there are frequently peri-orbital xanthelasma, excoriation marks, and signs of chronic liver disease. Serology demonstrates AMA in 95% and elevated serum IgM.

Ursodeoxycholic acid 13–15mg/kg/d PO slows progression and ameliorates pruritus, beyond which therapy there is no evidence to guide therapeutic decisions in those with progressive disease. Some experts recommend additional colchicine 600μg PO bd if LFT remain abnormal or liver histology is not improving at 6 months, together with methotrexate (0.25mg/kg weekly PO) in those with persistently severe disease. Preliminary evidence also suggests budesonide 6mg PO od may be beneficial in non-cirrhotic patients. For severe uncontrolled pruritus, colestyramine 4g PO qds is also effective. Ultimately, liver transplantation may be required.

:O: Ischaemic hepatitis

- Occurs with significant hypotension or hepatic arterial occlusion.
- Predisposing factors include congestive cardiac failure and hypoxia.
- In its mildest form, manifests as mildly deranged LFT (hepatitic picture, increased INR); at its most severe, with acute liver failure. LFT rise over hours and fall over days.
- Look for evidence of hypoxia ± hypotension (may have normalized by time of assessment: check previous observation and anaesthetic charts if available), signs of arteriopathy (abdominal bruits from hepatic arterial occlusion), and signs of right ventricular failure.
- May cause hepatic encephalopathy.
- Arterial compromise may be demonstrated by Doppler US or CT angiogram. Exclude other causes of hepatitis.
- Most cases respond to correction of the underlying aetiology. Correct hypotension and give supplemental oxygen.
- If the hepatic artery or coeliac axis is occluded, prognosis is poor (and correlates with extent of hepatic necrosis). Discuss with interventional radiologist whether angiographic revascularization possible.
- Usually associated co-morbidities and extent of disease preclude salvage surgery.
- Discuss with specialist centre if acute liver failure. Most patients are not fit enough for liver transplantation.

:O: Obstructive jaundice

The differential diagnosis for jaundice due to biliary tree obstruction is given in 'Assessment and causes of jaundice' (see 📖 pp. 208–10). Obstructive jaundice is frequently associated with pruritus, as irritant bile acids are deposited in subcutaneous tissues where they can persist for weeks. The classic description of pale stools and dark urine (due to absent conjugated bilirubin excretion into the GI tract) is, in fact, less helpful in differentiating obstructive/cholestatic from hepatitic disease. Abdominal pain suggests the presence of bile duct stones, whereas progressive painless jaundice implies malignant obstruction (although the history is often imprecise). LFT typically demonstrate high ALP and γGT, but marked elevation of transaminases can occur (particularly with choledocholithiasis). Fever, rigors, and elevated inflammatory markers (CRP, ESR) suggest developing cholangitis, which can rapidly progress to septicaemia (see Chapter 9). If suspected, obtain blood cultures, start broad-spectrum antibiotics (e.g. co-amoxiclav 1.2g IV tds), and expedite further investigations.

If biliary tree obstruction is possible, request an urgent US or CT to look for duct dilatation. US has >90% sensitivity and specificity for detecting gallbladder stones, but only 50% sensitivity for those in the CBD.

When to do an MRCP

MRCP should be performed in patients with evidence of biliary duct dilatation on initial assessment (although it may be prudent to proceed direct to therapeutic ERCP in patients with high clinical suspicion of large duct obstruction on US so as not to delay definitive management); or if choledocholithiasis suspected despite normal US. For indications and contraindications, see Chapter 13.

When to do an ERCP

ERCP with a side-viewing duodenoscope allows selective cannulation of the biliary and pancreatic ductal systems and their delineation by radio-opaque contrast injection. Its role as a primary diagnostic technique is rare with the development and availability of MRCP; it also has more limited capacity to visualize the biliary tree proximal to the site of obstruction. Current indications include:

- Relief of biliary obstruction by stenting of strictures.
- Removal of CBD stones.
- Biopsy ± brush cytology of biliary tree lesions.
- Biliary manometry in suspected sphincter of Oddi dysfunction.

Most contraindications are relative and include altered surgical anatomy rendering ductal access difficult or impossible (e.g. Roux-en-Y anastomosis; requires percutaneous approach), and coagulopathy (aim for INR ≤1.3 and platelets >50, particularly if sphincterotomy anticipated). Discontinue clopidogrel if possible (discuss with cardiologist first), and withhold warfarin for 5d pre-procedure (but with LMWH cover if high risk of clotting such as a metallic heart valve); check INR on day of procedure.

Complications of ERCP

The overall complication rate is 5–10% (see also Appendix, 📖 p. 360). Complications are more frequent in units performing <200 procedures/y and with endoscopists performing <40 procedures/y, although patient-related factors probably exert even greater influence.

- Pancreatitis (3–5%). Severe in 30%, with mortality of 0.5%. Risk factors include young age, female patient, suspected sphincter of Oddi dysfunction, normal serum bilirubin, previous ERCP-related pancreatitis, difficult CBD cannulation, contrast injection into the pancreatic duct, and performance of sphincterotomy or balloon sphincter dilatation.
- Cholangitis (2%). Generally arises when intrahepatic ducts have been filled with contrast but effective biliary drainage not obtained. Managed with broad-spectrum IV antibiotics and further attempts to establish effective drainage (e.g. via percutaneous transhepatic approach).
- Bleeding. Usually related to sphincterotomy and typically settles spontaneously. Endoscopic haemostasis is occasionally required but embolization or surgery rarely necessary.
- Retroperitoneal perforation (<1%). Presents acutely with surgical emphysema and pain in the absence of a rise in amylase. Diagnosed by CT. Mostly settles with conservative management; keep NBM and provide broad-spectrum antibiotics. However, close observation is required in view of the risks of retroperitoneal sepsis and abscess formation; these may necessitate percutaneous or surgical drainage.

Direct cholangioscopy

This technique is now available in a few centres in the UK and used for further assessment of indeterminate biliary strictures and direct electro-hydraulic lithotripsy of impacted bile duct stones.

Percutaneous transhepatic cholangiography

The liver is punctured under fluoroscopic guidance to enter the periph-eral intrahepatic bile duct system, and contrast medium injected. This is particularly useful to image lesions proximal to the common hepatic duct and when altered surgical anatomy restricts use of ERCP, but requires significant expertise to perform.

When to drain biliary obstruction

The management of gallstone disease and cholangitis is detailed in Chapter 9. Biliary drainage is indicated for actual or threatened cholangitis. The fol-lowing measures are useful for ameliorating pruritus:
- Ursodeoxycholic acid 13–15mg/kg/d PO.
- Colestyramine 4g PO qds (provide other medication 1h before or 4h after).
- Antihistamines (e.g. chlorphenamine 4mg PO qds).
- There is growing evidence that parenteral opioid antagonists (e.g. naloxone 400µg IV tds) are useful adjuncts for treatment of cholestasis-related pruritus not responsive to first-line measures.

Acholuric jaundice

Jaundice with absence of bilirubin in the urine is caused by either haemo-lysis or a congenital disorder of hepatic conjugation.

Haemolytic jaundice

Plasma bilirubin levels are related to the half-life of circulating erythro-cytes. Haemolytic jaundice is most frequently encountered with the inher-ited haemoglobinopathies, especially during 'crises'. Causes are shown in Box 14.1.
- Ask about a personal or family history of haemolytic anaemia, autoimmune or connective tissue disease.
- Enquire about recent illness and any foreign travel.
- Take a detailed medication history, including over-the-counter, herbal, and traditional remedies.
- Determine whether the patient has recently had a blood transfusion or exposure to blood products.
- Examine for splenomegaly and for evidence of an underlying connective tissue disease.

Patients with inherited haemolytic anaemias are also prone to pigment gallstones, which can obstruct. Those with sickle cell disease may also develop conjugated hyperbilirubinaemia due to hepatic infarction second-ary to microvascular occlusion.

Investigations

If bilirubin alone is abnormal amongst the LFT, determine whether it is pre-dominantly conjugated or unconjugated. If unconjugated, request a reticulo-cyte count and serum haptoglobin. If these are normal, they usually exclude haemolysis severe enough to cause jaundice, and a familial unconjugated hyperbilirubinaemia (e.g. Gilbert's syndrome) is likely. If abnormal, request:

- FBC, serum LDH, and blood film.
- Direct antibody test (Coombs test). Positive result suggests autoimmune haemolytic anaemia.
- Blood cultures, Monospot test, or malaria film, depending on clinical picture.
- Cold agglutinins (surrogate marker for *Mycoplasma* infection).
- Urine haemosiderin concentration. Present if intravascular haemolysis.
- Haematology opinion with the above results.

Hepatic conjugation defects

If the haemolytic screen is negative in a patient with isolated unconju-gated hyperbilirubinaemia, a hepatic conjugation defect is probable. The most common is Gilbert's syndrome, which affects ~5% of the population. Jaundice becomes more prominent on fasting, with intercurrent illness, or physiological stress (particularly infection or surgery), although bilirubin rarely rises >80µmol/L. The diagnosis can be confirmed by observing increased serum bilirubin following a 48h fast (restrict calories to <400/d) or a challenge with nicotinic acid 50mg IV, although these are almost never required clinically. No specific treatment is indicated, and the patient can be reassured that they do not have significant liver disease.

Box 14.1 Causes of haemolytic jaundice

Congenital
- Haemoglobinopathies:
  - Sickle cell disease (HbSS and HbSC genotypes).
  - β-thalassaemia major (jaundice usually trivial in thalassaemia minor).
- Red cell membrane disorders (hereditary spherocytosis, elliptocytosis, ovalocytosis, and stomatocytosis).
- Red cell enzyme defects:
  - Glucose-6-phosphate deficiency (favism).
  - Pyruvate kinase deficiency.

Acquired
- Autoimmune (positive direct antibody test):
  - Warm autoimmune haemolytic anaemia (idiopathic, SLE, haematological malignancy).
  - Cold autoimmune haemolytic anaemia (idiopathic, *Mycoplasma*/ EBV infection, paroxysmal cold haemoglobinuria).
  - Blood transfusion incompatibility reaction (ABO, rhesus, minor antigens).
  - Drug-induced immune-mediated haemolysis (high-dose penicillin, methyldopa).
  - Haemolytic disease of the newborn (rhesus incompatibility).

(Continued)

Box 14.1 *(Continued)*
- Acquired membrane disorders (paroxysmal nocturnal haemoglobinuria).
- Ineffective erythropoeisis (red cell aplasia, B12 deficiency).
- Drug-induced (e.g. sulfasalazine, ribavirin).
- Trauma (particularly shearing from mechanical heart valves).
- Microangiopathic haemolytic anaemia (MAHA):
  - HUS (see 🕮 p. 70).
  - Thrombotic thrombocytopaenic purpura (TTP).
  - DIC.
  - HELLP syndrome (see 🕮 p. 314).
- Infections (particularly malaria).
- Toxins (e.g. snake venom).

The Crigler–Najjar syndrome, which results from defects in the UDP-glucuronosyltransferase enzyme, causes more severe unconjugated hyperbilirubinaemia. The rarer type I is autosomal recessive and presents in neonates, causing kernicterus and death within 1y if not treated early with phototherapy and orthotopic liver transplantation. Type II is more common and benign, with a more complex inheritance pattern (either autosomal dominant with incomplete penetrance or autosomal recessive). Persistent, mild jaundice is usually noticed during childhood but rarely causes clinical problems. If required, phenobarbital reduces serum bilirubin concentrations, and drugs that displace unconjugated bilirubin from albumin (penicillin, salicylates, and sulphonamides) should be avoided.

Conjugated isolated hyperbilirubinaemia

Two familial syndromes of non-haemolytic, conjugated hyperbilirubinaemia in the absence of cholestasis have been recognized. Dubin–Johnson syndrome causes relapsing-remitting jaundice in the absence of pruritus, deranged serum transaminases, or elevated serum bile acids. Scintigraphic studies (e.g. HIDA scan) demonstrate no excretion into the biliary tree, and liver biopsy shows accumulation of black pigment within the parenchyma. No specific treatment is required.

Rotor syndrome is similar but without the histological findings on liver biopsy.

Sepsis

Jaundice is common in the septic patient (see Chapter 17) and may arise through a number of mechanisms. Its evaluation should proceed along the lines described in 'Assessment and causes of jaundice' (see 🕮 p. 208), and management is of the underlying infection. The presence of jaundice does not appear to influence prognosis, and it typically resolves completely once infection is controlled.

Jaundice

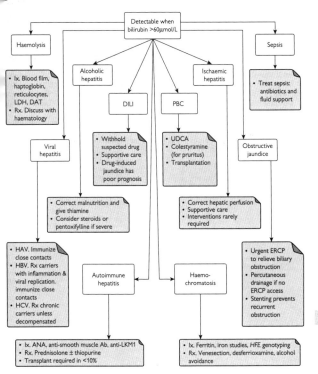

Further reading

Bloom S, Webster G, Marks D (2012) *Oxford Handbook of Gastroenterology and Hepatology, 2e.* Oxford University Press, Oxford.

European Association for the Study of the Liver (2010) EASL Clinical Practice Guidelines for HFE hemochromatosis. *J Hepatol* **53**: 3–22.

European Association for the Study of the Liver (2011) EASL Clinical Practice Guidelines: management of hepatitis C virus infection. *J Hepatol* **55**: 245–64.

European Association for the Study of the Liver (2012) EASL Clinical Practice Guidelines: management of chronic hepatitis B virus infection. *J Hepatol* **57**: 167–85.

Kamal SM, Ismail A, Graham CS, *et al.* (2004) Pegylated interferon alpha therapy in acute hepatitis C: relation to hepatitis C virus-specific T cell response kinetics. *Hepatology* **39**: 1721–31.

Manns MP, Woynarowski M, Kreisel W, *et al.* (2010) Budesonide induces remission more effectively than prednisone in a controlled trial of patients with autoimmune hepatitis. *Gastroenterology* **139**: 1198–206.

Thomas DL, Thio CL, Martin MP, *et al.* (2009) Genetic variation in IL28B and spontaneous clearance of hepatitis C virus. *Nature* **461**: 798–801.

Whitfield K, Rambaldi A, Wettersley J, *et al.* (2009) Pentoxifylline for alcoholic hepatitis. *Cochrane Database Syst Rev* **4**: CD007339.

Acute liver failure

⦿ Definitions of acute liver failure

Acute liver failure (ALF) is defined as potentially reversible severe liver injury with impaired synthetic function (INR >1.5) and hepatic encephalopathy, developing within 28d from the onset of jaundice, in the absence of pre-existing liver disease or with well-compensated chronic liver disease (O'Grady et al., 1993). Progression can be very rapid (see Table 15.1): one-third of patients die within 3wk and about one-third require liver transplantation. Approximately two-thirds of patients survive without transplant following paracetamol overdose, whereas only ~25% do so following liver failure due to other drug reactions (Ostapowicz et al., 2002).

Table 15.1 Characteristics of hyperacute, acute, and subacute liver failure

	Hyperacute	Acute	Subacute
Jaundice to encephalopathy (wk)	0–1	1–4	4–12
Increase in INR	Marked	Moderate	Mild to moderate
Severity of jaundice	Moderate	Moderate	Severe
Intracranial hypertension	Severe	Moderate	May occur
Survival without liver transplantation	Good	Moderate	Fair
Typical causes	Paracetamol, HAV, HEV	HBV	Non-paracetamol DILI

Reprinted from The Lancet, 376, 9736, Bernal et al., 'Acute liver failure', pp. 190–201, Copyright 2010, with permission from Elsevier.

Aetiology

Causes of acute liver failure in the UK include:
- Drug-induced hepatitis (68%):
  - Paracetamol overdose.
  - See Chapters 14 and 18 for other causes of DILI.
- Viral hepatitis (9%) (see Chapter 14).
- Toxins (2%):
  - *Amanita phalloides*.
  - Herbal remedies, khat (see Chapter 19).
- Malignancy (1%):
  - Lymphoma.
  - Malignant infiltration. Often associated with high ALP.
- Vascular (1%):
  - Budd–Chiari syndrome.
  - Veno-occlusive disease.
  - Ischaemic hepatitis.

- Miscellaneous (2%):
  - Wilson's disease. Not strictly acute as many patients are cirrhotic, but similar in other clinical respects.
  - Autoimmune hepatitis.
  - Malignant hyperthermia (including secondary to the drug 'ecstasy').
  - Pregnancy-related liver disease (see Chapter 19).
  - Reye's syndrome.
- Unknown (17%).

Presentation

History

Ask specifically about:
- Recent viral illnesses.
- Paracetamol.
- Alcohol and drug history.
- Travel history and vaccinations.
- Abdominal pain, vomiting.

Examination

Often presents with a complication of liver failure:
- Signs of chronic liver disease suggest 'acute-on-chronic' liver failure (see 📖 p. 244).
- Splenomegaly rare but occurs with Wilson's disease, autoimmune hepatitis, and lymphoma.
- Paracetamol overdose causes severe abdominal pain and retching.

Investigation

- Blood tests on admission:
  - Viral serology: HAV IgM, HBsAg, HBcAb IgM, delta virus if HBsAg-positive, HEV IgM, EBV, CMV, HSV, HIV.
  - Blood ammonia level (arterial or venous drawn without tourniquet).
  - Drug screen (especially paracetamol).
  - Plasma caeruloplasmin and copper.
  - G & S/cross-match.
- Blood tests on admission and daily thereafter:
  - FBC, U & Es, LFTs, coagulation screen, calcium, PO_4^{3-}.
  - Glucose (with additional bedside testing every 2h).
  - ABG (including lactate).
- Bacteriology (even if afebrile):
  - Blood, urine, and sputum cultures.
  - Throat and vaginal swabs.
- Imaging:
  - US liver. Assess liver parenchyma, spleen size, adenopathy (lymphoma), hepatic and portal vein patency. A nodular liver on

US is often seen in subacute failure and frequently incorrectly diagnosed as chronic liver disease.

- CT brain (to exclude other causes of obtundation).
- CXR (on admission and daily). To look for chest infection and ARDS.

• ECG.

• Pregnancy test in all women of childbearing potential.

• EEG. Helpful in assessment of hepatic encephalopathy (slow, high-amplitude delta waves).

• Liver biopsy. If suspected lymphoma, malignancy, or atypical presentation.

Initial management

• *It is **vital** to discuss all cases of severe liver injury with the regional transplant centre.* Have a low threshold to transfer the patient *before* significant deterioration, as GCS at admission to the liver unit is related to survival.

• Transfer as soon as possible if a patient fulfils criteria for liver transplantation (see 'King's College criteria', p. 246); delay can result in death as >48h needed to source adequate graft. Any patient with hepatic encephalopathy should be sedated, intubated, and ventilated prior to transfer.

• All patients should be admitted to HDU or ITU. Nurse supine and keep patient in a peaceful environment, which minimizes increases in intracranial pressure (ICP).

• The causes of ALF do not respond well to medical therapy; treatment is supportive until the acute insult resolves. Only orthotopic liver transplantation has been proven to increase survival, with >80% of patients alive at 1y.

• Patients are usually dehydrated on admission. Rehydrate, using crystalloid (e.g. Hartmann's, which provides less renal Cl$^-$ load than saline, thus reducing risk of hyperchloraemic metabolic acidosis), colloid (e.g. Gelofusine®), or 4.5% human albumin solution (HAS). Avoid 5% glucose, as risk of causing hyponatraemia and cerebral oedema.

• Place urinary, central venous, and arterial catheters, unless patient responds rapidly to fluid challenge. Reassess fluid balance, keeping CVP 6–10cm above mid-axillary point with colloid, HAS, or blood. Use of vascular monitoring technologies (e.g. PiCCO/LiDCO) or oesophageal Doppler in ITU setting allows more accurate assessment of haemodynamic status and cardiac output, and optimization of filling pressures. Avoid over-hydration, which increases ICP. Pay strict attention to aseptic insertion of any intravascular device and ensure meticulous line care.

• Provide oxygen by mask if SaO$_2$ <90%. Ventilate if grade 3 or 4 encephalopathy. Avoid ET tube ties, which compress the internal jugular veins.

- Start prophylactic antibiotics and antifungals (e.g. cefotaxime 2g IV od and fluconazole 200mg IV od) if at least grade 2 encephalopathy, systemic inflammatory response syndrome (SIRS; see Box 15.1), or refractory hypotension. Reduce doses if GFR <30mL/min. Avoid nephrotoxic antibiotics (e.g. aminoglycosides).
- If encephalopathy is grade 1, 2, or 3, and there is no ileus, provide lactulose 10–15mL PO qds (avoid NGT in conscious patients to avoid gagging, which can raise ICP).
- Stop all hepatotoxic medications (e.g. NSAIDs) and those that worsen complications (e.g. ACE inhibitors, opioids).
- Correct electrolyte abnormalities (if required, monitor serum levels 8–12 hourly):
  - If serum Na^+ <120mmol/L, replace with crystalloid or colloid rather than fluid restrict (otherwise, hepatorenal syndrome may develop).
  - Correct hypokalaemia (add 40mmol KCl to each litre of fluid).
  - Correct hypophosphataemia. If PO_4^{3-} <0.4mmol/L, give 25–50 mmol/L IV phosphate Polyfusor® over 12–24h via a dedicated large bore peripheral cannula, then recheck levels. Provide 40–80 mmol in divided doses over 24h if PO_4^{3-} between 0.4–0.7mmol/L. Hypophosphataemia is more common with paracetamol poisoning.
  - Hyperphosphataemia in paracetamol overdose also carries prognostic significance, with worse outcomes if PO_4^{3-} >1.0mmol/L.
  - Respiratory alkalosis is common early in illness. Lactic acidosis is often present early, when it may rapidly correct with volume replacement. Where it persists or develops later, it carries a poor prognosis.
- Keep blood glucose >3.5mmol/L with continuous 10–20% glucose infusion.
- Give vitamin K 10mg IV as a single dose (usually has no effect on INR). Maintain platelets >20 × 10^9/L with transfusions.
- Prescribe ranitidine 50mg IV tds to prevent stress ulceration.

Box 15.1 Systemic inflammatory response syndrome (SIRS)

At least two of:
- Temperature >38.5°C or <35°C.
- HR >90/min.
- RR >20/min or $PaCO_2$ <32mmHg.
- WCC >12 × 10^9/L or <4 × 10^9/L, or >10% immature (band) forms.

Data from R.C. Bone et al., 'Definitions for sepsis and organ failure and guidelines for the use of innovative therapies in sepsis. The ACCP/SCCM Consensus Conference Committee. American College of Chest Physicians/Society of Critical Care Medicine', Chest, 101, 6, pp. 1644–1655, 1992, American College of Chest Physicians.

Subsequent management

- Progression of hepatic encephalopathy may be rapid, especially with hyperacute or acute presentations, resulting in rapid loss of airway control.
- Intracranial hypertension due to cerebral oedema may occur abruptly. Cerebral oedema develops in 75% of patients with grade 4 encephalopathy and overall accounts for 20–25% of deaths, although the incidence is decreasing:
  - Nursing staff should examine the pupils every 30min and look for spikes of hypertension and disconjugate eye movements. Papilloedema is rare.
  - Unless treated, raised ICP progresses to decerebrate posturing (back, arms and legs rigid; hands in flexion; opisthotonus) and brainstem coning.
  - ICP monitoring is used in >50% centres to guide therapy; epidural catheters have a low complication rate (4%) and so are most widely used. Place if worsening grade 3 or 4 encephalopathy. Aim to keep ICP <20mmHg and cerebral perfusion pressure (MAP minus ICP) >50mmHg.
  - If ICP >20mmHg or worsening encephalopathy, provide 20% mannitol (100mL as slow IV injection qds PRN for a 70kg patient). This may cause fluid overload and is less effective if renal failure (in which case remove 3–5 times the volume of mannitol infused by haemofiltration). Hypertonic 3% saline 500mL IV, or 10–20mL boluses of 30% saline, to maintain serum Na^+ at 145–150mmol/L are alternatives. Pentobarbital induced coma may be required.
  - There is no role for hyperventilation (compromises cerebral blood flow). Indometacin 25mg IV over 1min can acutely depress ICP. N-acetylcysteine (NAC) is second-line treatment.
  - Moderate hypothermia (to 32–34°C) can reduce ICP by modulating cerebral blood flow.
  - If hypertensive, treat by reducing raised ICP with mannitol (anti-hypertensives can cause coning).
  - Anti-epileptics are safe.
- Perform short Synacthen® test if persistent hypotension or need for vasopressor use (adrenal insufficiency is common).
- Provide nutrition. Request urgent dietetic review for parenteral feeding if ileus or grade 3/4 encephalopathy. Those with milder disease can be fed with low-protein, high-calorie feeds. Instigate within 24h if patients malnourished (see Chapter 10).
- NAC provided for 72h with a loading dose regime has been shown in one report to be effective in mild encephalopathy from non-paracetamol acute liver injury, with 40% vs 27% transplant-free survival.
- Specific management strategies have been used in certain settings (see also Chapter 14):
  - Anti-viral therapy in acute HBV infection.
  - Aciclovir IV in acute herpes virus infection.

- Activated charcoal and forced diuresis following *Amanita phalloides* mushroom poisoning. There is some evidence for high-dose benzylpenicillin ± silibinin 20–50mg/kg/d IV (prevents uptake of toxin by undamaged hepatocytes).
- TIPS, surgical decompression, or thrombolysis in acute Budd–Chiari syndrome.
- Steroids can be used in autoimmune hepatitis, although often the presentation is too late for them to be effective.
- Wilson's disease (see 📖 p. 243).
- Expedite delivery for ALF due to acute fatty liver of pregnancy or HELLP syndrome.
- ALF due to malignant infiltration has a dismal prognosis, although occasional patients with lymphomatous/leukaemic infiltration survive and then undergo successful chemotherapy. The majority are haematological malignancies, although metastatic breast, colon, gastric, and small cell lung carcinomas are also seen. Massive cytokine release is often the cause of ALF, especially with haematological malignancy, rather than tumour burden; HBV re-activation may also occur following chemotherapy. It is important to establish the diagnosis to prevent inappropriate listing for transplantation, and transjugular liver biopsy may be required. Malignant infiltration rarely causes cerebral oedema; jaundice is milder and hepatomegaly more common; splenomegaly occurs with leukaemia/lymphoma. Transaminases can be raised up to 100-fold.
- Artificial hepatic assist devices (e.g. MARS) are used in some clinical trial centres.
- Auxillary liver transplantation has been used to allow the native liver to regenerate, obviating the need for long-term immunosuppression. Xenotransplantation (using porcine liver) has been used occasionally, with the longest reported graft survival being 9mo.

Markers of disease severity

The main prognostic factors for survival are degree of encephalopathy (see 📖 p. 245), patient age (prognosis worse if <10y or >40y), cause of ALF (better prognosis with paracetamol, HAV, and HBV), and INR. As ALF progresses, the following problems can be encountered:
- Cerebral. Cushing's triad indicates cerebral oedema (spikes of systolic hypertension, bradycardia, and irregular respirations). Control seizures with low-dose benzodiazepines and phenytoin.
- Circulatory. Falling diastolic BP (vasodilated hyperdynamic circulation). Provide vasopressors/inotropic agents (noradrenaline as the primary vasopressor) if cardiac index <3.5L/min/m^2 despite apparent euvolaemia, aiming for MAP of 65–80mmHg.
- Respiratory. Non-cardiogenic pulmonary oedema occurs in ~10%. Assisted ventilation may be required, but avoid high positive end expiratory pressures, which can elevate ICP.

- Renal:
  - Dysfunction occurs in ~70% cases of paracetamol-induced ALF (~40% with other aetiologies). Mostly due to acute tubular necrosis. Avoid terlipressin in these individuals as effects unpredictable; instead seek early renal support for haemofiltration (not haemodialysis).
  - Progressive renal dysfunction can also result from type 1 hepatorenal syndrome (see Box 15.2). If present, terlipressin 2g IV qds and 4.5% HAS IV enhance renal perfusion. Preliminary reports suggest benefit providing 7.5–12.5mg tds midodrine and 100–200µg octreotide SC tds, or noradrenaline and albumin IV; both titrated to raise MAP >15mmHg. Seek early renal support with haemofiltration.
  - Less common causes include glomerulonephritis with HBV/HCV, drug-related nephrotoxicity, or direct kidney injury in leptospirosis.
  - Prognosis is grave if severe, therefore, proactively try to prevent by optimizing MAP, avoiding nephrotoxins, and treating sepsis early. Note rise in urea attenuated as liver production will have reduced.

Box 15.2 Hepatorenal syndrome

Diagnose if:
- Acute or chronic liver disease with hepatic failure.
- Creatinine >200µmol/L, or creatinine clearance <40mL/min.
- No sustained improvement with 1.5L volume expansion.
- Proteinuria <0.5g/d.
- Normal renal tract US.
- Other causes of renal impairment excluded.

- Coagulopathy. Increasing INR and low-grade DIC. Do not correct coagulopathy (factor concentrates can precipitate DIC and worsen cerebral oedema), unless necessary for an invasive procedure or significant bleeding (occurs in 5%, usually GI). Give platelet support if thrombocytopaenic and bleeding. Recombinant factor VIIα (40µg/kg IV bolus) has been used before invasive procedures if FFP contraindicated.
- Sepsis. Bacterial and fungal infections (septicaemia, pneumonia, peritonitis, UTIs, line infection) are more frequent due to impaired immune function and need for multiple invasive procedures. May be difficult to diagnose as usual clinical signs of infection can be absent. Suspect if worsening encephalopathy or kidney injury. Low threshold for culturing blood, urine, and sputum; obtaining repeat CXR; and performing diagnostic paracentesis if ascites present. Sepsis retards hepatic regeneration and reduces the rate of successful liver transplantation.

☺ Paracetamol overdose

The management of ALF applies to all causes of liver failure, including that caused by paracetamol. For the general management of paracetamol overdose, see 📖 p. 296. The following additional points apply to its management in the context of ALF:

- Causes 57% of ALF in the UK, 39% in the USA, but is rare in some countries (Germany 15%, India 0%).
- NAC may be beneficial for up to 48h following overdose. Early randomized trials suggested reductions in mortality from late administration of NAC. Intervention studies showed improvements in systemic and cerebral haemodynamics and oxygen uptake.

☺ Acute presentations of Wilson's disease

Wilson's disease is an autosomal recessive disorder, occurring in 1/30,000 individuals. Mutations in the *ATP7A* gene, encoding Wilson's disease protein (WDP), reduce excretion of copper in bile, resulting in its retention in the liver. Disease may present between the ages of 3–40y. Liver disease is the most common presentation in childhood; neuropsychiatric presentations are more usual in adolescence and early adulthood.

The diagnosis is rarely made unless actively considered, and unexplained liver disease in a young person with Coombs-negative haemolytic anaemia should raise suspicion (presenting feature in ~10% of patients).

- LFTs are non-specific, but ALT usually <1,500IU/L and ALP low.
- Coagulopathy tends to be non-responsive to vitamin K.
- May have rapidly progressive renal failure.
- Perform slit lamp examination for Kayser–Fleischer rings (but note can also be seen in other cholestatic disorders).
- Plasma caeruloplasmin is <200mg/L in 85%. Note that caeruloplasmin is an acute phase reactant and hence may be falsely normal in Wilson's disease if coexistent acute inflammatory response. May also be low in chronic liver disease of any aetiology due to reduced synthesis, though concentration <100mg/L is diagnostic of Wilson's disease.
- Serum copper is >200μg/L in untreated cases.
- 24h urinary copper >1.6μmol/L (100 μg) is suggestive of Wilson's disease, but a level 40–100μg does not exclude the diagnosis; levels >3μmol/L are seen in 65%. Penicillamine challenge is not recommended for diagnosis of Wilson's disease in adults.
- Liver biopsy shows hepatic copper >250μg/g dry weight (normal <50μg/g).
- Genetic analysis is diagnostic, although the three most common mutations in the UK account for only 30% of patients.
- For EASL guidelines, see Clinical Practice Guidelines (2012).

If Wilson's disease is suspected, liaise with haematology to perform plasma exchange with FFP replacement to reduce copper concentration by up to 12mg per session. Despite this being preferable to haemofiltration or dialysis, most patients require liver transplantation. Oral D-penicillamine 750–1,500mg/d + pyridoxine 25mg/d remove up to 2mg copper daily and should be provided once ALF has resolved/post-transplantation. Trientine 300mg tds is an alternative, and zinc 150–300mg/d may be used for maintenance. Avoid foods with high copper content (chocolate, shellfish). Family members must undergo screening.

① **Acute-on-chronic liver failure**

Patients with cirrhosis and chronic liver disease may present with acute decompensation due to a variety of causes (see Chapter 16), but bacterial infection is the most common.

Clinical features

Patients usually have signs of chronic liver disease. Examine specifically for features of hepatic decompensation: encephalopathy (confusion, asterixis), ascites, oedema, jaundice, and fever.

Investigations

Assuming that the cause of liver disease is known, the most important aspect of investigation is multiple cultures, looking for any evidence of infection. The main causes of acute decompensation are:

• Intercurrent infection, especially SBP.
• GI haemorrhage/hypovolaemia.
• Hypoxia.
• Hypoglycaemia.
• Drugs, particularly sedatives, narcotics, and diuretics.
• Hepatotoxic insult, particularly alcohol and paracetamol overdose (as little as 4g/d in regular alcohol users or those taking cytochrome P450 inducers).
• Metabolic, including electrolyte disturbance.
• Constipation.
• Major surgery.
• Rarely hepatoma, or hepatic or portal vein thrombosis.

Management

As for patients with ALF, the mainstay of treatment is supportive. The decision on how aggressively to manage the patient (i.e. admission to ITU and invasive monitoring) depends on the previous diagnosis, whether there is a reversible element to the acute insult, and whether the patient is a candidate for liver transplantation. If this is the first presentation of liver failure, manage aggressively initially but, for the sake of dignity, it is important to stop escalating treatment if prognosis is very poor. Start 'blind' antimicrobial treatment (as outlined in 'Initial management' (see 📖 p. 238) if there is fever, increased WCC, or a high CRP, then tailor according to culture results.

☤ Hepatic encephalopathy

Neuropsychiatric disturbance in patients with acute or acute-on-chronic liver disease. May initially present with subtle changes in awareness or attention span ('lone hepatic encephalopathy'), without the severe features that complicate ALF. Believed to be caused by cerebral ammonia derived from the gut lumen. Features are listed in Table 15.2. If the diagnosis is unclear, encephalopathy can be confirmed by EEG (slow, high-amplitude delta waves), psychometric tests, and measurement of blood ammonia concentration. In subacute liver failure, modest hepatic encephalopathy is a sign of poor outcome.

Table 15.2 Grading of hepatic encephalopathy

Grade	Clinical features
1	Drowsy but coherent, mood change, constructional dyspraxia (70%)
2	Drowsy, confused at times, inappropriate behaviour, asterixis (70%)
3	Stuporose but rousable, alternatively restless or screaming (50%)
4	Comatose (<20%)

Overall survival rates in ALF shown in brackets.

Management

- Identify causes if suspected chronic liver disease.
- Screen for causes of decompensation (see 'Aetiology', 📖 p. 236).
- Usually precipitated by (subclinical) sepsis: screen and have low threshold to treat presumed bacterial infection.
- Give 20mL lactulose PO qds: poorly absorbed in the small bowel, digested and fermented in the large bowel, lowering faecal pH, and increasing *Lactobacilli* species. Titrate to obtain 2–3 soft stools/d.
  - Place ET tube to protect airway in those with advanced encephalopathy prior to oral/NG administration.
  - Lactulose enemas can be given if NBM.
  - An alternative is lactitol ~60g/d, which is more palatable with fewer side effects.
  - Ornithine aspartate 20g IV od over 4h is an alternative if NBM.
  - Sodium benzoate 10g/d PO improves ammonia clearance by increasing nitrogen excretion and can be used with lactulose.
  - Conversion of ammonia to urea is zinc-dependent, and zinc acetate 600mg od has been shown to improve encephalopathy compared to placebo.
- Avidly correct hypokalaemia, which worsens encephalopathy.
- Ensure adequate calorie intake, orally once encephalopathy improving. Do not recommend dietary protein restriction; these patients are often malnourished and catabolic. Maintain protein intake at 1–1.5g/kg/d.

- Rifaximin (a non-systemic antibiotic) 400mg PO tds or 550mg PO bd has largely replaced neomycin 500mg PO tds (the latter also potentially nephrotoxic though systemic absorption very small).
- Phosphate enemas twice daily help purge the large bowel. Most useful after an acute protein load (e.g. GI bleeding).

Criteria for emergency liver transplantation

King's College criteria for selection of recipients for emergency liver transplants

The King's College criteria are the most established, and have positive and negative predictive value for mortality of 88% and 65%, respectively.

Paracetamol overdose
- Arterial pH <7.3 following adequate volume resuscitation, or
- Combination of:
  - Encephalopathy > grade 3.
  - Creatinine >300μmol/L.
  - INR >6.5 (PTT >100s).

Non-paracetamol overdose
- Any grade encephalopathy and INR >6·5 (PTT >100s), or.
- Three of:
  - INR >3·5 (PTT >50s).
  - Bilirubin >300μmol/L.
  - Age <10y or >40y.
  - Unfavourable cause (DILI, non-A non-B hepatitis).
  - Jaundice >7d pre-encephalopathy.

This criteria was published in *Gastroenterology*, 97, 2, John G O'Grady et al., 'Early indicators of prognosis in fulminant hepatic failure', pp. 439–445, Copyright American Gastroenterological Association, 1989.

UK criteria for registration for emergency liver transplantation in adults

As treatments have improved, the King's College criteria have been superseded by the following:

Paracetamol overdose
The sensitivity of the King's College criteria has been enhanced by accepting two out of the following three criteria alongside evidence of deterioration (e.g. increased ICP, increased FiO_2 requirements, increasing inotropic requirements in the absence of sepsis):
- Arterial pH <7.25 after fluid resuscitation (lower pH threshold reflects better ITU care and earlier use of CVVHF).
- Lactate >3.5mmol/L on admission or >3.0mmol/L after fluid resuscitation (at least 24h after overdose). Discriminates survivors at an early time point.

- Coexisting INR >6.5 (PTT >100s), serum creatinine >300µmol/L, and grade 3–4 encephalopathy.

Non-paracetamol overdose
- Seronegative hepatitis, HAV, HBV, or idiosyncratic drug reaction with INR >6.5 (PTT >100s) and any grade of encephalopathy.
- Seronegative hepatitis, HAV, HBV, or idiosyncratic drug reaction with any three of the following:
  - INR >3.5 (PTT >50s).
  - Jaundice to encephalopathy time >7d.
  - Serum bilirubin >300µmol/L.
  - Age >40y.
- Acute presentation of Wilson's disease or Budd–Chiari syndrome with both coagulopathy and encephalopathy.
- Post-liver transplantation with:
  - Hepatic artery thrombosis within 21d.
  - Graft dysfunction within 7d (two of: AST >10,000IU/L, INR >3, lactate >3mmol/L, or no bile production).
  - ALF after live liver donation.

Acute liver failure

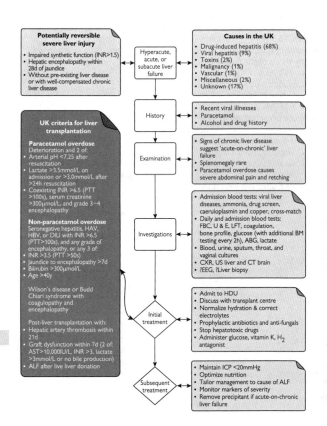

Potentially reversible severe liver injury
- Impaired synthetic function (INR>1.5)
- Hepatic encephalopathy within 28d of jaundice
- Without pre-existing liver disease or with well-compensated chronic liver disease

Hyperacute, acute, or subacute liver failure

Causes in the UK
- Drug-induced hepatitis (68%)
- Viral hepatitis (9%)
- Toxins (2%)
- Malignancy (1%)
- Vascular (1%)
- Miscellaneous (2%)
- Unknown (17%)

History
- Recent viral illnesses
- Paracetamol
- Alcohol and drug history

UK criteria for liver transplantation

Paracetamol overdose
Deterioration and 2 of:
- Arterial pH <7.25 after resuscitation
- Lactate >3.5mmol/L on admission or >3.0mmol/L after >24h resuscitation
- Coexisting INR >6.5 (PTT >100s), serum creatinine >300μmol/L, and grade 3–4 encephalopathy

Non-paracetamol overdose
Seronegative hepatitis, HAV, HBV, or DILI with INR >6.5 (PTT>100s), and any grade of encephalopathy, or any 3 of:
- INR >3.5 (PTT >50s)
- Jaundice to encephalopathy >7d
- Bilirubin >300μmol/L
- Age >40y

Wilson's disease or Budd Chiari syndrome with coagulopathy and encephalopathy

Post-liver transplantation with:
- Hepatic artery thrombosis within 21d
- Graft dysfunction within 7d (2 of: AST>10,000IU/L, INR >3, lactate >3mmol/L or no bile production)
- ALF after live liver donation

Examination
- Signs of chronic liver disease suggest 'acute-on-chronic' liver failure
- Splenomegaly rare
- Paracetamol overdose causes severe abdominal pain and retching

Investigations
- Admission blood tests: viral liver diseases, ammonia, drug screen, caeruloplasmin and copper, cross-match
- Daily and admission blood tests: FBC, U & E, LFT, coagulation, bone profile, glucose (with additional BM testing every 2h), ABG, lactate
- Blood, urine, sputum, throat, and vaginal cultures
- CXR, US liver and CT brain
- ?EEG, ?Liver biopsy

Initial treatment
- Admit to HDU
- Discuss with transplant centre
- Normalize hydration & correct electrolytes
- Prophylactic antibiotics and anti-fungals
- Stop hepatotoxic drugs
- Administer glucose, vitamin K, H_2 antagonist

Subsequent treatment
- Maintain ICP <20mmHg
- Optimize nutrition
- Tailor management to cause of ALF
- Monitor markers of severity
- Remove precipitant if acute-on-chronic liver failure

Further reading

Bernal W, Auzinger G, Dhawan A, et al. (2010) Acute liver failure. *Lancet* **376**: 190–201.

European Association for the Study of the Liver (2012) EASL Clinical Practice Guidelines: Wilson's disease. *J Hepatol* **56**: 671–85.

O'Grady JG, Schalm SW, Williams R (1993) Acute liver failure: redefining the syndromes. *Lancet* **342**: 273–5.

Ostapowicz G, Fontana RJ, Schiødt FV, et al. (2002) Results of a prospective study of acute liver failure at 17 tertiary care centers in the United States. *Ann Intern Med* **137**: 947–54.

Complications of cirrhosis and portal hypertension

① Causes and diagnosis of cirrhosis

Cirrhosis occurs following progressive hepatic fibrosis, with architectural distortion of the liver and nodule formation. It is a histological diagnosis. Late-stage cirrhosis is irreversible, at which point only liver transplantation is curative. Early-stage cirrhosis has been shown to improve following treatment and may be asymptomatic.

Decompensated cirrhosis is defined by the occurrence of serious complications, the prevention and treatment of which improve the morbidity and mortality associated with cirrhosis. Causes of decompensation are detailed in Box 16.1. Complications include:

- Ascites ± SBP.
- Hepatorenal syndrome.
- Variceal haemorrhage.
- Hepatic encephalopathy.
- Hepatopulmonary syndromes.
- HCC.

Box 16.1 Causes of decompensation of cirrhosis

- Progression of disease.
- Additional liver insult (e.g. alcohol, viral hepatitis).
- Acute upper GI bleed.
- Infection (particularly SBP).
- Dehydration.
- Constipation, including drug-induced (e.g. opiates).
- Portal vein thrombosis.
- Transformation to HCC.
- Increased portosystemic shunting (post-TIPS).

Aetiology

See Chapters 14 and 15, and Table 16.2. Despite extensive investigation, the cause remains uncertain in ~10% (termed cryptogenic cirrhosis), many of whom will have had unrecognized NASH.

History

Ask about:

- Fatigue, bruising, peripheral oedema, weight loss, pruritus, increasing abdominal girth, confusion, and sleep disturbance.
- Alcohol intake. It is estimated to require an average intake of 8U daily for 10y to develop cirrhosis.
- Personal or family history of hepatitis.
- IV drug use, blood transfusions, piercings, and tattoos.
- Sexual history.
- Previous obesity or diabetes mellitus.
- Presence of autoimmune diseases (including IBD, rheumatoid arthritis, and thyroid disease).
- Associated arthropathy and symptoms of hypogonadism in suspected haemochromatosis, COPD in suspected A1AT deficiency, and palpable purpura from type II cryoglobulinaemia in suspected HCV.

Examination

Look for:
- Jaundice.
- Hepatomegaly and splenomegaly.
- Stigmata of chronic liver disease: spider naevi; palmar erythema; Dupuytren's contracture; caput medusae (in which recanalization of the umbilical vein allows high-pressure portal flow to drain into abdominal wall veins, making them more prominent); muscle wasting; clubbing; Muehrcke's and Terry's nail changes (associated with hypoalbuminaemia); and, in males, gynaecomastia, feminizing hair distribution, and testicular atrophy.
- Parotid enlargement occurs in alcoholics.
- Ascites is often present, suggested by flank dullness (likelihood ratio for cirrhosis ≈ 7.2), although >1.5L is needed to detect clinically.
- Asterixis (bilateral, asynchronous flapping of outstretched, dorsiflexed hands) suggests encephalopathy.
- Kayser–Fleischer rings are present in ~50% patients with Wilson's disease but are usually only seen by slit-lamp examination.

Investigation

Blood tests

Request FBC, U & E, LFT, INR, and glucose (15–30% of cirrhotic patients have diabetes mellitus). The Bonacini discriminant score (see Table 16.1) can be used to indicate whether a patient is likely to have significant fibrosis: summated score <3 suggests mild fibrosis, whereas cirrhosis is present in 98% of patients with a score >7.

Table 16.1 Bonacini discriminant score

Score	0	1	2	3	4	5	6
Platelet count	>340	280–340	220–279	160–219	100–159	40–99	<40
ALT:AST ratio	>1.7	1.2–1.7	0.6–1.19	<0.6			
INR	<1.1	1.1–1.4	>1.4				

Adapted with permission from Macmillan Publishers Ltd: The American Journal of Gastroenterology, Bonacini et al., 'Utility of a discriminant score for diagnosing advanced fibrosis or cirrhosis in patients with chronic hepatitis C virus infection', 92, 8, pp. 1302, copyright 1997.

- Patients usually have hypoalbuminaemia due to reduced hepatic synthesis and poor nutrition. Exclude nephrotic syndrome and protein-losing enteropathy (see Chapter 10) if clinically indicated.
- The transaminases may provide a clue to aetiology but can be normal. Thus, alcoholic liver disease always has serum transaminases <400IU/L, often with AST > ALT. Suspect concomitant alcoholic hepatitis if transaminitis occurs with fever, jaundice, and anorexia (see 🕮 p. 221). High serum transaminases (>400IU/L) or ALT > AST suggest another cause (although the ratio can then reverse, as chronic hepatitis progresses to cirrhosis).
- High ALP (>3 × ULN) is common in PSC and PBC.
- Rising bilirubin suggests progressive cirrhosis and is related to prognosis in PBC.

- A very high γGT (out of proportion to the ALP) suggests alcoholic liver or biliary disease.
- PTT/INR reflects liver synthetic function.
- Thrombocytopaenia is the most common haematological abnormality. Leukopaenia and anaemia develop later, although anaemia may occur due to other reasons (GI bleeding, bone marrow suppression).
- *De novo* presentations should have a 'liver database' checked (see Table 16.2).

Table 16.2 Specific testing for common causes of cirrhosis

Cause	Tests
Alcohol	History, AST/ALT >2, γGT
Chronic HBV	HBsAg, αHBc Ab, HBeAg, HBV DNA
Chronic HCV	HCV antibody, HCV RNA
PBC	AMA, raised IgM, hyperlipidaemia
PSC	History of UC in 75%, MRCP/ERCP, stricture brushings
Autoimmune hepatitis	Raised IgG, ANA, smooth muscle Ab, anti-LKM1
Haemochromatosis	Iron studies, genotype
Wilson's disease	Caeruloplasmin, copper, liver biopsy
A1AT deficiency	A1AT level, phenotype studies if low
NASH	Hepatic imaging, liver biopsy
Chronic right heart failure	History, echocardiogram

Imaging

Radiography is used to detect complications of cirrhosis but is not accurate enough to (confidently) confirm its presence.

- Request an abdominal US, which often demonstrates a small, nodular liver with hypertrophy of the caudate and left lobes. Increased portal vein diameter, recanalization of the umbilical vein, or splenomegaly suggests portal hypertension.
- Ask for Doppler US to confirm portal and hepatic vein patency.
- Liver fibrosis is associated with increased stiffness, which can be assessed by sonographic techniques (e.g. FibroScan®) or elastography. These are accurate for advanced, but not mild, fibrosis.
- Use contrast-enhanced MR to characterize hepatic masses seen on US and to estimate the degree of iron overload in haemochromatosis.
- Liver biopsy is the gold standard for diagnosing cirrhosis (see Chapter 13). This should be performed if the diagnosis is unclear; use transjugular approach if the patient has coagulopathy or ascites. Have a lower threshold to request liver biopsy if metabolic causes are suspected (haemochromatosis, Wilson's disease, A1AT deficiency, NASH), especially if there is a family history of early-onset cirrhosis.
- Bone densitometry should be performed due to frequent association with osteoporosis.

Treatment

Treatment may be specific (see Table 16.3) or supportive. Supportive treatment comprises the following:

- Check serum antibody levels (HAV, HBV, pneumococcus, VZV). Vaccinate patients with chronic liver disease, as they are susceptible to infection. Ideally, do this prior to starting any immunosuppressant therapy. Recommend annual influenza vaccine.
- Advise abstinence from alcohol, especially in those with viral liver disease, and avoid >2g/d of paracetamol.
- Reducing portal pressure with non-selective β-blockade (see 📖 p. 17).
- Variceal banding or TIPS following index variceal bleed (see 📖 p. 16).
- Nutritional monitoring via dietetic services.
- Management of moderate ascites with paracentesis and diuretics.
- Treatment of encephalopathy (see 📖 p. 267).
- Biannual surveillance for hepatoma (see 📖 p. 270).
- Liver transplantation is the definitive treatment for end-stage cirrhosis and required in the minority. Only performed in ~650 patients/y in the UK, with no increase in frequency over the past 5y. Many patients are not eligible due to alcohol recidivism.

Prognosis

The Child–Turcotte score was designed to assess the risk of portocaval shunt surgery in cirrhotics, from which derives the modified Child–Pugh classification that is widely used today (see Tables 16.4 and 16.5).

Table 16.3 Specific treatments for common causes of cirrhosis

Cause	Treatment
Alcohol	Avoidance ± detoxification, vitamin B supplementation, nutrition
Chronic HBV	Anti-viral therapy (see Chapter 14). Vaccinate sexual partners and first-degree relatives
Chronic HCV	Anti-viral therapy if compensated cirrhosis
PBC	Colestyramine, antihistamines, UDCA 15mg/kg/d PO in divided doses, naltrexone, rifampicin, or colesevelam for pruritus (latter increases fat-soluble vitamin malabsorption), calcium/vitamin D as per serum levels ± bisphosphonate for metabolic bone disease, vitamin A 15,000U/d PO, vitamin K if INR prolonged, thyroxine if TSH raised
PSC	Dilate/stent dominant obstructing strictures. Potential role for prophylactic antibiotics

(Continued)

Table 16.3 (Continued)

Cause	Treatment
Autoimmune hepatitis	Treat if transaminases >10× ULN (>2× ULN if other adverse features), significant hepatitis or necrosis, or disease arises in children. Start prednisolone 60mg PO od and reduce by 10mg weekly to 20mg PO od, and continue for at least 3mo. Then add azathioprine 50mg PO od if TPMT level normal, and reduce prednisolone to 10mg PO od until remission. Survival at 10y independent of diagnosis of cirrhosis if treated (i.e. cirrhotics do well on treatment).
Haemochromatosis	Venesection decreases non-hepatic complications. Can reduce portal pressure and varices. Reduces hepatic fibrosis (but probably not cirrhosis).
Wilson's disease	Penicillamine, trientine, or zinc chelation. Plasmapheresis or transplant if ALF (see 📖 p. 243)
A1AT deficiency	Stop smoking, human α1-antiprotease IV, prompt treatment of chest infections
NASH	Correct obesity and hyperlipidaemia, tight glycaemic control, possible roles for vitamin E and metformin
Chronic right heart failure	Aim to reduce right heart pressures

Table 16.4 Modified Child–Pugh classification

Points	1	2	3
Ascites	Absent	Slight	Moderate
Bilirubin (µmol/L)	<34	34–51	>51
Albumin (g/L)	>35	28–35	<28
PTT (s > control) or INR	<4 or <1.7	4–6 or 1.7–2.3	>6 or >2.3
Encephalopathy	None	Grade 1–2	Grade 3–4

Score calculated as sum of points in each category, then grade determined as shown in Table 16.5. Reprinted from Liver and Portal Hypertension, Charles G. Child, pp. 50–64, Copyright 1964, with permission from Elsevier.

Table 16.5 Child–Pugh grading and outcomes

Grade	Score	1y survival (%)	2y survival (%)	Mortality (%)*
A	5–6	100	85	10
B	7–9	80	60	30
C	10–15	45	35	82

* Following abdominal surgery. Reprinted from Liver and Portal Hypertension, Charles G. Child, pp. 50–64, Copyright 1964, with permission from Elsevier.

The Model for End-stage Liver Disease (MELD) is a prospectively developed and validated prognostic model that is widely used, particularly to prioritize patients for liver transplantation. The score is derived from the following equation (bilirubin and creatinine in mg/dL):

$$MELD = 3.8 \times [Ln(Bilirubin)] + 11.2 \times [Ln(INR)] + 9.6 \times [Ln(creatinine)] + 6.4$$

Online calculators are available, specific to different types of liver disease (e.g. see 🔗 http://www.mayoclinic.org/meld/). Survival statistics at 3mo pre-transplant and 1y post-transplant, stratified by MELD score, have been calculated (see Table 16.6).

Table 16.6 Survival pre- and post-liver transplantation using MELD score stratification

MELD score	3mo pre-transplant survival (%)	1y post-transplant survival (%)
10	90	83
15	81	80
20	63	78
25	42	74
30	21	71

Reprinted from *Surgery*, 147, 3, Gleisner et al., 'Survival benefit of liver transplantation and the effect of underlying liver disease', pp. 147–392, 2010, with permission from Elsevier.

ⓘ Causes and diagnosis of non-cirrhotic portal hypertension

Aetiology

- Pre-hepatic:
  - Portal or splenic vein thrombosis.
  - Splanchnic arteriovenous fistula.
- Intrahepatic:
  - Pre-sinusoidal: schistosomiasis, PBC, sarcoidosis, PSC, congenital hepatic fibrosis, idiopathic portal hypertension.
  - Sinusoidal: vitamin A or arsenic toxicity, nodular regenerative hyperplasia.
  - Post-sinusoidal: veno-occlusive disease (including Budd–Chiari syndrome).
- Post-hepatic:
  - IVC obstruction.
  - Constrictive pericarditis.
  - Restrictive cardiomyopathy.

Presentation
- Usually well tolerated due to preserved liver function.
- Most common presentation is with variceal bleeding.
- Splenomegaly is common, with no stigmata of chronic liver disease.

Investigation
- Investigations to exclude main causes (see 🕮 p. 254).
- US often demonstrates splenomegaly and portal varices.
- Tests of liver fibrosis (e.g. FibroScan® or biopsy) often normal.

Treatment
- Treat varices (see Chapter 1).
- Enoxaparin 2mg/kg/d has been shown to both prevent and treat portal vein thrombosis in Child–Pugh B and C disease, and has been associated with lower mortality (Villa *et al.*, 2012).
- Bleeding complications are rare, although variceal eradication should occur prior to therapy.

Prognosis
Improved compared to patients with cirrhosis.

① Ascites

Ascites occurs commonly in end-stage cirrhosis (58% by 10y) due to portal hypertension and reduced renal perfusion, resulting in excess resorption of Na^+ and water. As homeostatic mechanisms fail, ADH secretion additionally promotes free water retention, resulting in hyponatraemia (despite total body Na^+ being increased). Ascites also frequently occurs in patients with Budd–Chiari syndrome or sub-fulminant hepatic failure. It does not occur in pre-hepatic (non-cirrhotic) portal hypertension (e.g. portal vein thrombosis, congenital hepatic fibrosis), as liver synthetic function is preserved. The main causes of ascites are shown in Table 16.7; more than one cause is present in ~5%.

Table 16.7 Causes of ascites in the UK

Cause	% of total
Cirrhosis (ALD) and/or alcoholic hepatitis	65
Cirrhosis (viral)	10
Cirrhosis (other)	6
Malignancy	10
Right ventricular failure (including constriction)	3
TB	2
Pancreatic disease	1
Other causes*	3

* Including Budd–Chiari syndrome, connective tissue diseases (particularly SLE), sarcoidosis, and familial Mediterranean fever.

History

In addition to questions related to cirrhosis (see 📖 p. 252), ask about:

• Weight loss.
• Bowel symptoms.
• Cardiac disease.
• Pancreatitis and abdominal pain radiating to the back.
• Contact with TB and travel history. Also note patient ethnicity (tuberculous peritonitis more common in Asians).

Examination

• Look for stigmata of chronic liver disease (see 📖 p. 253).
• Is the liver enlarged (steatosis, metastases), or hard and craggy (metastases, macronodular cirrhosis)? Cirrhotics usually have small, non-palpable livers. If ascites is tense, dip your fingers in and feel the liver before it floats away.
• Examine for abdominal masses, splenomegaly (portal hypertension, TB), and umbilical hernias.
• Is the patient encephalopathic? (see 📖 pp. 245, 267)
• Look for an elevated JVP, in which case consider a diagnosis of alcoholic cardiomyopathy or constrictive pericarditis rather than cirrhosis. Sit the patient upright, as a very high JVP may not be obvious in the semi-recumbent position. Avoid assessing hepatojugular reflux, which is uncomfortable.
• Assess fluid balance. Is there peripheral oedema? Weigh the patient (often overlooked but the easiest method to monitor fluid status).

Definitions

Ascites is graded as shown in Box 16.2.

Box 16.2 Grading of ascites

• Grade 1 (mild). Only detectable by US.
• Grade 2 (moderate). Moderate symmetrical distension of the abdomen.
• Grade 3 (severe). Marked abdominal distension; up to 25L can be present.

Reproduced from Kevin P. Moore et al., 'The management of ascites in cirrhosis: Report on the consensus conference of the international Ascites club', *Hepatology*, 38, 1, pp. 258–266, 2003, Wiley, with permission.

Uncomplicated ascites is uninfected and not associated with the hepato-renal syndrome (HRS). *Refractory* or *diuretic-resistant* ascites cannot be prevented by medical therapy alone and occurs in 5–10% of patients.

Investigation of patients with ascites

The cause is often self-evident but, when unclear, tests must be directed at both diagnosing the potential underlying liver disease and excluding other causes of ascites (such as malignancy or TB). Be wary of attributing ascites to alcoholic cirrhosis in heavy drinkers since only 20% develop cirrhosis.

Blood tests

- U & E. Hyponatraemia is common in cirrhotic ascites due to non-osmotic secretion of ADH. Hyponatraemia is an independent predictor of mortality in patients awaiting liver transplantation and improves prognostication when incorporated into the MELD score (see ℘ http://www.mayoclinic.org/meld/mayomodel8.html). Spontaneous or diuretic-associated renal impairment is also common. If serum creatinine is elevated, investigate as for HRS (see 🕮 p. 265).
- LFT. Occasionally, patients with PBC have marked ascites with little jaundice.
- Request FBC, glucose, amylase, PTT/INR, and blood cultures.

Urine tests

Measure urine Na^+ and K^+ on a spot sample (timed collections are not more sensitive). Without diuretics, secondary hyperaldosteronism results in a very low urine Na^+:K^+ ratio. Diuretic therapy should convert this to >1, in which case >90% of patients will be excreting >80mmol Na^+/d. This should result in salt and fluid excretion and consequent reduction in ascites *unless* they have a high salt intake or are non-compliant.

Ascitic fluid

SBP is present in 10–15% of patients admitted with cirrhotic ascites. It has a high mortality (30%). Hence:

- The most important test on ascitic fluid is *urgent* microscopy; >250 neutrophils/mm³ is diagnostic of SBP (see 🕮 p. 264). Sample is usually sent in a purple top (EDTA) FBC bottle. Organisms are only seen with Gram stain in 10% when their concentration is >1/mL. Suspect intestinal perforation if many organisms seen.
- The second most important test is to inoculate 10mL of ascites into blood culture bottles.
- Request cytology (send >100mL fluid to laboratory). Diagnostic in approximately two-thirds of malignant ascites (primary or secondary liver cancer and lymphomatous chylous ascites usually have negative cytology).
- The use of ascitic fluid protein to determine the cause of ascites is overrated. Conventionally, ascites is divided into an exudate or transudate, in which protein concentrations are >25g/L or <25g/L, respectively:
  - Patients with protein <10g/L are particularly susceptible to SBP.
  - The serum-ascitic albumin gradient (SAAG) has greater specificity. A gradient >11g/L is equivalent to a transudate and usually indicative of portal hypertension. Common causes are shown in Box 16.3.
- Ascitic glucose <2.8mmol/L and LDH higher than the serum ULN are suggestive of a perforated viscus (much rarer than SBP but requires emergency surgery) or malignant ascites. Ascitic:serum LDH ratio is ~0.4 in cirrhotic ascites, ~1 in SBP, and >5 with pancreatic ascites.
- Chylous ascites appears milky due to triglycerides >2.25mmol/L. This occurs in 1/200 cases, in 10% of whom it represents malignancy.
- Measure ascitic bilirubin if fluid is as 'brown as molasses'. If it is greater than the serum level, suspect a ruptured bile duct, gallbladder, or duodenum.

- Suspect intra-abdominal bleeding if *homogeneously* bloody. This occurs in 50% of patients with HCC and in ~25% of all cases of malignant ascites.
- Suspect TB ascites with predominantly mononuclear or lymphocytic infiltrates. Direct smear and ascitic culture have very low sensitivity. Peritoneoscopy with culture, histology, and PCR of a biopsied tubercle is the most rapid diagnostic method, with sensitivity approaching 100%.
- For EASL guidelines on investigation of ascites, see Clinical Practice Guidelines (2010).

Imaging
- CXR. May show sympathetic pleural effusion ± old rib fractures in an alcoholic.
- AXR. May show ground glass pattern with loss of psoas shadow.
- US. Request to confirm ascites (can detect >30mL), determine whether the liver looks cirrhotic, and exclude intrahepatic lesions. Request Doppler analysis to see if portal and hepatic veins patent (latter occluded in Budd–Chiari syndrome but widely patent in right ventricular failure).
- CT scan will yield similar information. Do not perform a CT scan with contrast in patients with incipient renal failure.

Box 16.3 Interpretation of serum-ascitic albumin gradient (SAAG)*

High SAAG (>11g/L)
- Cirrhosis (81%): alcohol (65%), viral (10%), cryptogenic (6%).
- Heart failure (3%).
- Pancreatic disease (1%).
- Rarer causes (3%):
  - Meig's syndrome.
  - Vasculitis.
  - Hypothyroidism.
  - Dialysis.
  - Budd–Chiari syndrome/veno-occlusive disease.
  - Constrictive pericarditis.
  - Nephrotic syndrome.
  - Kwashiorkor.
  - Serositis.
  - SBP.

Low SAAG (<11g/L)
- Peritoneal carcinomatosis or metastases (10%).
- TB (2%).

* Based on Runyon et al. (1992).

Treatment of patients with ascites

- Salt restriction. All patients should be placed on 'no-added' (rather than 'salt-poor') salt restriction and advised not to eat pre-packaged meals (since these contain a lot of salt). A no-added salt diet is equivalent to ~90mmol (2g) salt/d. Seek dietetic assistance. Poor compliance with diet is a frequent reason for hospital re-admission.

- Fluid restriction. Restrict to 1.0–1.5L/d if Na^+ <120mmol/L (do not perform if renal impairment). There is no net benefit to fluid restriction otherwise, or restriction to smaller volumes, as risk of development of HRS. Monitor with daily weights.
- Avoid renotoxins, particularly NSAIDs (which inhibit renal prostaglandins, causing renal vasoconstriction), ACE inhibitors, and aminoglycosides. Other anti-hypertensive agents should be used with caution.
- Correct hyponatraemia. If serum Na^+ is <120mmol/L, limit fluid intake to 1–1.5 L/d (unless clinically dry). Stop salt-losing diuretics. Consider vasopressin receptor antagonists (e.g. tolvaptan), which must be administered in hospital to avoid rapid Na^+ correction and central pontine myelinolysis (correct at a rate <10mmol/L/d). Hypertonic saline can be given to patients with neurologic manifestations thought to be due to severe hyponatraemia (e.g. 1L of 1.8% saline over 10h).
- Avoid hypokalaemia. Maintain K^+ between 3.5–5mmol/L (hypokalaemia increases renal NH_3 production, which can lead to encephalopathy).
- Renal impairment. If renal impairment (creatinine >120μmol/L), give colloid and crystalloid volume challenge (e.g. 500mL Gelofusine® IV over 1h followed by 1L 5% glucose IV over 4h), as opposed to fluid restriction. Paracentesis should be performed if grade 3 ascites to reduce intra-abdominal pressure. There is no hurry to commence diuretics; start once settled after paracentesis. More harm than good is done by diuresing patients who are hypovolaemic.
- Diuretics. Provided to enhance renal Na^+ loss (aiming to excrete >80mmol/d, assuming compliance with no-added salt diet). Start furosemide 40mg/d PO (prevents hyperkalaemia), and concurrently start spironolactone at 100mg/d PO as long as both Na^+ >125mmol/L and renal function normal. Gradually increase latter to 400mg/d, aiming for maximum weight reduction of 1kg/d or 0.5kg/d (with or without peripheral oedema, respectively). If the response is poor, furosemide can be gradually increased up to 160mg/d PO (avoid IV furosemide). Adjust these doses dependent on co-morbidity (e.g. hypokalaemia associated with alcoholic hepatitis, whereas hyperkalaemia associated with diabetic nephropathy and commonly seen in patients with cirrhosis due to NASH). Effective diuresis reduces risk of SBP by concentrating ascitic fluid opsonins.
- Paracentesis:
  - Perform if at least grade 2 ascites. Drain all fluid as quickly as possible (maximum 25L in 5h). Give 100mL of 20% albumin IV for each 3L (2L if renal impairment) ascitic fluid removed.
  - Paracentesis is a very safe procedure, even in patients with advanced liver disease with prolonged INR or thrombocytopaenia; <0.1% require transfusion because of the procedure (Grabau et al., 2004). Administration of clotting factors or platelets is NOT required unless patients have DIC.
  - Adjunctive abdominal US is only rarely required to identify a puncture point; usually insert the needle 3cm cephalad and 3cm medial to the anterior superior iliac spine.
  - Avoid performing close to surgical scars or in those with an ileus, to minimize risk of cannulating the bowel.

Special situations

- *Diuretic-resistant ascites in cirrhosis.* Occurs in 10%, indicative of pre-HRS. Confirm compliance with no-added salt diet (a spot urine Na^+/K^+ ratio <2.5 is expected with salt restriction). Patients with alcoholic, cirrhosis can become diuretic-responsive with complete abstinence from alcohol as can patients with cirrhosis due to autoimmune hepatitis treated with steroids and those with HBV cirrhosis treated with anti-virals. Other patients should be considered for TIPS or transplantation.
- *Malignant ascites.* Treatment of peritoneal carcinomatosis or chylous malignant ascites is palliative and includes total paracentesis to make the patient more comfortable. Albumin replacement is not required. There is no role for fluid restriction or diuretics in these patients. Patients with ascites due to massive hepatic metastases can have portal hypertension and should be treated similarly to those with cirrhosis.
- *Pancreatic ascites.* Usually associated with a pancreatic pseudocyst. Manage in consultation with surgical and hepatobiliary endoscopic colleagues.
- *Prophylaxis against SBP.* Prophylactic antibiotics reduce mortality by 30% in patients with ascites following variceal bleeding, those with ascitic protein <10g/L, and following SBP. Effective regimes include ciprofloxacin 750mg PO weekly, co-trimoxazole 960mg PO od for 5d each week, or norfloxacin 400mg PO od. National guidelines advocate only secondary prophylaxis at present.

Prognosis

The development of ascites in patients with cirrhosis indicates poor prognosis; 40% will be dead within 2y. Prognosis is worse for those with refractory ascites and those who develop SBP; it is less predictable in patients with alcoholic liver disease who stop drinking since there is considerable scope for some recovery. The MELD score risk-stratifies (see 📖 p. 257), and patients in a poor prognostic group should be considered for liver transplantation.

Complications

Para-umbilical herniae develop in up to 70% of patients with longstanding, recurrent tense ascites. There are often considerable risks when undertaking corrective surgery, which should only be performed as an emergency if there is intestinal rupture or incarceration, electively if there is thinning and weeping of skin overlying the hernia, or when liver transplant occurs. Aggressive management of ascites is necessary. Complications are shown in Box 16.4.

Box 16.4 Complications of ascites

- SBP.
- Para-umbilical herniae.
- Pleural effusions.
- HRS.
- Respiratory difficulties.
- Hyponatraemia.
- Hepatic encephalopathy (especially with SBP).

☼ **Spontaneous bacterial peritonitis**

Spontaneous bacterial peritonitis (SBP) is infection of pre-existing ascitic fluid in the absence of another intra-abdominal source. Exclude in all patients admitted with cirrhotic ascites as occurs in ~15% (but is rare in non-cirrhotic ascites). Predisposition occurs due to deficient immune function associated with advanced liver disease; risk is increased with low ascitic protein (reduction in opsonins). Most infections are caused by Gram-negative organisms (particularly *Enterobacteriaceae*), although Gram-positive infections are becoming increasingly frequent (Wiest et al., 2012).

History and examination

The presentation is protean and includes fever (>37.8°C is significant in patients with liver disease, who are usually mildly hypothermic), abdominal pain ± tenderness (present in minority), and subtly altered mental function. It may be asymptomatic. Signs are subtle, as ascitic fluid separates visceral and parietal peritoneal surfaces, preventing guarding.

Investigation

Confirm infection with diagnostic paracentesis:

- Diagnose SBP if microscopy shows >250 PMN/mm^3.
- Over 90% of patients will yield positive ascitic cultures when fluid is inoculated into blood culture bottles at the bedside.
- If culture is positive, but ascitic fluid contains <250 PMN/mm^3 (termed monomicrobial, non-neutrocytic bacterascites), repeat paracentesis and treat if >250 PMN/mm^3 on the repeat sample. Two-thirds of such infections resolve spontaneously, but treat empirically if the patient is unwell despite a low PMN count.
- Allow one 'spurious' PMN for every 250 RBCs if bloody tap obtained.
- Measure ascitic glucose and LDH to exclude secondary bacterial peritonitis. Suspect this diagnosis if multiple organisms are seen on Gram stain, with subsequent polymicrobial ascitic fluid cultures.

Treatment

Empiric treatment should be started as soon as samples for ascitic, urine, and blood analysis have been obtained; do not wait for the results if high clinical suspicion of SBP:

- Treat with broad-spectrum antibiotics for enteric organisms and Gram-positive cocci: cefotaxime 2g IV bd for 5d, piperacillin-tazobactam 4.5g IV tds for 5d, or ciprofloxacin 400mg IV bd for 2d then 500mg PO bd for 5d (third-line in those receiving quinolones prophylaxis).
- Add metronidazole 500mg IV tds if secondary bacterial peritonitis suspected, and obtain urgent surgical consult.
- Administering IV HAS 1.5g/kg on d1, and 1g/kg on d3, in those with rise in creatinine, reduces incidence of persistent renal impairment, and mortality (22% vs 41% at 3mo).
- Provide lifelong antibiotic prophylaxis on discharge (e.g. norfloxacin 400mg PO od).

- Primary prophylaxis is generally not advocated unless ascitic protein is 15g/L or there is severe renal impairment or liver disease likely to require urgent transplantation.

Prognosis

Most infections are successfully treated within 5d, in which case there is no need to repeat diagnostic paracentesis. In-hospital mortality following SBP relates to presence of renal dysfunction (67% if present vs 11% when absent). Irreversible renal impairment develops in one-third patients (10% if provided HAS); if significant, treat with a combination of octreotide and midodrine (see 🕮 p. 266). Medium-term prognosis is very poor, related to underlying liver disease; 2y mortality is ~50% if transplantation does not occur.

✺ Hepatorenal syndrome

Hepatorenal syndrome (HRS) is defined as acute renal failure in patients with advanced liver impairment. Splanchnic, and subsequently systemic, vasodilatation develop in response to portal hypertension (nitric oxide mediated), resulting in reduced renal perfusion. Increased cardiac output and renin-aldosterone-angiotensin activation are insufficient to overcome the extensive vasodilation.

Type 1 HRS occurs acutely, often associated with acute liver failure or decompensated cirrhosis. There is typically significant jaundice and coagulopathy. *Type 2* HRS is more chronic and usually seen in patients with refractory ascites.

Aetiology

Occurs due reduced renal perfusion secondary to:
- Haemodynamic changes occurring with cirrhosis.
- Severe alcoholic hepatitis.
- Fulminant hepatic failure.
- Hepatic dysfunction from metastases (rare).
- May be precipitated in the above patients by nephrotoxic agents (e.g. aminoglycosides), over-exuberant diuresis, GI haemorrhage, or sepsis.

Investigation

- Look for rising creatinine (actively consider diagnosis if >133µmol/L) and urea levels; these changes may be subtle and overestimate the true GFR due to decreased muscle mass (lowers creatinine) and reduced hepatic urea production. For more accurate assessment, measure 24h urine creatinine (although this can overestimate GFR by up to 40%). For EASL guidelines, see Clinical Practice Guidelines (2010).
- Consider an alternative diagnosis of acute tubular necrosis if the rise in creatinine is very rapid.
- Urine Na^+ is typically very low.
- Urine output is <500mL/d in ~65%; if possible, avoid urinary catheter to reduce risk of nosocomial infection.

- Benign urine sediment without dysmorphic red cells and red cell casts excludes glomerulonephritis.
- Request renal US to rule out obstruction.
- The diagnosis is one of exclusion and, therefore, other potential causes of renal dysfunction should be corrected. These include sepsis, intravascular volume depletion (administer HAS 1g/kg IV for 2d; for diagnosis of HRS, there should be no sustained improvement following 1.5L plasma expansion), and renotoxic drugs.

Treatment
- Patients are generally best managed in an HDU/ITU setting, with monitoring of urine output, and arterial and central venous pressures.
- Correct any hypovolaemia and stop all potentially renotoxic drugs. All diuretics should be stopped for the initial assessment of HRS (although furosemide may subsequently be useful to maintain urine output and treat central volume overload). There are no data as to whether continued administration of β-blockers is beneficial or detrimental.
- Drain ascites if tense.
- Midodrine 12.5mg PO tds (α1-agonist, causing systemic vasoconstriction) and octreotide 200µg SC tds (somatostatin analogue, which inhibits vasodilator release such as 5-HT) have been associated with improvement in renal function and survival, although short-term mortality is still >50%.
- Uncontrolled pilot data support use of noradrenaline and HAS, although this requires HDU support.
- Randomized trials assessing HAS and terlipressin 1–2mg IV qds (contraindicated if ischaemic heart disease) for up to 14d showed improved renal function in ~40% but no change in 3mo mortality, likely reflecting severity of underlying liver disease.
- One small study (12 patients) showed benefit of NAC administration.
- Two small studies have suggested benefit of TIPS, with gradual improvement in renal function over 6wk in some patients. Those with a MELD score >18 should not undergo this procedure, as their life expectancy of <3mo does not justify procedural morbidity.
- Dialysis can be considered in patients awaiting liver transplant or those with potentially reversible or treatable liver disease, but can be difficult due to labile haemodynamics.

Prognosis
Prognosis is very poor. Most patients die within weeks unless liver function improves (e.g. following alcohol abstinence) or transplant occurs.

Variceal haemorrhage

Acute mortality used to be 30% following variceal haemorrhage, with only 30% of patients alive after 1y. Survival has improved with modern techniques (splanchnic vasoconstriction, endoscopic banding, TIPS), but mortality remains high due to severe underlying liver disease, with ~20% dead at 6wk. See Chapter 1.

⊕ Hepatic encephalopathy

Aetiology

Reversible encephalopathy that occurs due to accumulation of nitrogenous compounds and other neurotoxins bypassing hepatic metabolism and entering the cerebral circulation. Often initiated by factors that cause decompensation. Type A is due to acute liver failure, type B to portal-systemic shunting but with normal liver function, and type C to intrinsic liver disease. Grading is shown in Table 16.8.

Table 16.8 Grading of hepatic encephalopathy

Grade	Clinical features
0	Normal
1	Clear consciousness, impaired higher cognitive functions (e.g. arithmetic), constructional dyspraxia (ask to draw five-pointed star), inversion of sleep-wake cycle
2	Disorientation and personality change. Asterixis
3	Confusion, increased somnolence
4	Coma

Risk factors for decompensation

Comprise hypovolaemia, bleeding, infection, alcohol intake, hypoxia, sedative medication, electrolyte disturbance (including zinc deficiency), non-compliance with treatment, constipation, recent TIPS (bypasses hepatic nitrogen metabolism), and emergence of HCC. Decompensation occurs more often with high BMI (43% of obese vs 15% of normal-weight individuals decompensated by 5y), high portal pressure, and low albumin (Berzigotti et al., 2011).

History and examination

Determine underlying cause of liver disease, precipitants, and grade (see Table 16.8). Transient neurological deficits can occur. Regularly assess GCS in those with grade 3/4 encephalopathy.

Investigation

- Exclude hypoglycaemia, uraemia, electrolyte disturbance (including zinc deficiency), and intoxication.
- Raised postprandial NH_3 levels can confirm the diagnosis (found in 75%) but are neither fully sensitive nor specific (see Chapter 13). It is often of little use, as diagnosis usually established clinically.
- CT brain may be required if diagnosis uncertain; EEG is rarely required (but may show slow, high-amplitude δ waves).
- Assess mental function using the Reitan trail test (see ♨ http://www.smjr.org/med/reitan.html); those without encephalopathy should complete it in fewer seconds than their age in years.

Treatment
- A precipitating cause is identified in >80%, so remove and prevent factors that can cause decompensation (see 📖 p. 267).
- Attentive nursing care in a well-lit environment is preferable to physical or chemical restraint. Avoid sedatives where possible but, if necessary, haloperidol is probably the safest.
- Supportive care is required for the patient with grade 3/4 encephalopathy. Assess safety of the airway, and consider ET intubation if not consistently maintained.
- Correct hypokalaemia (associated metabolic alkalosis increases the conversion of NH_4^+ to NH_3).
- Provide lactulose 30–60mL PO/NG tds/qds, aiming for 2–3 soft stools/d), in hospital and at discharge.
- Do not restrict diet, as patients are already malnourished.
- Rifaximin 550mg PO bd is effective for treating and preventing encephalopathy (Bass et al., 2010), although treatment is currently very costly. Other options include probiotics, acarbose, ornithine-aspartate (9g/d PO), sodium benzoate (10g/d PO), zinc acetate (600mg/d PO), flumazenil, and melatonin.
- Advise patient not to drive.

Prognosis
Most patients have, at least, subtle deficits in cerebration due to underlying liver disease. Minimizing precipitants is an important method to prevent recurrence. Liver transplantation is usually curative.

① Hepatopulmonary syndromes

Several pulmonary syndromes occur in the context of advanced liver disease:
- The hepatopulmonary syndrome (HPS) occurs when an increased alveolar-to-arterial gradient develops due to massive intrapulmonary capillary dilatation causing A-V shunting; consider this diagnosis with severe hypoxaemia (PaO_2 <60mmHg). It arises more often in those with spider naevi but is not closely related to liver disease severity. The diagnosis can be confirmed using bubble contrast echocardiography (saline bubbles bypass the lung filter and are seen in the left ventricle), nuclear scanning (technetium-labelled albumin bypasses the lung filter and is seen in brain or kidney), or high-resolution CT. The 5y survival is reduced with HPS (in one study from 63% to 23%) but, although oxygenation declines by ~5mmHg/y, patients tend to die from liver disease. Treat with long-term supplemental oxygen and expedite referral for liver transplantation.
- Ascites can cause diaphragmatic splinting with resultant V/Q mismatch.
- Pleural effusions (hepatic hydrothoraces) develop in ~5% of patients due to translocation of ascitic fluid through diaphragmatic defects and may occur in patients with no discernible ascites. The pleural effusions

are right-sided in 85%, left-sided in 13%, and bilateral in 2%. TIPS may be helpful in selected patients for recurrent symptomatic effusions.
• Portopulmonary hypertension occurs in 2% of patients with portal hypertension, presenting with breathlessness, chest pain, syncope, and peripheral oedema. Medical therapies are usually ineffective, and peri-operative (transplantation) mortality is high.

① **Hepatocellular carcinoma**

Hepatocellular carcinoma (HCC) occurs in all forms of cirrhosis, with a frequency of 4% per annum. Risk is higher in those with underlying viral hepatitis or haemochromatosis; cirrhosis due to autoimmune hepatitis or Wilson's disease carries lower risk.

History
Patients are often asymptomatic but may present with decompensated liver disease. Ask about RUQ pain, early satiety, and weight loss. Tumour secretion of vasoactive intestinal peptides causes diarrhoea in a minority.

Examination
Hepatomegaly, hepatic bruit, and jaundice are rare. Signs of chronic liver disease are common. Dermatomyositis may occur as a paraneoplastic phenomenon.

Investigation
• Check serum α-FP (also see Chapter 13); raised in 60%. Diagnostic when rising in context of suspicious nodule or if >500µg/L. Lower levels occur with chronic hepatitis, germ cell tumours, and pregnancy.
• Hypoglycaemia and hypercalcaemia may occur.
• US is the first-line imaging modality for screening and surveillance.
• Contrast MRI (or CT) required if nodule >1cm on US or if suspicious of multifocal disease in a severely cirrhotic liver. Nodule suggestive of HCC if hypervascular with increased T_2 signal. Occasionally, diagnosis requires interval scanning. Avoid percutaneous biopsy (3% seeding of needle tract) until treatment plan determined. Ten percent have metastatic disease at diagnosis (commonly lung, lymph nodes, bone, or adrenals).

Treatment
• Resectable lesions in Child–Pugh A (and possibly B) patients should undergo surgery, or radiofrequency ablation (RFA) if poor surgical candidate.
• Patients with unresectable lesions (>4 lesions <5cm, or 1 lesion >5cm) or with Child–Pugh C disease should be assessed for liver transplantation ± preoperative transarterial chemoembolization (TACE).
• If surgery or transplantation is not possible, consider TACE alone.

- Consider systemic chemotherapy or the tyrosine kinase inhibitor sorafenib (survival 11 vs 8mo; Llovet et al., 2008) in patients with metastases.
- For current EASL guidelines, see Clinical Practice Guidelines (2012).

Complications
See Chapter 21.

Prevention
National societies recommend liver US (± α-FP measurement, but at a cost of increasing false positive results) biannually. However, such a surveillance strategy has not consistently demonstrated reduced mortality, except in patients with HBV infection.

Prognosis
Median post-diagnosis survival is 6–20mo without treatment. Carefully selected patients who undergo resection or transplantation can have 5y survival rates as high as 90%. Up to 50–70% of patients are alive 5y after RFA, although this also, in part, reflects case selection.

Complications of cirrhosis and portal hypertension

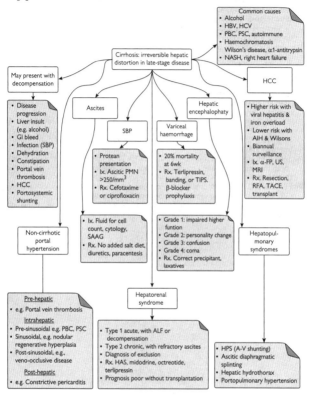

Common causes
- Alcohol
- HBV, HCV
- PBC, PSC, autoimmune
- Haemochromatosis
- Wilson's disease, α1-antitrypsin
- NASH, right heart failure

Cirrhosis: irreversible hepatic distortion in late-stage disease

May present with decompensation

HCC

- Disease progression
- Liver insult (e.g. alcohol)
- GI bleed
- Infection (SBP)
- Dehydration
- Constipation
- Portal vein thrombosis
- HCC
- Portosystemic shunting

Ascites

SBP

Variceal haemorrhage

Hepatic encephalopathy

- Higher risk with viral hepatitis & iron overload
- Lower risk with AIH & Wilsons
- Biannual surveillance
- Ix. α-FP, US, MRI
- Rx. Resection, RFA, TACE, transplant

- Protean presentation
- Ix. Ascitic PMN >250/mm³
- Rx. Cefotaxime or ciprofloxacin

- 20% mortality at 6wk
- Rx. Terlipressin, banding, or TIPS. β-blocker prophylaxis

- Ix. Fluid for cell count, cytology, SAAG
- Rx. No added salt diet, diuretics, paracentesis

- Grade 1: impaired higher funtion
- Grade 2: personality change
- Grade 3: confusion
- Grade 4: coma
- Rx. Correct precipitant, laxatives

Non-cirrhotic portal hypertension

Hepatopulmonary syndromes

Hepatorenal syndrome

<u>Pre-hepatic</u>
- e.g. Portal vein thrombosis
<u>Intrahepatic</u>
- Pre-sinusoidal e.g. PBC, PSC
- Sinusoidal, e.g. nodular regenerative hyperplasia
- Post-sinusoidal, e.g., veno-occlusive disease
<u>Post-hepatic</u>
- e.g. Constrictive pericarditis

- Type 1 acute, with ALF or decompensation
- Type 2 chronic, with refractory ascites
- Diagnosis of exclusion
- Rx. HAS, midodrine, octreotide, terlipressin
- Prognosis poor without transplantation

- HPS (A-V shunting)
- Ascitic diaphragmatic splinting
- Hepatic hydrothorax
- Portopulmonary hypertension

Further reading

Bass NM, Mullen KD, Sanyal A, et al. (2010) Rifaximin treatment in hepatic encephalopathy. N Engl J Med 362: 1071–81.

Berzigotti A, Garcia–Tsao G, Bosch J, et al. (2011) Obesity is an independent risk factor for clinical decompensation in patients with cirrhosis. Hepatology 54: 555–61.

Bonacini M, Hadi G, Govindarajan S, et al. (1997) Utility of a discriminant score for diagnosing advanced fibrosis or cirrhosis in patients with chronic hepatitis C virus infection. Am J Gastroenterol 92: 1302–4.

European Association for the Study of the Liver (2010) EASL Clinical Practice Guidelines on the management of ascites, spontaneous bacterial peritonitis, and hepatorenal syndrome in cirrhosis. J Hepatol 53: 397–417.

European Association for the Study of the Liver, European Organisation for Research and Treatment of Cancer (2012) EASL-EORTC Clinical Practice Guidelines: management of hepatocellular carcinoma. J Hepatol 56: 908–43.

Gleisner AL, Muñoz A, Brandao A, et al. (2010) Survival benefit of liver transplantation and the effect of underlying liver disease. Surgery 147: 392–404.

Grabau CM, Crago SF, Hoff LK, et al. (2004) Performance standards for therapeutic abdominal paracentesis. Hepatology 40: 484–8.

Llovet JM, Ricci S, Mazzaferro V, et al. (2008) Sorafenib in advanced hepatocellular carcinoma. N Engl J Med 359: 378–90.

Runyon BA, Montano AA, Akriviadis EA, et al. (1992) The serum-ascites albumin gradient is superior to the exudate-transudate concept in the differential diagnosis of ascites. Ann Intern Med 117: 215–20.

Villa E, Cammà C, Marietta M, et al. (2012) Enoxaparin prevents portal vein thrombosis and liver decompensation in patients with advanced cirrhosis. Gastroenterology 143: 1253–60.

Wiest R, Krag A, Gerbes A (2012) Spontaneous bacterial peritonitis: recent guidelines and beyond. Gut 61: 297–310.

Infections and the liver

Infections and the liver

The liver may be involved in direct infection or as part of a systemic illness. This chapter considers both processes. The viral hepatitides are covered in Chapter 14, and liver disease in HIV-infected patients in Chapter 12. Expert help is advised when managing tropical infections.

ⓘ Liver abscesses

Pyogenic abscess

Bacterial abscesses may arise from systemic infection or local portal phlebitis. They are more common in the older population, given the higher rates of predisposing co-morbidities. Common associations include obstructive biliary tree disease (30–40%, often causing multiple lesions), intra-abdominal infection (15–25%, particularly diverticulitis, appendicitis, IBD, and colonic malignancy), systemic infection (15–20%, including infective endocarditis), and direct trauma. Pre-existing liver lesions constitute a significant risk, especially with prior instrumentation or tumour necrosis (e.g. following chemoembolization or RFA of a HCC). Similarly, secondary bacterial infection of pre-existing amoebic abscesses or hydatid cysts can occur.

Infections are usually polymicrobial, with gut-derived anaerobes (*Bacteroides*), Gram-negative (*Escherichia coli*, *Klebsiella*), and Gram-positive (*Enterococci*, *Streptococcus milleri*) organisms. *Staphylococcus aureus* is common in IVDU. Melioidosis (caused by *Burkholderia pseudomallei*) is a rare cause of multiple small liver abscesses; it is most frequently acquired in South East Asia or Northern Australia.

Presentation

May be acute with RUQ pain and fever, or more indolent as a pyrexia of unknown origin (PUO). Jaundice and hepatomegaly are seen in 25%. A hepatic rub may be audible. Hepatic abscess should be considered in patients with cholangitis who remain septic despite relief of obstruction.

Investigation

- Blood tests:
  - Inflammatory markers (WCC, CRP, and ESR) are raised.
  - LFT. Typically show elevated ALP and reduced albumin.
  - Blood cultures. Positive in 50–80%.
  - Serology (CAP and ELISA) for *Entamoeba histolytica* should be performed in travellers from endemic regions.
- Radiology:
  - CXR. May demonstrate a raised right hemidiaphragm, pleural effusion, and/or right lower lobe consolidation.
  - US. Sensitivity 80–90%. The main differential is between an abscess and a simple cyst. Abscesses appear as hypoechoic masses with irregular borders. Also allows evaluation of the biliary tree.
  - Contrast CT. Helpful when diagnosis remains in question. Abscesses appear as hypodense ring-enhancing lesions. Sensitivity ~100%.

- Diagnostic aspiration. Performed if blood cultures negative and lesions fail to respond after 48h of antibiotics. Tinidazole 2g PO should be given to cover procedure if amoebic liver abscess possible. Similarly, be aware of the risks of aspirating an undiagnosed hydatid cyst (see 📖 p. 277).
- Identification of source. The primary site of infection should be carefully sought, with a low threshold for echocardiography and colonoscopy.

Treatment

Antibiotics should initially be given empirically to cover the broad-spectrum of organisms described in 'Pyogenic abscess' (see p. 274) (co-amoxiclav, cefuroxime + metronidazole, or piperacillin-tazobactam are appropriate). These can subsequently be adjusted according to culture results. Treatment should be continued for 2wk IV, then 2–6wk PO according to response.

Large solitary or multiple abscesses should be drained percutaneously under US or CT guidance, leaving a drain *in situ* for abscesses >5cm. Any biliary tree obstruction (see Colour plate 22) needs to be relieved. Surgery is rarely required but may be indicated for abscesses that are >5cm, multiloculated, or ruptured.

Complications

- Sepsis.
- Empyema.
- Peritonitis.

Prognosis

Treatment is successful in 80–90%, although abscesses can take weeks to months to resolve. Be guided clinically rather than radiologically, as changes in the latter lag behind. Mortality is high in children and the elderly, as well as those with severe co-morbidity or delayed diagnosis.

Amoebic liver abscess

Entamoeba histolytica is the major pathogenic amoebic species infecting humans. Acquisition is faeco-oral; cysts remain viable in the environment for up to 2mo. Incidence is highest in the Indian subcontinent, followed by South America, West Africa, and South East Asia. Cysts are ingested, from which trophozoites emerge and colonize the large bowel; the caecum and rectum are sites of predilection. Tissue invasion subsequently occurs, and organisms are thought to reach the liver via the portal vein. They then progressively and continuously expand, causing hepatocyte necrosis, liquefaction, and liver abscess.

Presentation

Fewer than 50% of patients give a history of preceding dysentery (see Chapter 6), and the latent period can be several months. The main symptoms are fever, sweating, liver or diaphragmatic pain, and weight loss. Onset is often abrupt, although may be insidious. Fever is characteristically intermittent with prominent evening spikes, associated with rigors and profuse sweating. Painful dry cough due to diaphragmatic irritation is common.

On examination, patients are often anaemic. Localized, tender hepato-megaly may occur; if involving the left lobe, this can present as an epigastric mass. There can be point tenderness over the abscess.

Amoebic brain abscesses are extremely rare (<0.1% of cases) but arise exclusively alongside hepatic disease. The usual presentation is with sudden onset headache, vomiting, changes in mental state, and seizures.

Investigation
- Blood tests:
  - Typically show normochromic normocytic anaemia, neutrophilia, elevated CRP and ESR.
  - LFT. Bilirubin and transaminases usually normal, although albumin is often very low.
  - Serology is >95% sensitive and specific. CAP distinguishes between current and past infection; IFAT does not. False negatives can occur early in infection, but rising titres will be seen on repeating the test.
- Radiology. As for pyogenic abscesses. Most lesions are solitary (70%), although multiple abscesses are commoner in children and patients with concurrent dysentery.
- Diagnostic aspiration. A therapeutic trial of an amoebicide (see 'Treatment', 📖 p. 276) is generally preferable to diagnostic aspiration. When performed, the classic description is of a pink-brown 'anchovy sauce' aspirate (although can be yellow or cream-coloured); this lacks the unpleasant smell of pus from pyogenic abscesses. White cells should not be seen on microscopy and, if present in a confirmed amoebic abscess, suggest secondary bacterial infection.
- GI investigations. Stool microscopy or colonoscopy may reveal unsuspected luminal involvement, even in the absence of dysentery. Microscopic examination of stool alone cannot differentiate cysts of *Entamoeba histolytica* from non-pathogenic *Entamoeba dispar* (although pathognomonic haemophagocytic trophozoites of the former may be seen on very fresh samples processed immediately). Use of stool ELISA can help clarify.

Treatment
Antibiotics are mandatory: tinidazole 2g PO od for 5d, or metronidazole 800mg PO tds for 10d. This should be accompanied by 10d of diloxanide 500mg PO tds to eliminate luminal bowel infection, as relapse is common unless parasitological cure is achieved. US monitoring of lesions is helpful, although no change is expected within the first 2wk.

Aspiration or surgery is required for abscesses that are very large where rupture is imminent (particularly if this would be into the pericardial sac, which carries 30% mortality), and where there is doubt concerning the diagnosis. Additionally, patients whose pain and fever do not subside within 72h have a high risk of rupture or antibiotic failure, and should generally undergo therapeutic aspiration. Caution is required with any attempt to aspirate, due to the potential for tracking and formation of an amoeboma on the skin.

Abscesses that rupture always require laparotomy. Those that extend into pleural or pericardial cavities necessitate drainage of these structures as well as the liver lesions.

Complications
- Obstructive jaundice, secondary to biliary tree compression.
- Extension into pleura, peritoneum, and pericardium.
- Extension to skin, with sinus formation.
- Subphrenic rupture.
- Empyema.
- Rupture into biliary tree, presenting as haemobilia.
- Hepatobronchial fistulation, presenting with 'anchovy sauce' sputum.
- Metastatic abscesses. Lung and (very rarely) brain.

Prognosis
Treatment is successful in 85% of patients with uncomplicated disease, but lower if complications have occurred. Most resolve rapidly, with evidence of improvement in <1wk and clinical resolution within 6wk. Radiological appearances take longer to resolve.

Hydatid disease

Cystic hydatid disease is a zoonotic infection caused by the tapeworm *Echinococcus granulosus* (or, more rarely, *Echinococcus multilocularis*). There are numerous endemic regions, and it is most common in rural communities. Adult tapeworms infest the small intestine of definitive hosts, usually canines. Eggs pass into faeces and contaminate soil, remaining viable for long periods before ingestion by intermediate hosts that include sheep, cattle, and man. They then hatch in the bowel into oncospheres, which penetrate the mucosa and disseminate through the bloodstream and lymphatics to generate cysts in liver (60%), lung (25%) and, rarely, bone, kidney, spleen, ovaries, and (exceptionally) brain.

Incubation is highly variable and may be prolonged for several years. Cyst growth is also unpredictable, ranging from static to >5cm/y.

Presentation
Most cysts are asymptomatic, although symptoms can arise from mass effects (palpable RUQ mass, abdominal pain, or obstructive jaundice) or complications (rupture with anaphylaxis or secondary infection). Extrahepatic cysts may present as:
- Lung: dyspnoea, cough ± haemoptysis, pneumothorax, or empyema.
- Peritonitis.
- Bone: pathological fracture or deformity.
- CNS: raised ICP, fits, spinal cord compression.

Investigation
- Blood tests. FBC may be normal. Eosinophilia is unusual unless the cyst is leaking. LFT may be normal or deranged. Serology is 90% sensitive.
- Imaging. CXR for coexistent lung lesions. US can delineate hepatic cysts, although CT is the gold standard, with 95% accuracy and high sensitivity for demonstrating characteristic daughter cysts.

Treatment
Generally requires a combination of medical and surgery therapy, as only 30% are cured using medical therapy alone (although some patients are managed expectantly). Surgical options include limited cystectomy or partial organ resection. Preoperatively, give albendazole 400mg PO bd for a

minimum of 14d (although, if clinical condition allows, prolonged therapy for several months associated with lower complication rate), and add in praziquantel 20mg/kg PO bd 2wk prior to intervention. During the procedure, sterilization of the cyst with 20% hypertonic saline or 90% alcohol and prevention of spillage by prior evacuation of contents are essential. Accidental release of scolices into the peritoneal cavity causes anaphylaxis ± secondary peritoneal hydatidosis.

An alternative in patients where surgery is unsuitable or for simple lesions is percutaneous aspiration, injection, and re-aspiration (PAIR). Cysts are punctured under US guidance and contents withdrawn. A protoscolicidal agent is injected (usually hypertonic saline), left for 15min, then re-aspirated. Albendazole 400mg PO bd should be given for at least 1mo over the peri-operative/procedural period. FBC and LFT should be monitored every 2wk. Prophylactic antihistamines are helpful.

If cyst rupture is suspected, give both praziquantel and albendazole.

Prognosis
Generally good, although recurrence in up to 30%.

ⓘ Bacterial infections

The liver may be involved during infection with mycobacteria, spirochaetes (*Leptospira* and *Borrelia*), actinomycetes, and Q fever.

Tuberculosis

Mycobacterium tuberculosis affects the liver in many forms (for discussion of atypical mycobacterial disease, see Chapter 12). There is a 2:1 male predominance, with most disease occurring in those aged 30–50y. Mycobacteria reach the liver through haematogenous spread or via the portal tract if there is GI disease. Four main pathological patterns are seen:

• *Miliary TB.* Occurs as part of systemic infection. Rarely has symptoms or signs directly related to the liver.
• *Granulomatous hepatitis.* Presents with unexplained fever, mild jaundice ± hepatomegaly. Biopsy shows caseating granulomas. There is improvement with anti-tuberculosis therapy.
• *Localized disease.* Includes tuberculomas, abscesses, and solitary or multiple nodules.
• *Cholangitis.* Secondary to portal lymphadenopathy or inflammatory strictures of intrahepatic ductal epithelium.

Hepatotoxicity may also be caused by anti-tuberculosis medication (see Chapter 18) or arise as an immune reconstitution inflammatory syndrome (IRIS) phenomenon when HIV-infected patients are commenced on HAART (see Chapter 12).

Presentation
Abdominal pain (mostly RUQ) is the main symptom of hepatobiliary TB. Nodular hepatomegaly is present in 45–100%, and splenomegaly in 25–57%. Jaundice occurs in 35% and is usually obstructive in nature.

The differential diagnosis is from other infections and granulomatous disorders, and neoplasia. Similar presentations can be seen in:

- Hodgkin's lymphoma.
- Sarcoidosis.
- Schistosomiasis (especially *Schistosoma mansoni*).
- Brucellosis.
- Syphilis.
- Toxoplasmosis.
- Leishmaniasis.
- Toxocara.
- Coccidioidomycosis.

Investigation

CXR demonstrates concurrent pulmonary abnormalities in 65%. AXR may show liver calcification (50%). US can delineate focal lesions. Percutaneous aspiration and biopsy may be radiologically guided for localized lesions, or blind for miliary or granulomatous hepatitis.

Treatment

Antibiotic therapy is similar to pulmonary disease, although often prolonged to 1y. Obstructive jaundice may require ERCP with stenting or percutaneous transhepatic drainage.

Prognosis

Two-thirds of patients respond well, but mortality is high in the remainder due to variceal bleeds related to portal hypertension, and cholangitis. Hepatic failure, in itself, is rarely fatal.

Leptospirosis (Weil's disease)

Weil's disease refers to the 10% of infections with *Leptospira icterohaemorrhagiae* that result in clinical hepatitis. The spirochaete is carried by rats, and is endemic in the tropics and a common cause of fever in Asia and Central and South America. Infection occurs through direct contact with soil or water contaminated with rat urine, entering skin through cuts or abrasions. Diagnosis requires a careful history to elicit possible exposures. Occupational and recreational risk factors include:

- Farm workers, veterinarians, and abattoir workers.
- Plumbers.
- Sewage workers.
- Military and naval personnel.
- Sports, including caving and those involving fresh water contact.

Presentation

A 7–14d incubation period is followed by a 4–7d septicaemic phase, characterized by flu-like symptoms (headache, myalgia, and dyspnoea). As organisms are cleared, there is a period of clinical improvement.

In a minority, there follows a second phase of illness during the following week, which is immune-mediated. Features include recurrence of fever, meningeal irritation, iritis, skin haemorrhagic lesions (petechiae, purpura, and ecchymoses), renal failure with acute tubular necrosis, and jaundice with hepatomegaly. The pathogenesis of jaundice remains unexplained; neither haemolysis nor hepatocellular necrosis are prominent, and it is difficult to demonstrate many organisms within the affected tissue.

On examination, there may be conjunctival suffusion, pharyngeal injection, hepatomegaly (60%), splenomegaly, and generalized lymphadenopathy.

Investigation
- Blood tests:
  - FBC. Hb and platelets usually low, with neutrophilia.
  - U & E. K^+ often low due to renal wasting.
  - LFT. Elevated bilirubin and ALT/AST > ALP. The degree of jaundice has no prognostic significance.
  - CK and aldolase are elevated during the first week in >50% with liver disease, as a consequence of coexistent muscle damage.
  - Spirochaetes may be demonstrable in blood samples during the first phase.
  - Serology is specific but has low sensitivity in early disease.
- Urinalysis. Frequently positive for protein, WBC, and RBC. Dark field microscopy of serially diluted urines for spirochaetes becomes positive in the second phase and remains so for several weeks. Yield is high, but culture usually takes too long to be useful clinically.
- Imaging. CXR may show patchy snowflake-like infiltrates in the peripheral lung fields.

Treatment
Antibiotics are highly effective if administered early. Treat moderate or severe disease with benzylpenicillin 1.2g IV qds. Use amoxicillin 500mg–1g PO tds or doxycycline 100mg PO od for 1wk for mild disease. Jarisch–Herxheimer reactions may occur, which should be managed supportively.

Complications
- Pulmonary haemorrhage. Consider prompt intubation and ventilation.
- Renal failure. Usually secondary to hypovolaemia that responds rapidly to IV fluids, but can develop interstitial nephritis. May require renal replacement therapy, as renal failure is the commonest cause of death.
- Coagulopathy. Bleeding principally occurs into skin or lung.
- Meningitis. Immune-mediated.
- Myopathy.
- Myocarditis. First-degree heart block is common and reversible.

Prognosis
Excellent if treated early, although overall mortality remains 5–10%, usually due to renal or cardiorespiratory failure. Liver involvement is rarely fatal, and patients demonstrate no residual liver dysfunction or pathological structural changes. Meningeal involvement is typically fully reversible.

Lyme disease
Lyme disease results from infection with *Borrelia burgdorferi*, transmitted via the *Ixodes* tick. There is a tick–vertebrate cycle, involving white-footed mice in North America but a variety of small mammals and birds in Europe. The disease is most prevalent in America, Canada, Northern Europe, and North Asia. It affects all ages, although incidences are highest in children aged 5–9y and adults >30y.

Presentation

Most cases are asymptomatic. When symptoms do arise, the illness is triphasic, starting with erythema migrans, a red macule or papule appearing at the site of a bite incurred 7–10 d earlier. This rash expands over days to week, with or without central clearing. Systemic involvement occurs with fatigue, myalgia, arthralgia, headache, fever, and regional lymphadenopathy. The second phase occurs weeks to months later, with cardiac and neurologic findings. The third phase occurs months to years later, with flitting large joint arthritis and cranial neuropathies and/or encephalopathy.

GI symptoms and signs are common during the early stages and include anorexia (20%), nausea (15%), vomiting (10%), abdominal pain (8%), hepatomegaly (5%), splenomegaly (5%), and diarrhoea (2%). Approximately 10% have symptoms suggestive of hepatitis, with biochemical evidence of mild hepatocellular injury in up to 30%. The usual pattern is mildly elevated transaminases, although these may also derive from myositis.

Treatment

Most manifestations resolve spontaneously, although antibiotics hasten recovery. Doxycycline 100mg PO bd or amoxicillin 500mg PO tds for 2–3wk are effective. Jarisch–Herxheimer reactions may occur.

Prognosis

Prognosis is excellent. Almost all manifestations resolve with antibiotics.

Actinomycetes

Actinomycoses are subacute to chronic granulomatous suppurative infections, with slowly progressive formation of multiple abscesses. They are caused by polymicrobial infection with various facultative anaerobes, principally *Actinomyces* (most commonly *A. israelii* or *A. gerencseriae*) and *Propionibacterium*. There is frequently co-infection with other gut organisms. Many actinomycetes derive from commensal oral flora. Patients are usually immunosuppressed.

Presentation

Abdominal actinomycoses are rare and usually originate from perforating disease, e.g. appendicitis, diverticulitis, or trauma. Most present as slow-growing tumours and can directly extend into other organs, including the liver. Haematogenous liver abscesses are also seen, particularly accompanying genital actinomycoses (associated with salpingitis and long-term use of intrauterine devices or vaginal pessaries).

Investigation

Diagnosis relies upon bacteriological examination of pus or affected tissue, and demonstration therein of pathognomonic sulphur granules. Radiology is non-diagnostic but may delineate organ invasion.

Treatment

Infection is always polymicrobial, so antibiotics should cover all causative and concomitant organisms. Suitable regimes are:

- Co-amoxiclav/benzylpenicillin + metronidazole + gentamicin.
- Ampicillin + clindamycin + clarithromycin.

Treatment needs to be prolonged (~3mo). Surgical drainage may be indicated for non-resolving abscesses or acute compression of adjacent structures.

Prognosis

Good with early diagnosis, but complications can otherwise be severe.

Q fever

Caused by *Coxiella burnetii*, an obligate intracellular bacterium. It is a zoonotic infection with a tick reservoir; person-to-person spread is rare. The incubation period is 2–3wk. A history of exposure to cattle, sheep, or goats is useful, but contact may be indirect and not recognized. Risk occupations include farmers, vets, animal transporters, and abattoir and tannery workers.

Presentation

Q fever can be acute or chronic. The most common clinical presentation is an influenza-like illness, with varying degrees of pneumonia and hepatitis. The diagnosis is often missed, as symptoms vary and are non-specific. Common manifestations include fever ± rigors, retro-orbital headache, myalgia, and rash (in 5–20%, usually maculopapular but can cause erythema nodosum). Hepatomegaly and elevated serum transaminases are common (51% and 85%, respectively), but frank hepatitis and jaundice are rare (<1%). Cardiac involvement can be fatal: myocarditis occurs acutely in <1%, but chronic 'culture-negative' endocarditis is more common. Q fever is associated with spontaneous abortion in pregnant women.

Investigation

- Blood tests:
  - FBC. WCC usually normal. Thrombocytopaenia in 25%.
  - LFT. Serum transaminases often elevated but raised bilirubin rare.
  - Serology. Mainstay of diagnosis, although significant titres may take 3–4wk to appear (therefore, treatment usually started on clinical suspicion).
  - Culture is technically difficult and not routinely available.
- CXR. Changes of Q fever pneumonia are non-specific, with diffuse bilateral infiltrates. Respiratory disease is usually mild, although ARDS can occur.
- Echocardiogram. Transthoracic (± transoesophageal if high risk) echocardiography should be performed to look for Q fever endocarditis.
- Liver biopsy. Rarely required. Fibrin-ring 'doughnut' granulomas are characteristic but not specific.

Treatment

Although acute disease is usually self-limiting, Q fever should be treated if suspected/identified due to the risk of secondary complications. Doxycycline 100mg bd for 14d is effective. Longer courses are required for those with endocarditis.

Prognosis

Generally very good, although a long-term association with chronic fatigue syndrome has been reported. Overall case fatality is 1–2%, predominantly due to cardiac involvement.

① Parasitic infections

The hepatobiliary system may be involved in a number of parasitic infections, including visceral leishmaniasis, schistosomiasis, fascioliasis, clonorchiasis, and ascariasis.

Leishmaniasis

The *Leishmania* parasite can cause visceral or cutaneous disease, depending on subspecies. The former results from infection with *Leishmania (L.). donovani* in India and Africa, and the latter from *L. major* in the Middle East, Asia, and Mediterranean littoral. Epidemics may also occur, usually in 15–20y cycles, particularly around the Ganges and Brahmaputra rivers in India and Bangladesh. Parasites are carried by sandflies, which live in rodent burrows.

It is estimated that for every clinical case of visceral leishmaniasis, ~30 are subclinical and undiagnosed. The disease shows a male predominance of 4:1 and, although all ages are affected, children <5y are particularly predisposed. Risk occupations include hunters and soldiers. Disease in tourists is rare. In immunocompromised individuals, leishmaniasis can develop as an opportunistic infection, in which presentations may be atypical.

Presentation

The incubation period is 2–8mo. Onset is typically insidious, although can be rapid in non-immune tourists during epidemics. The main initial presentation is with fever that classically spikes twice daily. Abdominal LUQ pain and distension result from massive splenomegaly; rupture is a rare but critical complication. The liver is moderately enlarged in one-third, although clinically relevant disease is unusual. Malabsorption leads to weight loss and diarrhoea. Hypoalbuminaemia can be profound, accompanied by oedema and leukonychia.

The clinical picture can vary according to geographic location. In Africa, generalized lymphadenopathy is common. In India, 20% of patients experience increased pigmentation (kala-azar) of the face and extensor surfaces during recovery. This may resemble lepromatous leprosy.

Investigation

- Blood tests. FBC typically shows normochromic normocytic anaemia (without reticulocytosis) leukopaenia, and thrombocytopaenia secondary to hypersplenism. Albumin is often <20g/L, although other LFT are usually normal. Serology is nearly 100% sensitive in the absence of HIV infection.
- Parasitology. Definitive diagnosis is made by identifying the organism by microscopy, culture, or PCR within affected reticuloendothelial tissues. Splenic aspiration is the most sensitive (95%), although complications are serious. Alternative sources are liver biopsy or bone marrow aspirate.

Treatment

The treatment of choice is liposomal amphotericin 3mg/kg IV od for 7–10d. This is costly, however, in endemic regions where alternatives include the antimony compounds sodium stibogluconate and megluminate antimoate.

The dose is 10–20mg/kg antimony for 21d. LFT and amylase must be monitored, along with ECG (long QT and non-specific T wave changes). Response is best determined clinically by monitoring fever, spleen size, Hb, albumin, and weight. Parasitological proof of cure is not required but helpful to determine relapse.

Nutritional deficiencies and intercurrent infections should be treated as they arise. Transfusion is rarely necessary.

Prognosis

Mortality in untreated cases is 15–25%, although there is generally a rapid response if treated early with cure rates >90%. Relapse is not uncommon, particularly amongst HIV-infected individuals. Monitoring for parasites at 6wk and 6mo aids early detection.

Schistosomiasis

Schistosoma (S.) mansoni, *S. intercalatum*, *S. japonicum*, and *S. mekongi* are amongst the commonest causes of hepatic infection worldwide. They are endemic in Africa (*S. mansoni*, *S. intercalatum*), South America (*S. mansoni*), the Middle East (*S. mansoni*), China (*S. japonicum*), and South East Asia (*S. japonicum*, *S. mekongi*). Parasites are acquired from fresh water where they reproduce in snails. They penetrate the skin to enter the bloodstream and mature and migrate to bowel. They can subsequently enter the portal system where eggs induce an immune response, peri-portal granuloma formation, and subsequently fibrosis, the severity of which correlates with disease duration and parasite load.

Presentation

A pruritic rash (cercarial dermatitis) occurs at the entry site within 24h. A hypersensitivity reaction can also manifest with a pruritic maculopapular eruption, lasting up to 2wk, and can be more intense with repeat exposures.

In primary infection, an acute toxaemia can arise (Katayama fever). Patients present with fever, urticaria, myalgia, and lethargy. This may mimic a viral illness, and the diagnosis is often missed. Serology and parasitological investigations are negative at this stage, although peripheral blood eosinophilia is typical. A history of exposure to contaminated water is key.

Chronic infection leads to GI symptoms and signs. Abdominal discomfort and diarrhoea are most common, although severe dysentery is rare. On examination, there may be tender hepatomegaly (particularly left lobe), with or without signs of portal hypertension, splenomegaly, and generalized lymphadenopathy. The lungs and CNS (including spinal cord) can also be involved; renal involvement is rare.

Co-infection with hepatitis B or C is associated with particularly aggressive hepatic disease.

Investigation

- Blood tests. May show anaemia and eosinophilia. LFT are typically normal. Serology may be helpful but is negative in early disease, and it may remain positive for some time after cure.
- Parasitology. Diagnosis is made by demonstrating eggs or schistosomes in stool, rectal snips, or affected liver.
- Imaging. US helpful for grading fibrosis and portal hypertension.

Treatment

The drug of choice is praziquantel, which is effective against all schistosomes affecting man. This may be given as a 40mg/kg single dose, or as two 20mg/kg single doses 4–6h apart.

Prognosis

Liver fibrosis is reversible if treatment is initiated early, although presentation is often delayed. Complete cure is achieved in 85%, and egg burden reduced by >95% in other patients. The most common cause of death is massive upper GI haemorrhage from oesophageal varices, present in ~80% with hepatic disease.

Fascioliasis

Fasciola hepatica is a trematode fluke. It has a worldwide distribution (including within the UK and Europe) but most common in South East Asia and Africa. The main hosts are sheep and cattle, although humans may consume cercaria from contaminated plants or water. Larvae excyst in the duodenum, migrate through the bowel wall and peritoneal cavity, and penetrate the liver. This migratory stage may last 3–4mo. Mature flukes can then move through the liver into large hepatic and common bile ducts.

Presentation

- The principal presentation is with fever, abdominal pain, and eosinophilia, although up to 50% of infections are asymptomatic.
- There may be tender hepatomegaly in the acute phase.
- Large worms obstructing the biliary tree may cause biliary colic, obstructive jaundice, cholangitis, or pancreatitis.

Investigation

- Blood tests:
  - FBC. Usually shows leukocytosis with eosinophilia.
  - LFT. When abnormal, most commonly cholestatic.
  - Serology.
- Stool. Microscopy for ova and parasites may be diagnostic, although has limited sensitivity.
- Imaging:
  - US. Larval burrow tracks within the liver show as hypodense hypoechoic lesions. Large worms obstructing the biliary tree cause duct dilatation.
  - CT/MRI. Demonstrate inflammatory lesions if US equivocal.
- ERCP. Required if evidence of biliary tree obstruction.

Treatment

Responds to triclabendazole 10mg/kg PO, two doses over 24h.

Clonorchiasis

Clonorchis sinensis is a liver fluke, most frequently acquired in China and South East Asia from eating infected fish. Cysts are digested in the duodenum, from which larvae are released. These may enter the biliary tree where they mature into adult worms. Unlike *Fasciola* and *Ascaris*, *Clonorchis* does not migrate.

Presentation
- Most infections are asymptomatic.
- Acute infection may present with fever, eosinophilia, and urticarial rash.
- Worms in the biliary tree can cause biliary colic, cholangitis, and pancreatitis.
- Chronic infection is a risk factor for developing cholangiocarcinoma.

Investigation
- Blood tests:
  - FBC. May show eosinophilia.
  - LFT. Often normal but can be cholestatic. Check amylase if clinical suspicion of pancreatitis.
  - No serological test available.
- US. Perform if clinical suspicion of biliary tree obstruction.
- ERCP. Indicated if there is evidence of cholangitis or pancreatitis.

Treatment
Infections respond to praziquantel 30mg/kg PO. Provide three doses, each 6h apart. ERCP is indicated for cholangitis and pancreatitis, at which worms can be mechanically extracted.

Ascariasis

Ascaris lumbricoides is a nematode worm acquired from ingestion of contaminated soil. It has a widespread geographic distribution but is most prevalent in rural tropics. Disease is relatively more common in children, who also carry higher worm loads.

Eggs hatch in the small intestine, then penetrate the intestinal wall into the portal circulation. From the liver, they are carried haematogenously to the lungs, from where they migrate up the bronchial tree and over the epiglottis back into the digestive tract. They can also migrate to ectopic sites in patients in whom the GI tract has been disrupted, e.g. by drugs, anaesthesia, or surgical manipulation.

Adult worms have a lifespan of 1y, after which they are spontaneously expelled from the bowel.

Presentation
Most cases are asymptomatic, although presentations may include fever, malaise, nausea, vomiting, intestinal colic, or diarrhoea. The migratory phase can cause a hypersensitivity eosinophilic pneumonitis, with urticaria and bronchospasm (Loeffler's syndrome) lasting on average 7–10d. In severe disease, a large number of worms can entangle to form obstructing boluses. Depending on location, these can cause intestinal obstruction, acute appendicitis, pancreatitis, or ascending cholangitis with obstructive jaundice. The latter is often associated with multiple liver abscesses, caused by disintegration of trapped worms or eggs, or biliary tree obstruction.

Investigation
- Blood tests and microscopy:
  - FBC. Usually normal. Eosinophilia during migratory phase.
  - LFT and amylase useful if obstruction of the biliary tree or pancreatic duct suspected.

- Stool microscopy diagnostic but false negatives within first 40d of infection.
- No serological test available.

Imaging:
- CXR. May show transient mottling or opacities during migratory phase but otherwise normal.
- AXR. Usually normal, although can show a large bolus of worms (particularly during contrast studies) or obstruction with extremely heavy loads.
- US. If suspect biliary obstruction or hepatic abscess.

ERCP. Indicated if there is evidence of cholangitis or pancreatitis for diagnosis and therapeutic removal of worms.

Treatment
Anti-helminth agents are indicated in all cases irrespective of presentation or worm load, as the consequences of a single episode of ectopic migration are severe. Suitable choices include:
- Albendazole 400mg PO bd for 3d.
- Piperazine 3.5g PO, single dose.

These agents are unsuitable for pregnant women and children, and expert advice should be sought in such cases. Piperazine is a paralysing agent and should not be used in intestinal obstruction as it may exacerbate the blockage.

Supportive treatment is required for other complications. ERCP is indicated for cholangitis or pancreatitis. Intestinal obstruction should be managed as described in Chapter 9 and may require surgical intervention.

Prognosis
Medical therapy is curative in >90% patients.

The liver in sepsis

Patients with bacterial sepsis frequently present with deranged LFT in the absence of evidence of direct liver infection. They account for up to 20% of jaundiced patients in hospital. Mechanisms are varied and include:

- Haemolysis.
- Drug reactions.
- Hepatic dysfunction. Down-regulated transporters and enzymes impair uptake and conjugation of bilirubin.
- Ischaemia. Hypoperfusion resulting from septic shock.
- Cholestasis. Reduced biliary tree exporters.

Jaundice is particularly common in patients with pneumococcal pneumonia. Typically, bilirubin is <100μmol/L, and liver transaminases and ALP are normal. The cause is unknown but possibly due to endotoxin and cytokine-mediated repression of hepatic transporters and enzymes. Deranged LFT are also a feature of Legionnaire's disease, in which AST, ALT, and ALP may all be elevated. Hyperbilirubinaemia is less common and tends to be seen only in patients who are severely ill.

Cholestasis of sepsis occurs primarily in children and adults with Gram-negative infections. Pruritus is not a major feature. LFT typically reveal a mild conjugated hyperbilirubinaemia (<100μmol/L) with elevated ALP (usually <3× ULN).

Evaluation of the jaundiced patient should follow the guidelines set out in Chapter 14 and is directed at excluding other treatable causes. Unconjugated hyperbilirubinaemia should prompt an evaluation for haemolysis, with a differential diagnosis of exacerbation of Gilbert's syndrome. Conjugated hyperbilirubinaemia requires imaging of the liver and biliary tree to rule out hepatic abscess and cholangitis. Liver biopsy is not helpful.

Management of the jaundiced patient with sepsis is of the underlying infection. There is no evidence to support any treatment aimed primarily at ameliorating liver dysfunction such as NAC or UDCA.

Neither the presence of jaundice nor its severity influence survival outcomes or overall prognosis. There is usually complete resolution.

nfections and the liver

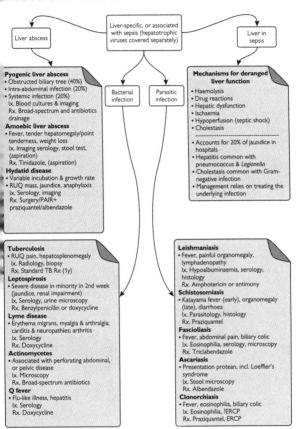

Liver-specific, or associated with sepsis (hepatotrophic viruses covered separately)

Liver abscess

Liver in sepsis

Bacterial infection

Parasitic infection

Pyogenic liver abscess
- Obstructed biliary tree (40%)
- Intra-abdominal infection (20%)
- Systemic infection (20%)
  Ix. Blood cultures & imaging
  Rx. Broad-spectrum and antibiotics drainage

Amoebic liver abscess
- Fever, tender hepatomegaly/point tenderness, weight loss
  Ix. Imaging serology, stool test, (aspiration)
  Rx. Tinidazole, (aspiration)

Hydatid disease
- Variable incubation & growth rate
- RUQ mass, jaundice, anaphylaxis
  Ix. Serology, imaging
  Rx. Surgery/PAIR+ praziquantel/albendazole

Tuberculosis
- RUQ pain, hepatosplenomegaly
  Ix. Radiology, biopsy
  Rx. Standard TB Rx (1y)

Leptospirosis
- Severe disease in minority in 2nd week (jaundice, renal impairment)
  Ix. Serology, urine microscopy
  Rx. Benzylpenicillin or doxycycline

Lyme disease
- Erythema migrans, myalgia & arthralgia; carditis & neuropathies; arthritis
  Ix. Serology
  Rx. Doxycycline

Actinomycetes
- Associated with perforating abdominal, or pelvic disease
  Ix. Microscopy
  Rx. Broad-spectrum antibiotics

Q fever
- Flu-like illness, hepatitis
  Ix. Serology
  Rx. Doxycycline

Mechanisms for deranged liver function
- Haemolysis
- Drug reactions
- Hepatic dysfunction
- Ischaemia
- Hypoperfusion (septic shock)
- Cholestasis

- Accounts for 20% of jaundice in hospitals
- Hepatitis common with pneumococcus & *Legionella*
- Cholestasis common with Gram-negative infection
- Management relies on treating the underlying infection

Leishmaniasis
- Fever, painful organomegaly, lymphadenopathy
  Ix. Hypoalbuminaemia, serology, histology
  Rx. Amphotericin or antimony

Schistosomiasis
- Katayama fever (early), organomegaly (late), diarrhoea
  Ix. Parasitology, histology
  Rx. Praziquantel

Fascioliasis
- Fever, abdominal pain, biliary colic
  Ix. Eosinophilia, serology, microscopy
  Rx. Triclabendazole

Ascariasis
- Presentation protean, incl. Loeffler's syndrome
  Ix. Stool microscopy
  Rx. Albendazole

Clonorchiasis
- Fever, eosinophilia, biliary colic
  Ix. Eosinophilia, ?ERCP
  Rx. Praziquantel, ERCP

Drug-induced liver injury

① Drug-induced liver injury

Drug-induced liver injury (DILI) accounts for ~1% of general medical admissions, <5% of all cases of jaundice, but up to 30% of acute liver failure. It is associated with >1,000 medications and herbal products. The following principles apply:

• All drugs may cause acute liver injury.
• Most forms of DILI lead to an acute hepatitis with raised transaminases.
• Some drugs cause predominantly cholestatic liver injury.
• Some drugs can cause fatty change, or fibrosis and cirrhosis.
• One drug may cause multiple patterns of injury.
• Most drug reactions are idiosyncratic.
• The diagnosis is one of exclusion.
• Drug withdrawal does not always lead to improvement.
• Drug challenge is rarely justified.

Drug reactions typically begin within 5–90d of initial exposure or 1–15d following re-exposure. The majority are asymptomatic and identified on the basis of rising serum aminotransferases or ALP. These are mostly of no clinical significance (e.g. with lone rise in ALT <3x ULN) and resolve weeks to months after discontinuation of the drug. An aminotransferase level >5x ULN, or the combination of aminotransferase levels >3x ULN with jaundice, implies high risk of liver damage ('Hy's law'), with mortality of 9–12%. Some drugs (e.g. isoniazid) lead to adaptation, whereby elevated transaminases may return to normal despite continuation of the drug.

The drugs most commonly associated with liver injury are paracetamol and antibiotics (especially co-amoxiclav). Other drugs which cause significant liver injury include isoniazid and pyrazinamide, as well as many antidepressants. The most frequent patterns of injury are listed in Table 18.1. Recreational drugs (including ecstasy and cocaine) and herbal remedies are also frequent culprits. Drug reactions may be predictable or idiosyncratic. Many require conversion to toxic metabolites.

Risk factors include population variants in cytochrome P450, alcohol misuse, polypharmacy (through enzyme induction), female sex, and increasing age. There are few data to suggest that patients with chronic liver disease are more prone to DILI in general, although they tolerate injury less well. In such patients, it is important to establish baseline LFT. Drugs known to be more toxic in chronic liver disease are listed in Table 18.2.

It is important to recognize that some drugs (e.g. phenytoin, carbamazepine, and barbiturates) induce γGT, and this does not constitute DILI. It is also important to recognize that a drug which causes myositis will also elevate 'liver enzymes' in the absence of liver injury.

The most important intervention is immediate discontinuation of the causative drug. In patients receiving many different medications, the one started most recently is likely to be responsible, although stopping all drugs, where possible, followed by cautious re-introduction of low-risk agents is advocated. Repeated exposure usually causes more rapid and severe DILI. Patients with liver failure require transfer to a liver transplant

Table 18.1 Drug-injury liver disease

Pattern	Common drugs
Fulminant hepatitis	Paracetamol, halothane
Acute or chronic hepatitis	Co-amoxiclav (younger patients), anabolic steroids, anti-tuberculosis drugs, anti-retrovirals, aspirin, bupropion, disulfiram, ketoconazole, lisinopril, losartan, methyldopa, nitrofurantoin, sodium valproate, SSRIs, statins
Subclinical liver disease	Antibiotics, antidepressants, isoniazid, lipid-lowering drugs, sulfonamides, salicylates, sulfonylureas, quinidine
Granulomatous hepatitis	Allopurinol, carbamazepine, diltiazem, hydralazine, phenytoin, quinine, sulphur-containing drugs
Hepatic fibrosis	Vitamin A, methotrexate
Steatosis (macrovesicular)	Amiodarone, tamoxifen, valproate
Steatosis (microvesicular)	Nucleoside reverse transcriptase inhibitors, sodium valproate, tetracycline
Hepatic neoplasia	Anabolic steroids, oestrogens
Budd–Chiari syndrome	Oestrogens
Hepatic sinusoidal obstruction	Azathioprine, busulfan, mercaptopurine, tetracycline, vitamin A
Cholestasis	Anabolic steroids, azathioprine, carbamazepine, chlorpromazine, clopidogrel, co-trimoxazole, diclofenac, efavirenz, erythromycin, ezetimibe, ketoconazole, nevirapine, oestrogens, penicillins (e.g co-amoxiclav in elderly patients), phenytoin, rifampicin, rosiglitazone, co-trimoxazole, tricyclics
Mixed patterns	Phenytoin, quinolones

Table 18.2 Drugs that are more toxic in chronic liver disease

Drug	Risk factor
Anti-retrovirals	Hepatitis B, hepatitis C
Anti-tuberculosis drugs	Hepatitis B, hepatitis C
Ibuprofen	Hepatitis C
Methimazole	Hepatitis B
Methotrexate	Alcoholic liver disease, steatohepatitis
OCP	Liver tumours
Rifampicin	PBC
Vitamin A	Alcoholic liver disease

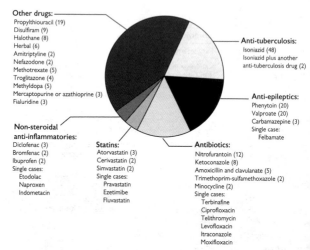

Fig. 18.1 Non-paracetamol-based drugs causing acute liver failure in patients requiring emergency liver transplantation in the USA, 1987–2006.

Reprinted from The Lancet, 376, William Bernal et al., 'Acute liver failure', pp. 190–210. Copyright 2010, with permission from Elvsevier. Data from Ayse L. Mindikoglu et al., 'Outcome of liver transplantation for drug-induced acute liver failure in the United States: Analysis of the united network for organ sharing database', *Liver Transplantation*, 15, 7, pp. 719–729, 2009, Wiley.

unit (for indications, see Chapter 15); DILI-associated acute liver failure has 80% mortality.

Treatment is largely supportive, as there are no specific treatments for DILI other than:

- NAC for paracetamol toxicity (see 📖 p. 296).
- L-carnitine for valproate toxicity. Loading dose of 100mg/kg IV (to maximum of 6g) over 30min, followed by 15mg/kg every 4h over 10–30min until clinical improvement occurs.

Acute DILI

Acute DILI is the most common form, accounting for 10% of all cases of acute hepatitis. Histologically, it can present as an acute hepatitis, cholestatic injury, mixed patterns, or acute steatosis. Extrahepatic manifestations can occur (hypersensitivity reactions with penicillin, mononucleosis-like illness with phenytoin). The vast majority of DILI simply cause asymptomatic elevation in transaminases, which may resolve despite continuation of the drug.

Acute hepatitis
Clinically, acute drug-related hepatitis may be indistinguishable from viral hepatitis, with jaundice, elevated serum aminotransferases (ALT >1,000U/L strongly suggests drug-induced, viral, or ischaemic hepatitis), and prolonged PTT. An allergic-type presentation may rarely be present, with fever, rash, lymphadenopathy, and peripheral blood eosinophilia; steroids may be helpful in such patients. Histologically, there is a spectrum from mild focal necrosis to massive hepatocyte damage.

Acute cholestasis
Acute cholestasis presents with jaundice, pale stools, and dark urine. LFT show elevated ALP and γGT. Transaminases can be mildly elevated. US excludes biliary obstruction. Pruritus may be intense but often responds to colestyramine, antihistamines, or UDCA. Cholestasis tends to resolve slower than other forms of liver injury (over months), but overall prognosis is better than with hepatocellular injury.

Acute steatosis
A number of drugs cause acute hepatic steatosis but, nonetheless, this remains uncommon. Jaundice is mild, and transaminases lower than in hepatocellular disease. Suspect if the patient is unwell (e.g. severe haemorrhage, shock, hypoglycaemia, or coma). Severe presentations have high mortality. Liver biopsy is diagnostic, showing microvesicular steatosis related to inhibition of mitochondrial fatty acid oxidation.

Chronic DILI
Defined as abnormal liver enzymes for >6mo. Accounts for 10% of DILI, more often following acute cholestasis. Resembles other causes of chronic liver disease such as autoimmune hepatitis or alcoholic liver disease. Often diagnosed following liver biopsy.

Chronic hepatitis
Generally occurs with long-term use of the offending drug. Can resemble autoimmune hepatitis, including positive serological markers.

Chronic cholestasis
May evolve from acute DILI. Usually resolves (>3mo) on stopping the drug but may progress to cirrhosis. Consider in a patient suspected to have PBC without serum AMA.

Chronic steatosis
Macrovesicular, due to impaired release of lipids from hepatocytes. Presents with hepatomegaly but minimal LFT derangement. Consider when diagnosing NAFLD or NASH in a patient taking suspect medication. Occasionally progresses to cirrhosis in weeks to months, thence chronic liver failure.

☢ Paracetamol

Paracetamol (acetaminophen) remains the commonest cause of DILI. Liver damage in overdose relates to the toxic action of one of its metabolites. In therapeutic doses, the drug is principally conjugated to glucuronide and sulphate forms. Less than 10% is oxidized to N-acetyl-p-benzoquinoneimine (NAPQI), a highly reactive species that is normally immediately conjugated to glutathione, then excreted. In overdose, the main conjugation pathways become saturated and NAPQI formation increases. Liver glutathione stores rapidly deplete, leading to unrestrained NAPQI reactions and hepatocellular necrosis.

Clinical presentation

Toxicity, including the extent and rate of liver damage, is dose-related. Most patients are usually asymptomatic for the first 24h, although nausea, vomiting, and abdominal pain may occur. Liver damage is usually biochemically detectable from 18h, with hepatic tenderness from 48h. Maximum liver damage occurs between 72–96h after ingestion, with jaundice and encephalopathy. In patients who do not provide a reliable history of drug exposure, a very high AST (>5,000IU/L) is suggestive of paracetamol-induced liver injury.

Patients may also present having taken repeated supratherapeutic ingestions of paracetamol (staggered overdose). The time courses of metabolic derangements in these individuals are less well defined, and nomograms less sensitive in predicting outcomes. Staggered overdoses are associated with higher rates of fulminant hepatic failure, liver transplant, and mortality (Craig et al., 2012). These may arise either as direct consequences of the mode of administration or due to delays administrating NAC.

Investigation and prognostication

One challenge in managing paracetamol overdose is to predict which patients are at risk of significant DILI. This needs to be achieved early, as treatment is most effective before LFT become deranged.

Always measure serum paracetamol if overdose suspected. A dose of 7.5–10g is potentially serious in most adults. A single measure of plasma paracetamol concentration is an accurate predictor of liver damage if taken >4h after overdose (unless drugs slowing gastric emptying, such as opiates or anticholinergics, are co-ingested). Levels can be interpreted according to the modified Rumack–Matthew nomogram (see Fig. 18.2), with 60% of patients above the line likely to sustain liver damage unless protective treatment is given. Plasma concentrations are still of value with presentations >12h after ingestion, particularly in conjunction with PTT. Certain patients are at greater risk, including those with:

- Pre-existing liver disease.
- The elderly.
- Chronic alcohol misuse (*acute* ingestion may be protective).
- Malnutrition.
- CYP450-inducing medications (phenytoin, carbamazepine, sodium valproate, oxcarbazepine, topiramate, phenobarbital, rifampicin, ritonavir, efavirenz, modafinil, St. John's wort).
- HIV.

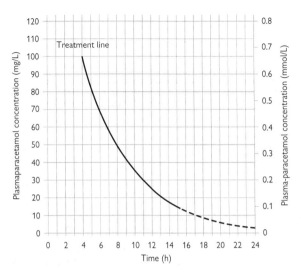

Fig. 18.2 Paracetamol toxicity nomogram.

This Crown copyright material is reproduced by permission of the Medicines and Healthcare products Regulatory Agency (MHRA) under delegated authority from the Controller of HMSO.

Baseline and daily monitoring should include FBC, U & E, LFT, coagulation screen, lactate, and glucose. PTT and pH are of particular prognostic value: PTT >20s or pH <7.3 at 24h are indicators of poor outcome. Serum aminotransferases may become markedly elevated within 48–72h (e.g. >3,000IU/L) but are less helpful than clotting and clinical state. Lactate >3.5mmol/L at 24h after overdose or >3.0mmol/L after fluid resuscitation is an indication for transplantation (Neuberger et al., 2008).

Management

Activated charcoal (1g/kg, max 50g) is of value within 1h of ingestion to limit absorption (up to 4h with co-administered drugs that delay gastric emptying). IV fluids are indicated for patients in pre-renal failure or those with significant losses through vomiting.

The next treatment goal is to replenish glutathione stores by infusion of NAC, or oral methionine. Treatment regimens are:

• NAC IV: 150mg/kg over 1h in 200mL 5% glucose, then 50mg/kg in 500mL 5% glucose over 4h, then 100mg/kg in 1L 5% glucose over 16h. Repeat latter infusion twice in large overdoses, especially if PTT prolonged or transaminases remain >1,000IU/L. The loading dose is often associated with flushing and other anaphylactoid

symptoms. If this occurs, stop the infusion, treat with antihistamine (e.g. chlorphenamine), and restart at a lower infusion rate.
• Methionine PO: 2.5g initially, then 2.5g 4-hourly for three doses, to total dose of 10g over 12h.

Treatment is effective within 10h of overdose (with no deaths reported in any of the large studies). NAC is still advocated in patients who present later with significant overdose, in all those who have taken a staggered overdose, or when the history is unreliable, although the evidence base for these is weaker.

A number of other supportive measures are helpful. Late presenters, or those with deteriorating liver function, should receive 10% glucose IV to prevent hypoglycaemia. PPIs reduce risk of GI bleeding from stress ulcers, which can be catastrophic if there is coagulopathy. There is no evidence that correcting deranged clotting empirically alters prognosis. FFP should not be given, except in severe haemorrhage, unless the patient has been listed for transplantation; nor should it be given for 'invasive procedures' without explicit consent from the local transplant centre. There is no role for forced diuresis or haemofiltration to aid elimination of paracetamol, although renal replacement therapy may be required if acute renal failure supervenes.

Liver transplantation may be required in patients with fulminant hepatic failure. Contact the specialist liver unit early, especially if any of the following are present:
• PTT >30s or INR >3.
• Arterial pH <7.3 (mandates transfer to a liver unit).
• Serum creatinine >200µmol/L.
• Hypoglycaemia.
• Encephalopathy.

Other complications
• Renal failure (25%), usually due to acute tubular necrosis. May occur independent of liver failure.
• Severe thrombocytopaenia.
• Metabolic acidosis.
• Hypoglycaemia.
• Hypophosphataemia.
• GI haemorrhage.
• Cerebral oedema and coma.
• Mortality (5%).

① Statins

Statins are amongst the most commonly prescribed drugs. Raised aminotransferases >3x ULN are seen in 3%, and generally transient. There are very few documented incidences of severe liver injury, particularly given their widespread use, and no evidence that these drugs are less safe in chronic liver disease. Acute liver failure is idiosyncratic, occurring in 1 per 10^6 patient-years, equivalent to the background rate of idiopathic liver failure.

Autoimmune hepatitis has been described in case reports. This is rare but should be considered when there are deranged LFT associated with rash, positive ANA or anti-smooth muscle antibodies, or failure to resolve despite drug discontinuation. Prednisolone is helpful.

A number of current guidelines advocate LFT monitoring at 12wk and annually thereafter. There is no evidence that this strategy prevents significant DILI, and false positives may lead to discontinuation of beneficial cardiac drugs.

① NSAIDs and aspirin

The incidence of reported NSAID-induced liver injury ranges from 3–23/100,000 (Rubenstein and Laine, 2003); it constitutes ~10% of recognized DILI (Bessone, 2010), and several NSAIDs have been withdrawn from the market due to hepatotoxicity. That said, the overall risk is low, given the prevalence of NSAID use: 6% of the adult population receive prescription NSAIDs annually, and 24% use over-the-counter products (although the latter typically for short durations). Risk factors for DILI include dose and duration of use, age, pre-existing hepatic steatosis, and metabolic syndrome.

Aspirin

Liver toxicity is dose-dependent, although patients with juvenile rheumatoid arthritis or hypoalbuminaemia and SLE are more susceptible. Non-specific focal necrosis, hepatocellular degeneration, and hydropic changes are commonly seen.

Aspirin can also cause Reye's syndrome in children, a mitochondrial dysfunction disorder that leads to free fatty acid hepatic accumulation and massive steatosis. Clinically, it presents with metabolic acidosis, encephalopathy, hypoglycaemia, coagulopathy, and azotaemia.

Diclofenac

Diclofenac is the most widely used NSAID. Hepatotoxicity is rare and may only emerge after a prolonged latent period. In those developing DILI, jaundice is common (75%), and LFT most frequently show a mixed hepatocellular/cholestatic picture.

Ibuprofen

Ibuprofen is also extensively used and widely available over the counter. It possesses the best liver safety profile of all NSAIDs, with very low rates of hepatic toxicity. This is probably attributable to its short plasma half-life and lack of secondary pathological metabolites. Although there are a few case reports of liver disease associated with ibuprofen use, it is generally a very unlikely causative agent. Risk may be marginally elevated with chronic HCV.

Sulindac

Liver toxicity is 5–10 times more common with sulindac than other NSAIDs. Patients >50y are at particular risk, and the male:female ratio is 1:3.5. Cholestatic patterns of injury are twice as frequent as hepatocellular patterns, and hypersensitivity mechanisms implicated in 60%.

Other non-selective COX inhibitors

Indometacin and naproxen are frequently used non-specific COX inhibitors, with favourable adverse effect profiles. Hepatotoxicity is infrequent, although various patterns have been described.

Hepatotoxicity due to piroxicam is uncommon but may result in severe hepatocellular necrosis. This reaction appears to be idiosyncratic and dose-independent.

Coxibs

These are NSAIDs designed to selectively inhibit COX-2. They gained popularity due to a lower incidence of GI side effects, but this has been partially offset by recognition of increased cardiovascular morbidity and mortality. Coxib-induced DILI occurs in 1/100,000, with variation between agents. Raised serum transaminases are observed in 0.6% of patients taking celecoxib, 1% with etoricoxib, 2% with rofecoxib, and 3% with lumiracoxib (since withdrawn from the market).

Nimesulide

Nimesulide is a COX-2 selective NSAID with a unique chemical structure. There have been numerous reports of severe hepatotoxicity, leading to its market withdrawal in many countries. Nonetheless, it is still available in several European countries, although the European Medicines Agency recommends restricting length of therapy to 15d, with maximum dosage of 100mg/d. There is a broad spectrum of hepatotoxicity, including acute hepatitis, cholestasis, mixed pictures, and massive and submassive hepatocellular necrosis. Approximately 17% of nimesulide-related DILI are severe.

① Anticonvulsants

Hepatotoxicity with anticonvulsants is well recognized and cause 6–8% of DILI. Liver injury is frequently due to toxic metabolites.

Phenytoin

Acute and chronic hepatotoxicity may occur with phenytoin use. There is no correlation between its serum concentration and DILI, or between liver and CNS toxicity. Liver injury usually reverses following drug cessation, although overall mortality is ~13%. Multiple patterns are described:
• Increased ALP and γGT. Occur as part of hepatic adaptation.
• Hypersensitivity reactions. Associated with fever, rash, and eosinophilia.
• Acute hepatitis. Rare but can be severe. Symptoms develop 1–6wk after initiating treatment.

- Chronic liver injury. Usually reported when phenytoin is not discontinued in the face of abnormal LFT.

Carbamazepine

As with phenytoin, carbamazepine DILI does not correlate with its serum concentration. At least 10% of patients develop asymptomatic rises in serum transaminases and ALP, and up to 60% an elevated γGT. These are generally not of sufficient magnitude to recommend drug cessation, although severe reactions may occur (most frequently in children). Acute liver failure is rare but occasionally fatal. Patterns of injury include:

- Cholestasis.
- Hepatic necrosis.
- Granulomatous hepatitis.
- Hypersensitivity reactions.
- Vanishing bile duct syndrome.

Sodium valproate

Reversible increases in serum aminotransferases occur in 10–40% of patients taking sodium valproate during the first few months of treatment. These will often normalize despite continuation of therapy. Clinically significant DILI occurs in 1/15,000 (more frequent in children). Three main subtypes are recognized:

- Toxic hepatitis with submassive/zonal hepatocyte necrosis. Occurs in 1/37,000, mostly within 2–3mo of starting therapy. Valproate use is associated with carnitine depletion (an essential co-factor in mitochondrial fatty acid β-oxidation). Outcomes of severe hepatotoxicity are better with L-carnitine supplementation (38% increased survival).
- Hyperammonaemia. Valproate inhibits carbamyl phosphate synthetase, impairing the transformation of carbamyl phosphate and ornithine into citrulline and thus disrupting the urea cycle. Hyperammonaemia may occur with normal LFT. The prevalence is high (up to 50%), and thus this rarely causes clinically significant disease. It may, however, occasionally be responsible for encephalopathy, particularly in patients with underlying urea cycle disorders. L-carnitine supplementation is helpful.
- Reye-like syndrome, with associated microvesicular steatosis.

Certain groups are recognized to be at high risk (incidence 1/500) of severe valproate-associated hepatotoxicity. These include patients with:

- Age <3y.
- Past medical or family history of:
  - Mitochondrial enzyme deficiencies (urea cycle disorders or long-chain/medium-chain fatty acid oxidation defects).
  - Reye's syndrome.
  - Friedreich's ataxia.
- Sibling affected by sodium valproate hepatotoxicity.
- Multiple drug therapies.

Lamotrigine

Used in the treatment of partial and generalized seizures. There are a few reports of acute hepatitis and isolated cases of fulminant hepatic failure.

Topiramate

Add-on therapy in patients with partial and generalized epileptic seizures, and Lennox–Gastaut syndrome. Isolated cases of acute liver failure with hepatocellular injury have been reported.

Other anticonvulsants

There are a few case reports of DILI with oxcarbazepine and phenobarbital. Clinically significant hepatotoxicity has not been reported with levetiracetam, tiagabine, benzodiazepines, or ethosuximide.

① Antidepressants

Use of antidepressant medication is increasing. Significant DILI is rare but has been reported with multiple classes of these agents.

Selective serotonin reuptake inhibitors (SSRIs)

Most frequently prescribed antidepressants. Abnormal LFT are observed in up to 0.5% of patients on long-term therapy. Severe hepatotoxicity is rare, although acute hepatitis has been described with fluoxetine, paroxetine, sertraline, and duloxetine. Cholestasis has also been reported, particularly with use of sertraline.

Tricyclic antidepressants

Principally cause cholestatic injury but are rarely associated with hepatocellular damage or vanishing bile duct syndrome.

Monoamine oxidase inhibitors

These drugs are less commonly employed now than previously. Acute hepatitis is a feature in 1%, particularly with iproniazid (now withdrawn in the UK).

Serotonin-noradrenaline reuptake inhibitors (SNRIs)

Venlafaxine and nefazodone have been associated with severe hepatocellular injury and, occasionally, fulminant hepatic failure requiring transplant.

Trazodone

Serotonin antagonist and reuptake inhibitor. Has been implicated in cases of acute and chronic hepatocellular injury, and cholestasis. The latent period to emergence of DILI can be up to 18mo.

① Amiodarone

Amiodarone is an iodinated drug frequently used in the acute and chronic management of cardiac dysrhythmias. Asymptomatic elevations in transaminases occur in up to 25% of patients on long-term therapy. Symptomatic

DILI arises in <1%; both acute fulminant hepatitis and chronic hepatitis with cirrhosis can develop. Liver injury results from inhibition of mitochondrial β-oxidation and, possibly, phospholipidosis.

ⓘ Anti-tuberculosis drugs

A number of drugs employed in the treatment of TB have the potential to cause DILI. Approximately 10% of patients receiving anti-tuberculosis treatment will develop deranged serum aminotransferases, of whom 10% are at risk of severe hepatic necrosis.

Monthly LFT monitoring is required in those with abnormal baseline results, those with liver disease (hepatitis B or C, or alcohol abuse), in pregnancy and for 3mo post-partum, and in those receiving pyrazinamide. All patients should be educated about symptoms of potential DILI (anorexia, nausea, vomiting, jaundice, rash, pruritus, fatigue, fever, abdominal discomfort, bruising, arthralgia) and, if present, LFT should be performed at 2–4 weekly intervals.

In general, hepatotoxicity manifests with ALT >5x ULN or >3x ULN with symptoms (most smaller rises resolve spontaneously). In such circumstances, all anti-tuberculosis drugs should be temporarily stopped. Exclude other causes of liver disease (perform a full liver screen), as DILI is a diagnosis of exclusion. To restart, it is generally recommended to commence with rifampicin, followed by ethambutol. If these are tolerated for at least 7d, isoniazid can be re-introduced. If DILI recurs, remove the last drug added. Avoid pyrazinamide if hepatotoxicity is prolonged or severe. Some experts provide second-line agents to avoid treatment cessation (e.g. an aminoglycoside, ethambutol, and moxifloxacin); seek advice.

Rifampicin

May cause dose-dependent interference with bilirubin uptake, resulting in subclinical unconjugated hyperbilirubinaemia without hepatocellular damage. Also potentiates hepatotoxicity of other drugs. ALT elevated in 20% and is >2x ULN in 2.5%. Hepatocellular injury is, however, rare; consider with disproportionate rise in bilirubin and ALP. It appears to be a hypersensitivity reaction, which may be more common with large intermittent doses. May be associated with renal dysfunction, haemolytic anaemia, and a flu-like syndrome. Conjugated hyperbilirubinaemia can result from inhibition of bile salt exporters.

Isoniazid

Isoniazid is predominantly cleared via acetylation by N-acetyltransferase-2 to toxic monoacetyl hydrazine, then to non-toxic diacetyl hydrazine. Genetic polymorphisms correlate with fast, slow, and intermediate acetylator enzyme action. Most cases of presumed isoniazid hepatotoxicity are associated with pyrazinamide use.

Many patients (10–20%) get increased serum aminotransferases within weeks to months of initiation. These are usually modest and transient, with only 0.1–2.0% developing clinical hepatitis and/or liver failure. There is ethnic variation, with lower risk in Afro-Caribbean individuals. Rifampicin enhances isoniazid hepatotoxicity (2.6% higher than with single-agent therapy). Hepatitis B and C increase risk, although HIV does not.

The influence of acetylation rate is controversial. Early studies identified rapid acetylators as at greater risk of hepatotoxicity, but these relied on phenotypic characterization of acetylation status. This may have been confounded due to differences in absorption. As fast acetylators clear monoacetyl hydrazine more quickly, slow acetylators may actually have greater cumulative exposure. Recent studies based on enzyme genotyping have shown that slow acetylators experience transaminase elevations >3x ULN more frequently and to higher peaks than fast acetylators. The significance remains unconfirmed.

Pyrazinamide

Pyrazinamide is frequently used in combination therapy, and many believe this drug is actually responsible for much of DILI attributed to isoniazid. It may exhibit both dose-dependent and idiosyncratic hepatotoxicity, and there is crossover with previous reactions to isoniazid. It may also induce hypersensitivity reactions with eosinophilia, and granulomatous hepatitis. It is usually not restarted if thought to have caused DILI.

Other anti-tuberculosis drugs

- *Rifabutin*. Hepatotoxicity is uncommon at usual doses, and it causes less induction of hepatic microsomal enzymes than rifampicin. Elevated transaminases have been reported with high doses, especially in combination with macrolides. In AIDS patients treated for disseminated atypical mycobacterial infection with such a regimen, hepatotoxicity is 8%.
- *Ethambutol*. There is one report of cholestatic jaundice, not clearly attributable to the drug.
- *Fluoroquinolones*. Ciprofloxacin and moxifloxacin are partly metabolized by the liver. Reversible transaminase elevation occurs in 2–3%, and severe hepatocellular injury and cholestasis in <1%.

① Co-amoxiclav

Co-amoxiclav is one of the most widely prescribed antibiotics and the most frequently reported to cause DILI. Liver injury is presumed to result mostly from the clavulinic acid component. Symptomatic hepatitis occurs in 3–17/100,000. Jaundice is most commonly cholestatic, usually developing 1–4wk (but reported up to 8wk) after drug cessation. Pathologically, it is associated with ductopaenia (vanishing bile duct syndrome). It typically follows a benign course and resolves within 2mo.

A hepatocellular injury picture is rare but can present in the first week. It is more frequent in younger patients, in comparison to cholestatic injury that typically affects older individuals. Hepatotoxicity is usually mild with subsequent complete recovery. Occasionally, the outcome can be severe or protracted, with 3% dying or requiring liver transplant and up to 7% sustaining persistent liver damage.

ⓘ Minocycline

Minocycline is a tetracycline antibiotic widely used in young patients for treatment of acne vulgaris. It is associated with three patterns of DILI:

- Dose-related direct hepatotoxicity with severe microvesicular or macrovesicular steatosis. Mostly reported with IV administration.
- Allergic idiosyncratic reaction. Hepatitis with fever, rash, lymphadenopathy, and eosinophilia. Onset 3–4wk after commencing therapy.
- Autoimmune hepatitis. Often accompanied by arthralgia/arthritis, fever, fatigue, and rash. Mean onset ~15mo post-exposure. Blood tests show absence of eosinophilia, and 90% are strongly positive for ANA. Liver biopsy demonstrates peri-portal inflammation with piecemeal necrosis, reflecting chronic active hepatitis.

Treatment involves drug discontinuation ± steroids (for unresolving allergic/autoimmune subtypes).

ⓘ Oral contraceptive pill

DILI with oral contraceptive pills (OCPs) is very rare, but a number of patterns have been reported:

- *Budd–Chiari syndrome.* The risk of venous thromboembolism is increased 2-fold with oestrogen-containing OCPs, particularly during the first year of use, due to acquired activated protein C resistance. Thrombosis of the hepatic vein or terminal IVC can occur. Its importance may have been overemphasized, as most reports derive from the 1990s when the oestrogen dose was higher.
- *Hepatic sinusoidal obstruction (veno-occlusive disease).* Gives rise to a syndrome of jaundice, painful hepatomegaly, and ascites. It is particularly associated with norethisterone. Histology shows diffuse centrilobular damage with marked sinusoidal fibrosis, peri-central hepatocyte necrosis, and narrowing of central veins.
- *Peliosis hepatis.* Rare. Biopsy shows blood-filled cavities within liver.
- *Neoplasia.* Hepatic adenomas, adenomatosis, and HCC have been attributed to OCP use in 4/100,000 individuals.

ⓘ Khat

Chewing khat leaves (*Catha edulis*) is common in East Africa and the Arabian Peninsula. The leaves contain cathine and cathinone, which have amphetamine-like effects. Khat can cause fulminant hepatitis. Its use should be suspected when patients from ethnic communities where khat consumption is prevalent present with otherwise unexplained liver injury.

① Herbal remedies

The use of herbal remedies is increasingly common. These agents can cause most patterns of liver injury (see Table 18.3). An accurate history is required, although information concerning their use may be withheld. Patient education is important, including the notion that 'natural' does not always equate with 'safe': compounds may consist of mixtures that are often impure, and botanicals may be misidentified or contaminated. They should be advised to report symptoms potentially deriving from DILI.

In the absence of a history, their use should be suspected with unusual patterns of liver injury. These include zonal necrosis, necrosis with steatosis or bile duct injury, and veno-occlusive disease.

Table 18.3 Herbal remedies causing liver injury

Remedy (component)	Reported DILI
Bajiaolian (podophyllotoxin)	Deranged LFT
Camphor	Deranged LFT
Carp capsules (cyprinol)	Deranged LFT
Cascara sagrada (anthracene glycosis)	Cholestasis, hepatitis, portal hypertension
Chaparral leaf (*Larrea tridentate*)	Necrosis, chronic hepatitis, cholestasis
Chinese herbal tea (*T'u san-chi'i*)	Veno-occlusive disease
Comfrey tea (Pyrrolizidine alkaloids)	Veno-occlusive disease
Dai-saiko-to	Acute hepatitis
Germander (*Neoclerodane diterpenes*)	Necrosis, fibrosis, cirrhosis
Glue thistle (*Atractylis gummifera*)	Diffuse necrosis
Greater celandine (*Chelidonium majus*)	Hepatitis, fibrosis
Impila (*Callilepsis laureola*)	Necrosis
Jin Bu Huan (*Lycopodium serratum*)	Acute and chronic hepatitis, fibrosis, steatosis
Kava	Diffuse hepatocellular necrosis, intrahepatic cholestasis, fulminant hepatic failure
Kombucha mushroom	Deranged LFT
Licorice (*Glycyrrhizin*)	Vanishing bile duct syndrome, antagonizes spironolactone
Ma-huang (ephedrine)	Acute hepatitis
Margosa oil (*Azadirachta indica*)	Reye's syndrome
Maté tea (pyrrolizidine alkaloids)	Veno-occlusive disease

(Continued)

Table 18.3 *(Continued)*

Remedy (component)	Reported DILI
Oil of cloves (eugenol)	Acute liver damage
Pennyroyal oil (pulegone)	Necrosis
Prostata (saw palmetto)	Hepatitis, fibrosis
Sassafras albidum	Carcinogenic in animals
Sho-saiko-to (*Scutellaria*)	Necrosis, fibrosis, microvesicular steatosis
Teucrium polium	Necrosis, fibrosis, acute liver failure
Venencapsan	Acute hepatitis, focal steatosis

Drug-induced liver injury

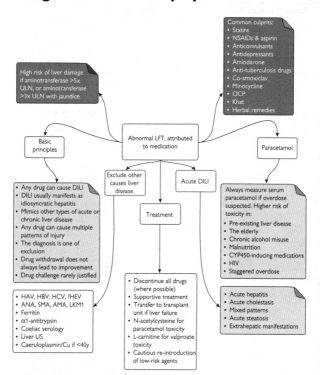

Common culprits:
- Statins
- NSAIDs & aspirin
- Anticonvulsants
- Antidepressants
- Amiodarone
- Anti-tuberculosis drugs
- Co-amoxiclav
- Minocycline
- OCP
- Khat
- Herbal remedies

High risk of liver damage if aminotransferase >5x ULN, or aminotransferase >3x ULN with jaundice

Abnormal LFT, attributed to medication

Basic principles

Paracetamol

Exclude other causes liver disease

Acute DILI

Treatment

- Any drug can cause DILI
- DILI usually manifests as idiosyncratic hepatitis
- Mimics other types of acute or chronic liver disease
- Any drug can cause multiple patterns of injury
- The diagnosis is one of exclusion
- Drug withdrawal does not always lead to improvement
- Drug challenge rarely justified

Always measure serum paracetamol if overdose suspected. Higher risk of toxicity in:
- Pre-existing liver disease
- The elderly
- Chronic alcohol misuse
- Malnutrition
- CYP450-inducing medications
- HIV
- Staggered overdose

- HAV, HBV, HCV, ?HEV
- ANA, SMA, AMA, LKM1
- Ferritin
- α1-antitrypsin
- Coeliac serology
- Liver US
- Caeruloplasmin/Cu if <40y

- Discontinue all drugs (where possible)
- Supportive treatment
- Transfer to transplant unit if liver failure
- N-acetylcysteine for paracetamol toxicity
- L-carnitine for valproate toxicity
- Cautious re-introduction of low-risk agents

- Acute hepatitis
- Acute cholestasis
- Mixed patterns
- Acute steatosis
- Extrahepatic manifestations

Further reading

Bernal W, Auzinger G, Dhawan A, et al. (2010) Acute liver failure. *Lancet* **376**: 190–201.

Bessone F (2010) Non-steroidal anti-inflammatory drugs: what is the actual risk of liver damage? *World J Gastroenterol* **16**: 5651–61.

Craig DG, Bates CM, Davidson JS, et al. (2012) Staggered overdose pattern and delay to hospital presentation are associated with adverse outcomes following paracetamol-induced hepatotoxicity. *Br J Clin Pharmacol* **73**: 285–94.

Mindikoglu AL, Magder LS, Regev A (2009) Outcome of liver transplantation for drug-induced acute liver failure in the United States: analysis of the United Network for Organ Sharing database. *Liver Transpl* **15**: 719–29.

Neuberger J, Gimson A, Davies K (2008) Selection of patients for liver transplantation and allocation of donated livers in the UK. *Gut* **57**: 252–7.

Rubeinstein JH, Laine L (2004) Systematic review: the hepatotoxicity of non-steroidal anti-inflammatory drugs. *Aliment Pharmacol Ther* **20**: 373–80.

The liver in pregnancy

Liver disease in pregnancy

A number of liver disorders are unique to, or more likely to occur in, pregnancy. These should be considered alongside the other causes of liver disease that occur in non-pregnant patients. Transient mild derangements of LFT are common and rarely require further assessment beyond repeat monitoring to ensure normalization. However, liver disorders in pregnancy often present non-specifically and, therefore. all patients merit formal clinical assessment.

Table 19.1 highlights the relationship between liver disorders and foetal gestational age. US and MRI (without gadolinium contrast) are the imaging modalities of choice, as they avoid ionizing radiation. Where LFT are abnormal, it is prudent to check HBV and HCV serology (if not already performed), as measures can be instituted to limit vertical transmission. Expert obstetric advice should be sought when managing pregnant women with liver disease.

Table 19.1 Liver disorders specific to pregnancy

First trimester	Second trimester	Third trimester
Hyperemesis gravidarum	Obstetric cholestasis	Obstetric cholestasis
(Obstetric cholestasis)	(Pre-eclampsia)	Pre-eclampsia
	(HELLP)	HELLP
		Acute fatty liver of pregnancy
		Hepatic rupture

Parentheses indicate occurrence in this trimester possible but unusual.

Liver function tests in pregnancy

Normal physiological changes in pregnancy result in minor derangements in LFT, secondary to haemodilution or altered hepatic synthetic function (see Table 19.2). ALP is produced by the placenta and, although organ-specific isoenzymes can be measured, this is rarely necessary. Increased serum bilirubin or aminotransferases are, however, pathological and require investigation. Serum total bile acid concentrations should be measured in cholestatic disorders, as levels predict adverse foetal outcomes; similarly, high serum urate predicts adverse outcomes in the hypertensive disorders (pre-eclampsia, eclampsia, and HELLP syndrome).

Palmar erythema and spider naevi can be normal in pregnancy.

Table 19.2 LFT derangement in normal pregnancy

LFT	Alteration	Trimester	Mechanism
Bilirubin	None		
AST	None		
ALT	None		
γGT	None		
ALP	Increased	3	Placenta
Albumin	Decreased	2	Haemodilution
Fibrinogen	Increased	2	Increased synthesis

① Hyperemesis gravidarum

Intractable severe vomiting causing dehydration, ketosis, and loss (>5%) of body weight. Occurs in 0.3–2% of pregnancies, arising during the first trimester, and typically resolves by 18wk gestation. It is more common in younger women, non-smokers, primiparas, and multiple or molar pregnancies. A 2-fold, reversible increase in serum aminotransferases occurs in 50% (although can be as high as 20× ULN), with minor elevation of ALP and bilirubin in 10%. The aetiology of deranged LFT is unclear, as is their significance. Management is detailed in Chapter 4, and involves correction of fluid and electrolyte deficiencies, and the use of thiamine to prevent Wernicke's encephalopathy and anti-emetics. Pregnancy outcomes are usually unaffected, although severe malnutrition is associated with foetal growth retardation.

① Obstetric cholestasis

Acute intrahepatic cholestasis accounts for 20% of cases of jaundice in pregnancy and affects 0.5–1% of all pregnancies. The cause is unknown but may relate to impaired conjugation of bile salts caused by the high oestrogen state. It occurs in 50% of patients who have previously developed cholestasis due to OCP use and may arise in the ovarian hyperstimulation syndrome. It is relatively benign for the mother but has negative consequences for the foetus: prematurity is increased 3-fold, and rates of foetal distress and stillbirth are higher.

Onset can be at any time, although third trimester is most common. The main presentation is generalized pruritus, particularly severe on the palms and soles. Subclinical steatorrhoea may be detectable, with fat malabsorption and vitamin K deficiency. Jaundice is present in <10% and typically occurs 1–4wk later, associated with pale stools and dark urine. LFT show mild elevation in bilirubin, moderately raised aminotransferases (occasionally >1,000IU/L), rises in ALP (although also produced by placenta), but only marginally increased γGT. Serum bile acids rise (cholic acid > chenodeoxycholic acid); foetal complications correlate with their concentrations and are not seen with levels <40µmol/L. US is necessary to exclude gallstone disease; MRCP helpful if diagnostic doubt. Liver biopsy is not required.

Treatment is symptomatic with UDCA (10–15mg/kg/d) for the duration of pregnancy, which relieves pruritus and may improve foetal outcomes. Colestyramine should be used with caution, as it can exacerbate vitamin K deficiency. In general, elective delivery is recommended by 38wk to minimize foetal complications, although some advocate careful observation and induction of labour only if foetal distress intervenes.

Perinatal mortality is 3–5%. Cholestasis recurs in up to 60% of subsequent pregnancies.

☼ Acute fatty liver of pregnancy

Acute fatty liver of pregnancy is a microvesicular steatosis caused by mitochondrial dysfunction that complicates 1 in 14,000 pregnancies. It predominantly occurs during the third trimester (particularly between wk34–37), although may manifest earlier or post-partum. Risk factors include nulliparity, or having a male foetus or twin pregnancy. Up to 40% have associated pre-eclampsia or HELLP syndrome.

Initial symptoms include headache, fatigue, nausea, vomiting, and abdominal discomfort. In severe cases, jaundice (conjugated bilirubin >100µmol/L) develops within 2wk. Urine is bile-stained and stools are pale. Progression to acute liver failure may be rapid, with encephalopathy and death within days. Serum aminotransferases are usually elevated to <750IU/L. Hypoglycaemia is common, and blood film commonly shows neutrophilia, normoblasts, thrombocytopaenia, target cells, and giant platelets. DIC is relatively common. Upper GI haemorrhage, acute renal failure, pancreatitis, and transient diabetes insipidus may occur. Hyperuricaemia is present in 80%. US may reveal steatosis, although CT is more sensitive. For Swansea diagnostic criteria, see Box 19.1. Foetal and maternal mortality is 10–20%.

Box 19.1 Swansea diagnostic criteria for acute fatty liver of pregnancy*

- Vomiting.
- Abdominal pain.
- Polydipsia/polyuria.
- Encephalopathy.
- Bilirubin >14µmol/L.
- Glucose <4mmol/L.
- Urate >340µmol/L.
- WCC >11 × 10^9/L.
- Ascites or bright liver on US.
- AST or ALT >42IU/L.
- NH_3 >47µmol/L.
- Creatinine >150µmol/L.
- PTT >14s or APTT >34s.
- Microvesicular steatosis on liver biopsy.

* ≥6 required for diagnosis, in the absence of alternative explanation.

Reproduced from *Gut*, C L Ch'ng et al., 'Prospective study of liver dysfunction in pregnancy in Southwest Wales', 51, 6, pp. 876–880, copyright 2002, with permission from BMJ Publishing Group Ltd.

Liver biopsy may rarely be required to differentiate from acute viral hepatitis or pre-eclampsia, which is important for assessing prognosis in future pregnancies. Histology demonstrates microvesicular fat deposition, with rare hepatocyte necrosis and minimal inflammation, similar to Reye's syndrome.

Definitive management involves early delivery. Extreme caution with careful monitoring is advised if expectant management is employed, as deterioration can be sudden and unpredictable. Careful fluid balance is required, as the risk of pulmonary or cerebral oedema is increased. Hypoglycaemia is prevented by IV glucose. Aggressive correction of coagulopathy has been recommended. Liver transplantation has rarely been required. With specialist care, maternal mortality is <1% and peri-natal mortality 7%. These values are higher without close monitoring and early intervention. Risk of recurrence is <15%.

Although most cases are idiopathic, acute fatty liver of pregnancy may arise in heterozygous mothers carrying foetuses with long-chain 3-hydroxyacyl-CoA dehydrogenase (LCHAD) deficiency. These infants may present after birth with non-ketotic hypoglycaemia, Reye's syndrome, or sudden infant death. Diagnostic testing for the *G1528C* mutation is therefore recommended in all mothers with this presentation.

⊙ Pre-eclampsia

Pre-eclampsia (pre-eclampsic toxaemia, PET) refers to hypertension (BP >140/90mmHg or >30/15mmHg above baseline) with proteinuria, and occurs in 5–10% of pregnancies. Peripheral oedema may also be seen but is no longer required for the diagnosis. Eclampsia is defined by the presence of seizures in addition to these features.

Pre-eclampsia arises from the end of the second trimester. Risk factors include being primagravida, extremes of age, multiple gestation, and family history. Deranged LFT occur in 25% of mild and 80% of severe presentations; the most common abnormality is raised serum aminotransferases, usually <150IU/L. Jaundice complicates severe cases. US and CT demonstrate a combination of parenchymal infarcts and haemorrhage. The management of liver disease is similar to that for pre-eclampsia, with urgent delivery alongside BP control (labetalol, hydralazine, and nifedipine are first-line drugs) and magnesium sulphate to prevent convulsions. LFT then typically improve, although a late cholestatic phase with rise in ALP and γGT is common.

☼ HELLP syndrome

The syndrome of haemolysis, elevated liver enzymes, and low platelets (HELLP) is a thrombotic microangiopathy, affecting 0.2% of pregnancies. It occurs in 20% of patients with severe pre-eclampsia, although can be diagnosed in its absence. Risk factors include older age, Caucasian ethnicity, and multiparity. Four diagnostic criteria required:
- Haemolysis on peripheral blood film.
- LDH >600IU/L.
- ALT or AST >70IU/L.
- Platelets <100 × 10^9/L.

Symptoms begin between wk28 and wk36 but can occur post-partum. Malaise and fatigue are followed by headache, epigastric and RUQ pain, nausea, and vomiting. Massive LFT derangement and right shoulder tip pain are ominous signs. These indicate liver infarction or haematoma with impending rupture, confirmed by US or CT.

In addition to the laboratory abnormalities described above, the blood film picture is of a microangiopathic haemolytic anaemia (MAHA), with schistocytes, echinocytes and spherostomatocytes, and depleted serum haptoglobin. MAHA may also be seen in haemolytic uraemic syndrome (HUS) and thrombotic thrombocytopaenic purpura (TTP), and it is important to distinguish these diagnoses from HELLP. Severity may be graded using the Mississippi classification (see Table 19.3). Haematological and LFT abnormalities usually resolve from 2d post-partum. Liver biopsy is rarely indicated.

Table 19.3 Mississippi classification of HELLP

Class	Severity	Platelet count
I	Severe	<50 × 10^9/L
II	Moderate	50–100 × 10^9/L
III	Mild	>100 × 10^9/L

Reprinted from *American Journal of Obstetrics and Gynaecology*, 180, 6, James N. Martin *et al.*, 'The spectrum of severe preeclampsia: comparative analysis by HELLP (hemolysis, elevated liver enzyme levels, and low platelet count) syndrome classification', pp. 1373–1384, Copyright 1999, with permission from Elsevier.

Maternal complications occur in up to 50%, often requiring blood transfusion and correction of coagulopathy. Up to 25% develop DIC (high D-dimer predicts severity), and 20% pleural effusions or pulmonary oedema. Renal failure secondary to acute tubular necrosis arises in up to 8%. Thrombocytopaenia predisposes to placental abruption (16%), subcapsular liver haematomas (1%), wound haematomas following Caesarian section, and retinal detachment (1%). Eclampsia is twice as common in these patients.

Although conservative supportive treatment has been advocated in mild disease, indications for urgent delivery include maternal or foetal distress, and persistent severe RUQ pain or shoulder tip pain with hypotension. Dexamethasone may temporally improve maternal disease and promote foetal maturation, reducing complications of premature delivery. Maternal mortality is 1% but peri-natal mortality up to 30%. Raised urate is an independent predictor of poor outcome. Liver transplantation has been used successfully.

Close observation is required for at least 48h following delivery. HELLP recurs in 5% of subsequent pregnancies.

☠ Spontaneous hepatic rupture

Spontaneous rupture of the liver complicates 1 in 100,000 pregnancies, almost exclusively in the late third trimester. It is potentially life-threatening. Approximately 80% arise in association with severe pre-eclampsia or HELLP, and 20% with acute fatty liver of pregnancy, hepatic neoplasia, or liver abscess. The right lobe is most commonly affected.

The classic presentation is sudden onset RUQ pain, nausea and vomiting, hypotension, and abdominal distension. Peritonitis may ensue. Increased serum transaminase concentrations >3,000IU/L are frequently seen. The diagnosis can be confirmed by US or CT; differential diagnoses include aortic dissection and diaphragmatic rupture.

Management involves haemodynamic and volume support ± blood products as required; consider activating 'major haemorrhage protocol' (see Appendix, 📖 pp. 360–1). Definitive treatment is angiography with hepatic artery embolization, or laparotomy and surgical haemostasis. Delivery should be by Caesarean section.

① Gallstone disease

Gallstones develop in 10% of pregnancies, and existing stones grow more rapidly. Less than 0.3% are symptomatic, and presentation and management are described in Chapter 9. ERCP with sphincterotomy or stenting is indicated for CBD stones, which can be sensitively and safely detected by US or MRCP without risk of radiation to the foetus. Surgery can usually be deferred until after delivery, although those presenting early risk recurrence. Laparoscopic cholecystectomy can be considered in the second trimester, although ERCP with sphincterotomy is safer for choledocholithiasis. Ensure an experienced endoscopist performs the ERCP (if necessary, refer patient to tertiary centre). The radiation dose is at least 10-fold less than that associated with congenital malformation when delivered in the first trimester, and even less thereafter; despite which, the foetus must be shielded from radiation. A technique for non-radiation ERCP has been described (Shelton et al., 2008).

☼ Pancreatitis

Pancreatitis occurs most frequently in the third trimester and immediate post-partum period. Management is described in Chapter 9. Most cases in pregnancy result from gallstone disease or iatrogenic post-ERCP. Diagnosis can be more difficult, as there is a physiological increase in serum amylase during pregnancy, although a rise >1,000U/L is still essentially diagnostic. Serum lipase may be helpful. Nutritional support should be considered to protect the foetus.

✪ Budd–Chiari syndrome

High oestrogen states increase pro-thrombotic tendency, related to diminished concentrations of anti-thrombin III. This can be associated with thrombosis of the hepatic veins or IVC. RUQ pain, hepatomegaly, and maternal ascites should suggest the diagnosis, which is confirmed by US with Doppler.

Anticoagulation with therapeutic dose of LMWH SC bd should be commenced. In patients who do not respond, further treatment options include hepatic venous balloon dilatation or insertion of a TIPS, although data on their use in pregnancy are limited. Maternal mortality is high (up to 70%).

① Viral hepatitis

Acute viral hepatitis remains the commonest cause of jaundice in pregnancy. The presentation, course, and management are largely unchanged by pregnancy (see Chapter 14). There is no protective effect in terms of transmission to the newborn from C-section as opposed to vaginal delivery.

Hepatitis B

Vertical transmission occurs in 50% of cases of acute hepatitis, rising to 70% in the third trimester. Transmission is less common with chronic carriage, but varies with viral replication and is up to 90% in patients with high level of viraemia. This can be interrupted by use of hepatitis B IV Ig at birth, and vaccination within the first week post-partum and boosters at 1, 2, and 12mo. Lamivudine may be safely given in the third trimester.

Hepatitis C

Transmission in chronic carriers occurs in up to 8% of patients, correlating with viral load. Seroconversion of infants may take up to 1y to appear, although detection of viral RNA by PCR allows earlier recognition. Ribavirin is teratogenic and absolutely contraindicated.

Hepatitis E

RNA virus that causes acute hepatitis. It occurs predominantly in the Middle East and Asia, often in water-borne epidemics, and is transmitted via the faeco-oral route. In pregnancy, maternal mortality is up to 20% due to fulminant liver failure in the third trimester. Spontaneous abortion or intrauterine death occur in 12%. Vertical transmission is rare. Diagnosis is by IgM anti-HEV serology, and treatment supportive.

Herpes simplex virus

Pregnant women are more susceptible than the general population to HSV-1 and HSV-2 hepatitis. Patients present with elevated serum transaminases. Leukopaenia, thrombocytopaenia, and coagulopathy are common, although bilirubin is often normal. Mucocutaneous lesions are only present in 50% and, therefore, the diagnosis should be considered in any pregnant woman with liver failure. CT shows multiple low-density areas of necrosis, and liver biopsy is definitive. Treatment with aciclovir (5mg/kg IV qds for severe disease; 800mg PO 5 times/d for mild-to-moderate infections) should be initiated on clinical suspicion and not delayed whilst confirmatory tests are pending, as maternal mortality is up to 40%.

Pre-existing cirrhotic liver disease

Pregnancy in cirrhotic women is rare due to associated subfertility. When successful, rates of miscarriage, prematurity, and perinatal death are higher. Maternal mortality is up to 10% and correlates with degree of hepatic dysfunction rather than its underlying aetiology.

Portal hypertension worsens in pregnancy because of increased IVC compression by the gravid uterus. As such, all cirrhotic women should have endoscopic screening for upper GI varices. Banding of high-risk lesions before pregnancy is appropriate. Propranolol may be used but can cause foetal growth restriction, bradycardia, and hypoglycaemia. Terlipressin may be required in an emergency, but there are concerns regarding effects on placental perfusion and risk of abruption.

The liver in pregnancy

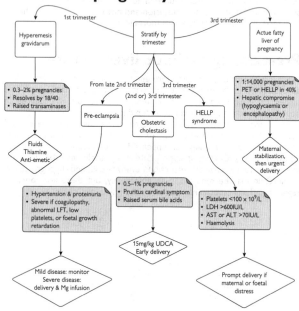

Further reading

Shelton J, Linder JD, Rivera-Alsina ME, Tarnasky PR Commitment, confirmation, and clearance: new techniques for nonradiation ERCP during pregnancy (with videos). *Gastrointest Endosc.* 2008 Feb; **67**(2): 364-8. doi: 10.1016/j.gie.2007.09.036.

Chapter 20

Hepatic trauma

General principles of management

The liver is the most frequently injured organ following blunt trauma to the abdomen. Management initially follows Advanced Trauma and Life Support (ATLS) guidelines for emergency resuscitation and assessment; further intervention is then determined by the degree of haemodynamic instability.

Mechanisms of injury

The most common mechanisms of injury are deceleration (particularly road traffic accident and falls) and direct blows to the abdomen. Deceleration injuries disrupt the liver capsule and parenchyma at sites of attachment to the diaphragm, with shear forces that propagate along the major hepatic venous branches. Direct trauma (see Colour plate 23) or penetrating injuries (see Colour plate 24) may lacerate the parenchyma whilst leaving the capsule intact. Contusion can result from compression of the liver against fixed bony structures such as the ribs or spine. Injuries to gallbladder or bile ducts are rare.

Liver injury occurs more readily in children than adults, as ribs are more flexible (thus transmitting greater force), and the developing liver has a weaker connective tissue framework.

Initial resuscitation and assessment

Resuscitation should proceed according to ATLS guidelines using the ABCDE approach (see Fig. 20.1), with the airway as the initial priority. Patients with hepatic trauma have frequently been involved in high-risk injuries, and immobilization of the cervical spine in a semi-rigid collar is often appropriate until this can be formally assessed. The chest should then be examined for immediately life-threatening injuries, including open or tension pneumothoraces, flail chest, or massive haemothorax; these should be treated if present.

The main cause of preventable post-injury death is haemorrhage. Hypotension should be assumed to relate to blood loss until proven otherwise. Site two large-bore (12G or 14G) IV lines, and resuscitate with either crystalloid or colloid. If the patient does not respond, give type-specific or O-negative blood (consider activation of 'major haemorrhage protocol', as this has been shown to reduce mortality; see Appendix, pp. 360–1). Further management of suspected hepatic trauma then depends upon haemodynamic stability (defined as systolic BP >90mmHg, and pulse rate <100/min) following these measures.

Associated injuries are common, involving the thorax (50%), spleen (22%), bony pelvis (20%), kidney (9%), bowel (4%), and pancreas (2%).

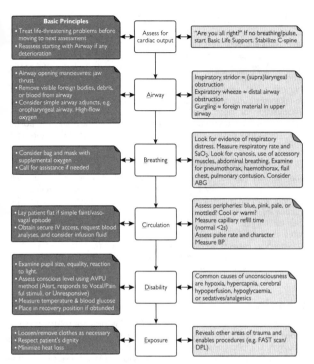

Fig. 20.1 Resuscitation: ABCDE. Data from Resuscitation Council (UK) 2010 Resuscitation Guidelines (see ✆ http://www.resus.org.uk/pages/guide.htm).

Haemodynamically unstable

Trauma to the RUQ, thoraco-abdominal area, or flank, in association with hypotension or abdominal distension, is high risk for major liver injury. Haemodynamically unstable patients with abdominal trauma should ideally have a focused assessment with sonography for trauma (FAST) scan, or diagnostic peritoneal aspiration (DPA) if this is not available, with the aim of detecting intraperitoneal haemorrhage. If either test is positive, immediate emergency laparotomy to control any bleeding point is indicated; otherwise, investigation should proceed to CT. Emergency bedside US should also be used to exclude haemothorax and haemopericardium.

☼ Borderline haemodynamic stability

In patients in whom haemodynamic stability is marginal (e.g. those who have transient response to fluid resuscitation), urgent contrast CT is required to rapidly detect and quantify any haemoperitoneum, active haemorrhage or vascular disruption, and to grade severity of hepatic injury. Extra-luminal contrast or intraparenchymal contrast blush are neither completely sensitive nor specific for ongoing haemorrhage but should be taken seriously, and they do predict high risk of requiring angiographic embolization or laparotomy. Causes of a false positive CT angiogram include pseudoaneurysm or fistula between the hepatic artery and portal vein. These may persist, thrombose, regress, or enlarge and rupture and should, therefore, not be ignored.

① Haemodynamically stable

The majority (up to 85%) of patients with blunt abdominal injury will be stable or only mildly hypotensive and can be managed expectantly. If stable with GCS 15/15, no abdominal pain or tenderness, and no distracting injuries, they can be observed in the emergency department and then discharged. The presence of any of these features, however, mandates abdominal CT and admission for a minimum of 24h observation. Additionally, patients who have high-risk injuries (e.g. death of another passenger in the same vehicle in a road traffic accident) but remain stable should be observed for 24h.

Imaging

The gold standard is contrast-enhanced CT. The aims are to detect intraperitoneal blood, delineate the nature and severity of any liver injury, recognize complications of hepatic trauma early, and exclude damage to other intra-abdominal viscera or pelvic structures. Major hepatic vein injury should be suspected with lacerations or haematomas that extend into the dome of the liver or those near the IVC. These constitute severe injuries, with a 6.5-fold increased risk of requiring hepatic surgery. Their presence must be known by the surgeon conducting exploratory laparotomy, as mobilization of the liver predisposes to massive haemorrhage.

The liver injury scale is the most widely used classification (see Table 20.1). Although originally developed to prognosticate and guide surgical intervention, it is criticized for lacking sensitivity (65%) and specificity (85%). The best indicators for surgical management are haemodynamic instability, or active extravasation or sentinel clot (high attenuation clot at the site of bleeding) on CT. The scale also does not emphasize the presence of arterial bleeding, which is amenable to angiographic embolization. Its main current use is for comparison of baseline to subsequent images to quantify recovery and detect complications (see Fig. 20.2).

CT has a number of other pitfalls, which should be appreciated. It is poor at detecting small, superficial capsular lesions (especially those adjacent to the falciform ligament) or subtle subcapsular bleeds (particular if image slices are too thick). Otherwise, false negative images are rare, although false positives are not infrequent, usually if peri-portal oedema

Table 20.1 Liver injury scale

Grade	Injury	Description
I	Haematoma	Subcapsular, <10% surface area
	Laceration	Capsular tear <1cm parenchymal depth
II	Haematoma	Subcapsular, 10–50% surface area, or intraparenchymal <10cm diameter
	Laceration	1–3cm parenchymal depth, <10cm length
III	Haematoma	Subcapsular, >50% surface area, or expanding or ruptured subcapsular or intraparenchymal >10cm
	Laceration	>3cm parenchymal depth
IV	Laceration	Parenchymal disruption involving 25–75% hepatic lobe or 1–3 Couinaud's segments within a single lobe
V	Laceration	Parenchymal disruption involving >75% of hepatic lobe or >3 Couinaud's segments within a single lobe
	Vascular	Juxtahepatic major venous injury
VI	Vascular	Hepatic avulsion

Increase grade by 1 in the presence of multiple injuries, up to grade III. Reproduced from Ernest E. Moore et al., 'Organ injury scaling: spleen and liver (1994 revision)', *The Journal of Trauma: Injury, Infection, and Critical Care*, 38, 3, pp. 323–324, copyright 1995, with permission from Wolters Kluwer.

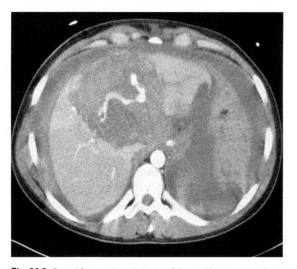

Fig. 20.2 Central fracture through the liver following blunt trauma with active arterial haemorrhage and haemoperitoneum. Reproduced with kind permission from John Karani.

or blood tracking along tissue planes are present. There are discrepancies between CT and direct angiography for arterial bleeding, with high CT false positives due to venous extravasation. CT may also misinterpret the nature of a peritoneal collection. In general, progressive growth of peri-hepatic or intraparenchymal collections with low attenuation suggest a biloma; collections with gas bubbles or fluid levels indicate probable abscess formation; and persistent or increasing low attenuation free fluid within the peritoneal cavity with enhancement and peritoneal thickening imply biliary peritonitis.

Definitive management

In most patients, non-operative treatment with close monitoring is the accepted standard of care, particularly if the following criteria are met:
• No peritonism.
• Signs restricted to the RUQ.
• Early CT reported by an experienced radiologist as grade I/II injury.
• No other associated intra-abdominal injuries requiring operation.
• <4U blood transfusion related to hepatic injury.
• 24h access to surgical review, operating theatres, and intensive care facilities.

Most patients with defined injuries and borderline haemodynamic instability can be successfully managed by arterial embolization. If local resources are insufficient, discuss with a specialist liver unit for advice ± transfer if indicated and the patient is stable. Haemodynamically unstable patients with large volumes of intra-abdominal fluid or active hepatic haemorrhage require laparotomy for surgical control of bleeding points. Splenectomy may be indicated if concomitant injury present. Hepatectomy or vascular isolation/shunting are reserved for the most advanced injuries, as these procedures are associated with high mortality. After surgery, further CT should be performed to identify any continuing haemorrhage, which may be amenable to embolization.

Close supervision post-intervention in HDU allows early detection of re-bleeding. Monitoring should include regular vital signs, repeated abdominal examination, and serial FBC. In contrast to splenic injuries, patients with continued haemorrhage typically present with gradual reductions in Hb or Hct, and increased transfusion requirements rather than acute compromise. Such patients require immediate angiography or laparotomy, depending on severity. Sudden development of abdominal pain or distension, haematemesis, or melaena suggest haemobilia.

Routine follow-up is not cost-effective after successful intervention without early complications, unless clinical symptoms and signs develop.

:✪: Complications

- Delayed haemorrhage (3.5%); <20% require transfusion.
- Haematoma.
- Bile duct injury:
  - Biloma (3.0%).
  - Bile leakage.
  - Fistulation.
  - Haemobilia.
- Infection:
  - Abscess (0.7%).
  - Biliary peritonitis.
- Abdominal compartment syndrome.

Haematomas may be asymptomatic but should usually be embolized due to risk of rupture. This can occur into the liver, peritoneum, duodenum, or biliary tract, presenting with haemobilia. It should be suspected with a sudden drop in Hb and RUQ pain, or haematemesis or melaena.

Distal bile leakage is usually transient without clinical significance. Proximal leaks can cause bilomas, abscesses, or peritonitis, which most commonly develop slowly over weeks. Bile duct injury is diagnosed by MRCP or radionuclide imaging with ^{99m}Tc-iminodiacetic acid. First-line treatment is CT-guided drainage, except for biliary peritonitis in which case laparoscopy is indicated. Persistent bile leakage requires ERCP. All patients should have follow-up MRCP to confirm resolution.

Overall mortality is 10%, although only 2% is attributable to liver injury itself, with most of the remainder due to associated head injuries or sepsis.

Hepatic trauma

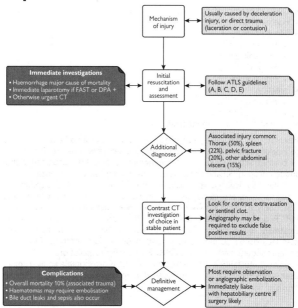

Mechanism of injury → Usually caused by deceleration injury, or direct trauma (laceration or contusion)

Immediate investigations
• Haemorrhage major cause of mortality
• Immediate laparotomy if FAST or DPA +
• Otherwise urgent CT

Initial resuscitation and assessment → Follow ATLS guidelines (A, B, C, D, E)

Additional diagnoses → Associated injury common: Thorax (50%), spleen (22%), pelvic fracture (20%), other abdominal viscera (15%)

Contrast CT investigation of choice in stable patient → Look for contrast extravasation or sentinel clot. Angiography may be required to exclude false positive results

Complications
• Overall mortality 10% (associated trauma)
• Haematomas may require embolisation
• Bile duct leaks and sepsis also occur

Definitive management → Most require observation or angiographic embolization. Immediately liaise with hepatobiliary centre if surgery likely

Further reading

Moore EE, Cogbill TH, Jurkovich GJ, et al. (1995) Organ injury scaling: spleen and liver (1994 revision) *Trauma* **38**: 323–4.

Hepatic, neuroendocrine, and general oncological emergencies

Emergency presentation of hepatic malignancy

Hepatocellular carcinoma (HCC) is the fifth most common cancer worldwide. It usually develops on the background of cirrhosis, most frequently as a result of chronic hepatotropic viral infection. Untreated, the majority of patients die within 1y of diagnosis. However, there are now a number of potentially curative options for patients diagnosed with early stage disease, and overall 5y survival is between 50–70% in specialist centres.

Pancreatic adenocarcinomas and cholangiocarcinomas typically present with obstructive jaundice. Surgical cure is only possible in 10–15% of cases, although chemotherapy and radiotherapy can delay progression.

The liver is a common site for metastases from primary tumours at other sites. This section concentrates on the management of complications of HCC, although similar principles apply to hepatic metastases (albeit these carry worse prognosis due to more advanced disease stage).

Spontaneous rupture

HCC rupture with intraperitoneal haemorrhage occurs in 3–15% of patients. Acute mortality is high (25–75%), as is liver failure (12–42%). Tumour rupture is the mode of presentation in up to 50% of patients with benign hepatic adenomas. The mechanism of spontaneous rupture is not fully understood but may involve rapid tumour growth with necrosis, splitting of the overlying parenchyma, vascular erosion, or increased hepatic venous pressure due to extrinsic compression by the tumour. Tumour size, degree of extrahepatic protrusion, and portal vein thrombosis are predictors of rupture. Hepatic haematoma and rupture also occur in HELLP syndrome (see Chapter 19).

Clinical presentation

The most common symptom is sudden onset abdominal pain, often accompanied by anaemia, abdominal distension, or hypovolaemic shock. Diagnosis is principally established by demonstrating haemoperitoneum on US or CT, which can also determine portal vein patency; diagnostic peritoneal lavage can help confirm if equivocal. In up to one-third of patients, the diagnosis is made at emergency exploratory laparotomy. Elevated serum bilirubin, haemorrhagic shock on admission, and poor pre-rupture performance status are adverse prognostic factors.

The goals of management are to restore circulating volume, achieve haemostasis, and maximize preservation of functioning liver parenchyma.

Stabilizing the patient

- Ensure airway protected.
- Assess haemodynamic stability (HR, BP, peripheral temperature).
- Restore circulating volume:
  - Insert two large-bore cannulae (14–16G).
  - If shocked, infuse 1L of 0.9% saline or 500mL colloid (e.g. Gelofusine®) stat. Repeat according to response.
  - Obtain blood samples for FBC, U & E, LFT, clotting, calcium, and G & S. If shocked on admission, cross-match 8U blood. Consider

activating 'major haemorrhage protocol' (see Appendix,
📖 pp. 360–1), transfusing O-negative blood, and emergency
laparotomy if no response to initial fluid resuscitation.
- Correct coagulopathy:
  - If INR >1.5, give FFP 10–15mL/kg + vitamin K 0.5–1mg IV (or 10mg
    if no prospect of repeated anticoagulation).
  - For specific guidance regarding reversal of warfarin and heparin, see
    Chapter 1.
  - If platelets <50 × 10⁹/L, transfuse 1–2 pools.
- Consider inserting urinary catheter.

Achieving haemostasis

- Trans-arterial embolization. Initial approach in patients with preserved
  liver function without complete portal vein thrombosis. Rarely
  effective in prolonging survival if bilirubin >50µmol/L. Success rate
  53–100%, with 30d mortality 0–37%. Tumour re-ruptures in 0–35%,
  which carries extremely poor prognosis. Complications include
  post-embolization syndrome (occurs in 26–85%; consists of fever,
  abdominal pain, nausea, and elevation of LFT; usually resolves
  spontaneously within 1–2wk) and liver failure (12–33%; most common
  cause of death after embolization).
- Surgical haemostasis. Achieved by using a combination of packing,
  electrocauterization, hepatic artery ligation, or alcohol injection.
  Mortality higher than angiographic techniques.
- Surgical liver resection. Achieves both haemostasis and definitive
  treatment of the underlying HCC with a single operation. However,
  emergency resection is associated with poor outcomes; tumour stage
  and liver functional reserve are often unknown, and presence of
  haemorrhagic shock impairs liver function more than during an elective
  procedure. In-hospital mortality with emergency resection ranges from
  17 to 100%; as such, this procedure should be reserved for patients
  with small, easily accessible tumours and non-cirrhotic livers. These
  challenges may be overcome by performing staged liver resection,
  which has superior in-hospital mortality (0–9%) and 1y survival
  (54–100%), or conducting initial staging laparoscopy.
- Conservative management. Involves correction of coagulopathy and
  close monitoring (including imaging). Appropriate in stable patients,
  but have a low threshold for proceeding to definitive haemostatic
  techniques if any deterioration. Consider admitting to a Level 1 ward/
  HDU. Also appropriate for moribund patients with an inoperable
  underlying tumour; mortality >90% with this approach.

① Jaundice

Jaundice develops in 19–40% of HCC patients. In the majority, it is caused
by diffuse tumour infiltration of liver parenchyma, hilar invasion, or progressive terminal liver failure due to underlying advanced cirrhosis.

Obstructive jaundice is uncommon in HCC (1–12%), but frequently the
presenting feature of pancreatic adenocarcinoma or cholangiocarcinoma.
It may arise through cystic duct invasion, haemobilia, bile duct thrombus
(blood from intra-tumoural haemorrhage), pus, sludge, or extrinsic compression by involved lymph nodes. There may be associated cholangitis.

Investigation
- Blood tests. LFT to determine whether jaundice hepatitic or cholestatic (see Chapter 13). Check for coagulopathy.
- Doppler US imaging is modality of choice.
- If jaundice hepatic, proceed to CT to delineate parenchymal lesions.
- If jaundice obstructive, proceed to CT and MRCP:
  - Presence of intra-luminal soft tissue in the bile duct with arterial phase enhancement is typical of HCC with tumour thrombi.
  - Biliary strictures from HCC are typically short and smooth, and confined to the porta hepatitis.
  - Strictures in cholangiocarcinoma usually multiple and long, with segmental dilatations producing a characteristic 'rat tail' appearance.
- Brush cytology at ERCP can differentiate HCC from cholangiocarcinoma.

Management
Treatment of hepatitic jaundice is similar to other causes of acute liver failure (see Chapters 14 and 15), and of the underlying HCC. Obstructive jaundice requires bile duct decompression. This may be achieved at ERCP with sphincterotomy ± stenting, which can also be palliative. HCC invading the bile ducts, or bile duct thrombi, may require operative intervention with removal of debris ± T-tube drainage; this can include lobectomy aimed at curing the underlying tumour.

Liver capsular pain
- Effective pain control can be achieved using the WHO analgesic ladder:
  - Step 1. Non-opioid analgesia (e.g. paracetamol 1g qds, or NSAIDs such as ibuprofen 400mg tds).
  - Step 2. Mild opioids (e.g. codeine 30–60mg qds, or tramadol 50–100mg qds).
  - Step 3. Strong opioids (morphine 5–10mg 4-hourly PO). Halve the dose if administering parenterally. Slow-release preparations (e.g. fentanyl 25–100µg hourly via transdermal patch, changed every 72h) useful for chronic pain. Provide laxatives/anti-emetics to minimize side effects.
- NSAIDs are often particularly effective in this setting.
- Dexamethasone 4–8mg PO bd is a useful adjunct.
- Paravertebral nerve blocks occasionally required for intractable pain.

Ascites
Malignant ascites is usually refractory to diuretic medication and may require repeated paracentesis (see 📖 p. 262) for symptom relief if tense. The procedure should be US-guided if there is fluid loculation or peritoneal involvement. There is no rationale for IV plasma expansion with HAS unless liver synthetic function is compromised. Aim to drain to dryness, but remove drain within 12h to prevent infection. Diuretics are only useful in patients with portal hypertension (SAAG >11g/L); consider with massive hepatic metastases or HCC-associated cirrhosis.

Emergency presentation of neuroendocrine tumours

A number of neuroendocrine tumours (NETs) are relevant to the GI tract and liver. Emergency presentations relate to effects of secreted hormones or those of the mass lesion (which may be painful or bleed, perforate, or obstruct the bowel; see Chapter 9). Diagnosis depends on localizing the tumour and demonstrating hormonal excess (see Box 21.1). NETs may occur as part of a multiple endocrine neoplasia (MEN) syndrome, so be observant for synchronous lesions and their consequences (especially hypercalcaemia). Patients should be referred to specialist centres.

⚙ Phaeochromocytomas

Tumour of the adrenal medulla (90%) or sympathetic nervous system ganglia (10%). Secrete catecholamines, predominantly noradrenaline and adrenaline. Emergency presentation with hypertensive crises. There is no categorical BP threshold at which this becomes an emergency, but systolic BP >220mmHg or diastolic BP >120mmHg are generally accepted limits.

Clinical features

- Hypertension. May be accelerated phase or malignant (associated with retinal haemorrhage, papilloedema, encephalopathy, or intracerebral haemorrhage). Ensure fundoscopy performed, and consider CT head.
- Palpitations/tachycardia.
- Headache.
- Sweating.
- Pallor.
- Paraesthesia and cold extremities.

The classic triad of headache, palpitations, and sweating in the presence of hypertension is 91% sensitive and 63% specific for the diagnosis (even when these present without intercurrent hypertension, they should prompt investigation). Lone paroxysmal hypertension and adrenal incidentalomas also require investigation, albeit with low likelihood of disease. High-risk patients include MEN2 and von Hippel–Lindau families, or those with previous phaeochromocytoma. Episodes are paroxysmal and can last from minutes to hours. Crises may be precipitated by raised intra-abdominal pressure due to external compression, straining, or exercise.

Diagnosis

- Blood tests:
  - Chromogranin A. Elevated hormone output suggests NET but is not specific to phaeochromocytoma. Useful for monitoring progression, response to treatment, and recurrence.
  - Metanephrines.
- 24h urinary catecholamines, vanillylmandelic acid (VMA) and homovanillic acid (HVA), and/or fractionated metanephrines.
- MRI to characterize anatomy.
- FDG CT-PET is of limited use for identifying metastatic disease.

- Radionuclide scanning. ^{111}Indium pentetreotide (octreotide scan) or metaiodobenzylguanidine (MIBG) scans sensitive and specific. Used when cross-sectional imaging negative but disease likelihood high, or for planning radionuclide targeted therapy.

Box 21.1 Measurement of gut hormone profiles

Demonstration of elevated serum chromogranin A and relevant gut peptide concentrations are critical to diagnosis of several NETs. However, results may be invalid if samples are not obtained and handled correctly:
- Stop PPIs 3wk before testing.
- Stop H2 receptor antagonists 72h before testing.
- Fast patient overnight before test.
- Inform laboratory:
  - That you are taking the sample.
  - Of the concomitant serum urea and calcium.
  - Of current medications patient is receiving.
  - Of details of any previous gastric surgery.
- Take 10mL blood into a heparin tube, and mix by inversion.
- Place on ice, and transfer immediately to laboratory.
- Sample should be separated in a refrigerated centrifuge and frozen at $-20°C$ within 15min of collection.

Treatment
- Hypertensive crises:
  - If phaeochromocytoma is suspected, treatment of choice is IV α-blockade with phentolamine 1–5mg, repeated every 15min as required, or phenoxybenzamine 1mg/kg infused over at least 2h.
  - GTN infusion (0–10mL/h, titrated according to response) is a reasonable alternative.
  - β-blockers (e.g. labetalol infusion) may be used but always after α-blockade to prevent unopposed α-mediated vasoconstriction, which may worsen hypertension.
  - Avoid dropping BP too quickly (aim to achieve one-third reduction over 24h), as transient loss of auto-regulation of cerebral perfusion can result in watershed infarcts.
- Surgical cure with laparoscopic adrenalectomy possible in ~75%.

⊕ Neuroendocrine (carcinoid) tumours

The term 'carcinoid tumour' is now rarely used, and has been replaced by the term 'neuroendocrine tumour' of the identified primary site (e.g. gastric, ileal, bronchial). They arise from the 'diffuse endocrine system', and the classical cell is the enterochromaffin cell. Most arise within the GI tract, and 25% from the lung. They may secrete a range of hormones, including serotonin (5-HT), histamine, and bradykinin. 5-HT is metabolized in the liver to 5-hydroxyindoleacetic acid (5-HIAA) by monoamine oxidase; serotonin syndrome arises when the hormonal load exceeds enzyme capacity. The majority of such patients have liver metastases or extra-intestinal primaries that bypass the portohepatic circulation. These tumours are generally slowly progressive (>80% 5y survival in surgically reated patients; median survival >2y in those with metastatic disease). Most patients have non-functional tumours (i.e. no associated syndrome); however, 10% present with the classical carcinoid syndrome.

Clinical features
- Diarrhoea.
- Abdominal cramps.
- Episodic cutaneous flushing and telangiectasia.
- Wheeze.
- Right heart failure (secondary to endocardial fibrosis, causing pulmonary stenosis and tricuspid regurgitation).

Diagnosis
- Serum chromogranin A. Low specificity, so not used as a screening test (see comments under 'Phaeochromocytoma', 📖 p. 333).
- Elevated 24h urinary 5-HIAA suggests carcinoid (sensitivity 75%), although false positives occur after eating bananas, avocado, pineapple, walnuts, coffee, or chocolate. Not accurate for monitoring.
- Staging with contrast CT of thorax, abdomen, and pelvis. MRI is most sensitive for liver metastases.
- ^{111}Indium pentetreotide scan (octreotide scan) is the most sensitive imaging modality for metastatic disease. It is also used for predicting patients responsive to octreotide or radionuclide targeted therapy.
- MIBG scan is less commonly used in modern practice.
- FDG CT-PET is of little value in typical low-grade NETs but may be helpful in high-grade tumours (Ki67 proliferation index >20% on histology). ^{68}Ga octreotate PET is very sensitive for NETs.

Treatment
- Carcinoid syndrome:
  - Octreotide 50–200µg SC tds, titrated according to response.
  - Monthly long-acting preparations of somatostatin analogues are available (octreotide LAR IM, Somatuline Autogel® SC).
  - Salbutamol 2.5–5mg NEB PRN for wheeze.
  - Loperamide 2–4mg PO up to qds for diarrhoea.
  - Avoid precipitants (alcohol, spicy food, strenuous exercise).
- Carcinoid crisis:
  - Octreotide 100–200µg IV bolus, and then infusion of octreotide at 50µg/h. After 24h, switch to octreotide SC.
  - Octreotide infusion should also be used to prevent carcinoid crisis in patients undergoing procedures such as hepatic artery embolization and surgery.
  - In carcinoid crisis, also consider chlorphenamine 10mg IV and hydrocortisone 100mg IV.
- Surgical cure possible for isolated lesions or limited liver metastases.
- Reduce tumour load of hepatic metastases using hepatic artery embolization/chemoembolization, interferon-α, or peptide radionuclide targeted therapies, e.g. ^{131}I-MIBG or ^{90}Y- or ^{177}Lu-octreotide. Surgical debulking resection sometimes performed if complete resection impossible.

① **VIPomas**

These tumours are usually solitary and located in the pancreatic tail; >60% are malignant. Diagnosis is based on the presence of large-volume diarrhoea and raised serum VIP levels. Identified by CT in most cases.

Clinical features

- Profuse watery diarrhoea. Often >3L/day.
- Dehydration.
- Hypokalaemia, hypomagnesaemia, and hypochloraemia.
- Flushing.

Treatment

- IV fluid replacement. May need >5L/24h.
- K^+ and Mg^{++} supplementation.
- Octreotide 50–200µg SC tds, titrated according to response.
- Monthly long-acting preparations of somatostatin analogues are available (see 📖 p. 335).
- Surgery curative in ~30%.
- Chemotherapy may be considered, as may molecular targeted agents (e.g. mTOR inhibitors, tyrosine kinase inhibitors) or peptide radionuclide targeted therapies.

① **Insulinomas**

Most located within pancreas, equally distributed between the pancreatic head, body, and tail. Usually <5cm. Multiple lesions in 10% and <10% malignant. Clinical features relate to symptomatic hypoglycaemia, and patients may become morbidly obese due to compensatory overeating.

Diagnosis

- 72h fast with 3–6 hourly measurement of blood glucose, insulin, and C-peptide levels. Induces hypoglycaemia with disproportionately elevated insulin. Elevated C-peptide confirms endogenous source (as opposed to factitious disease from self-administration of insulin).
- Screen for illicit use of oral hypoglycaemic drugs.
- CT or MRI may localize lesion but <40% sensitive if <3cm.
- EUS and selective venous sampling may be required.
- ^{111}Indium pentetreotide scan (octreotide scan) is useful in malignant insulinomas but often negative with benign tumours.

Treatment

- Advise small, regular meals.
- Diazoxide 5mg/kg PO daily in 2–3 divided doses. Inhibits insulin release.
- Octreotide 50–200µg tds SC, titrated according to response. Controls symptoms in 60%.
- Surgery curative in 70–95%.
- Chemotherapy, mTOR and tyrosine kinase inhibitors, and peptide radionuclide targeted therapies, can be considered.

① Glucagonomas

Cause elevated glucose by stimulating glycogenolysis. Usually >5cm; 60% are malignant, associated with local invasion or metastases in 50–80%.

Clinical features

- Weight loss.
- Hyperglycaemia/diabetes mellitus (40–90%).
- Diarrhoea.
- Migratory necrolytic erythema. Often located on thighs, perineum, or extremities.
- Increased risk of DVT.

Diagnosis

- Serum glucagon >1,000pg/mL. May be episodic.
- CT/MRI/EUS reveal tumour within the pancreas.

Treatment

- Standard treatment of diabetes mellitus.
- Octreotide 50–200µg tds SC, titrated according to response. May improve weight loss, diarrhoea, and rash. Monthly long-acting preparations of somatostatin analogues are available.
- Loperamide for diarrhoea, 2–4mg PO up to qds.
- Surgery performed for local disease but cure in only 20%.
- Chemotherapy, mTOR and tyrosine kinase inhibitors, and peptide radionuclide targeted therapies, can be considered.

① Somatostatinomas

These tumours are very rare and may arise in the pancreas or duodenum; >70% are malignant. The predominant symptom is diarrhoea. Somatostatin syndrome consists of diabetes mellitus, cholelithiasis, achlorhydria, and steatorrhoea. The diagnosis is established by demonstrating markedly elevated serum somatostatin concentrations, alongside tumour localization using CT, MRI, or EUS.

Treatment

- Octreotide 50–200µg tds SC, titrated according to response.
- Loperamide for diarrhoea, 2–4mg PO up to qds.
- Surgical resection.
- Chemoembolization.
- Chemotherapy, mTOR and tyrosine kinase inhibitors, and peptide radionuclide targeted therapies can be considered.

① Gastrinomas

Seventy percent arise in the duodenum and 30% in the pancreas; 60–70% are malignant. Pancreatic lesions tend to be larger and more likely to have metastasized. Zollinger–Ellison syndrome consists of the triad of peptic ulcer disease, gastric acid hypersecretion, and gastrinoma.

Clinical features

- Epigastric pain. Reflects peptic ulceration.
- Diarrhoea ± steatorrhoea.
- Palpable abdominal mass (with larger tumours).

Diagnosis
- OGD demonstrating multiple peptic ulcers.
- Fasting serum gastrin >1,000pg/mL (in absence of achlorhydria):
  - If gastrin concentrations equivocal (115–1,000pg/mL), perform secretin provocation test (0.26µg/kg secretin IV). Take blood samples at 5, 10, and 30min following exposure; a rise in serum gastrin >200pg/mL is diagnostic.
  - Gastric pH <2.0 with >140mL gastric fluid production over 1h confirms hypersecretion (although rarely performed).
- Octreotide scan to localize primary tumour and metastases.
- CT, MRI, or EUS to characterize anatomy and plan surgery.

Treatment
- High-dose PPI (omeprazole 40–80mg/d, pantoprazole 80–160mg/d).
- Octreotide 50–200µg tds SC, titrated according to response. Monthly long-acting preparations of somatostatin analogues are available.
- Chemoembolization.
- Chemotherapy, mTOR and tyrosine kinase inhibitors, and peptide radionuclide targeted therapies can be considered.
- Curative surgical resection in localized tumours without metastases.

① General oncological emergencies

Febrile neutropaenia

Systemic chemotherapy is usually ineffective in HCC and thus rarely used, except for palliative treatment. It has a greater role in the management of cholangiocarcinoma, as well as for some causes of liver metastases. Most chemotherapeutic agents cause a nadir in peripheral blood neutrophil counts 10–14d after administration. Febrile neutropaenia comprises the presence of pyrexia >37.5°C, with a neutrophil count <0.5 × 10^9/L (or <1.0 × 10^9/L if downward trend). Neutropaenic sepsis is defined as febrile neutropaenia with associated tachycardia, hypotension, or other evidence of organ dysfunction.

- Advise any patient who might have febrile neutropaenia to attend hospital urgently; most will be stable, but there is potential for rapid deterioration. Avoid use of paracetamol at home, as this can mask fever and impede assessment.
- Perform a full history and examination to identify possible septic foci (although many infections derived from endogenous GI flora). The screen should exclude peri-anal abscesses, but digital rectal examination should not be performed due to risk of bacterial translocation.
- Examine any long-term indwelling lines or ports. Remove if cellulitic.
- Obtain IV access and administer fluids.
- Send blood tests, including FBC, U & E, LFT, coagulation screen, CRP, peripheral blood cultures, and blood cultures from each lumen if a central venous catheter is *in situ*. Mark the origin of each culture on the bottles.
- Request CXR and MSU (+ other cultures as guided by clinical findings).

- Admit all patients with febrile neutropaenia to a neutral or positive pressure side-room. Perform observations every 30min–4h, depending on haemodynamic stability. Request oncology review.
- Administer broad-spectrum antibiotics as soon as possible, guided by local protocols:
  - Piperacillin-tazobactam 4.5g IV tds + gentamicin 7mg/kg IV od is usually an appropriate initial regimen. Discuss with microbiology if previous penicillin allergy or renal dysfunction.
  - Add in teicoplanin 400mg IV (6mg/kg if >85kg) if suspicion of line sepsis. Administer bd for three doses, then od thereafter.
- When blood culture results available:
  - If positive, adjust antibiotics according to sensitivities.
  - If negative and patient improving, complete 5d course of piperacillin-tazobactam, but stop gentamicin after two doses.
  - If negative and patient still pyrexial despite 48h treatment, discuss changing agents with microbiology. Possible strategies include switching to a carbapenem, adding in a glycopeptide (if not already initiated), or extending cover to include fungi.
- Consider admitting to HDU/ITU if haemodynamic compromise.
- Discuss adjuvant use of G-CSF with oncology team.

☼ Spinal cord compression

Metastatic infiltration of the spinal cord must be recognized early to minimize long-term neurological sequelae. Clinical features include:
- Back pain.
- Spastic paraparesis.
- Dermatomal sensory level, with diminished sensation below this.
- Saddle anaesthesia, faecal incontinence, reduced anal tone, and urinary retention in cauda equina syndrome.

If cord compression possible:
- Organize urgent MRI of the whole spine (within 24h).
- Initiate dexamethasone 8mg IV bd empirically. Consider concomitant gastroprotection with a PPI. Monitor BMs.
- Provide thromboprophylaxis with LMWH and graduated compression stockings.
- Administer laxatives if constipated.
- Insert urinary catheter if in retention.
- Request an urgent oncology opinion, as may need to plan radiotherapy.
- Discuss with neurosurgery if cord compression confirmed as, if decompression possible, this offers the best chance of preserving ability to ambulate long-term.

① Cerebral metastases

Cerebral metastases may present with focal neurological symptoms or signs, or seizures, or be detected incidentally on cross-sectional imaging of the brain (for staging or other indications).
- Contrast CT is the initial imaging modality of choice if suspected.
- MRI is superior for posterior fossa or brainstem lesions.

- If lesions symptomatic or there is surrounding oedema, start dexamethasone 8mg PO/IV bd. Consider gastroprotection with PPI.
- Request neurosurgical and oncology opinion.

ⓘ Hypercalcaemia

The normal range of serum calcium is 2.15–2.60mmol/L. Of the calcium ions present in peripheral blood, about half are free, whereas most of the remainder are bound to albumin. Unadjusted lab values, therefore, need to be corrected for serum albumin concentrations, calculated by:

$$\text{Corrected [Ca]} = \text{Measured [Ca]} + \{(40 - [\text{albumin}]) \times 0.02\}$$

Clinical features

- Abdominal pain.
- Constipation.
- Anorexia.
- Depression, fatigue, and/or confusion.
- Acute pancreatitis.
- Nephrolithiasis.
- Renal failure.
- Nephrogenic diabetes insipidus.

Treatment

- Initial management of symptomatic hypercalcaemia >3mmol/L is by volume expansion with IV 0.9% saline; 3–6L over 24h may be required.
- Once adequately rehydrated, use IV bisphosphonates if serum calcium still >3mmol/L:
  - Administer 60mg pamidronate IV if calcium between 3.0–3.4mmol/L.
  - Administer 90mg pamidronate IV if calcium >3.4mmol/L.
  - The concentration of pamidronate should not be >60mg in 250mL 0.9% saline. It should be given as a slow infusion at a rate of 20mg/h.
  - It takes a few days for serum calcium concentrations to fall, and a response may not be observed for 48–72h. Trough concentrations are usually achieved by d5, and normocalcaemia maintained for 3wk.

Hepatic, neuroendocrine, and general oncological emergencies

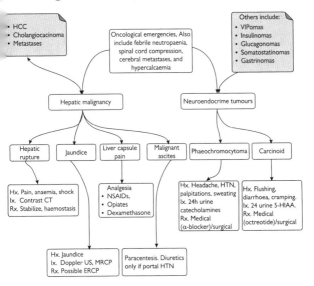

Liver transplant patients

Management of liver transplant patients with abnormal LFT

The management of chronic liver disease has been transformed by orthotopic and live-related liver transplantation. Early post-surgical outcomes are closely linked to preoperative performance status, quality of the donor organ, and surgical complexity. Advances in operative techniques and immunosuppressive therapies have improved survival to 90% at 1y, 70% at 5y, and 50% at 10y. The prevalence of long-term complications has correspondingly increased, many of which arise secondary to prolonged use of immunosuppressants.

All liver transplant patients presenting with worsening LFT merit investigation. These should be tailored according to the clinical picture, timing of illness in relation to initial surgery, and level of immunosuppression. Be aware that classical clinical manifestations of hepatobiliary disease may be absent, given denervation of the liver and post-surgical anatomy. While recommendations for investigating specific clinical problems are outlined in this chapter, in general, US with Doppler analysis is the initial imaging modality of choice. This may require follow-up (even if normal where clinical suspicion of a complication is high) with MRCP, ERCP, percutaneous cholangiography (via T-tube if indwelling), and/or liver biopsy. In patients receiving high level immunosuppression, perform a thorough infection screen (including herpesviridae, re-activation of hepatotropic viruses, and fungal studies according to clinical presentation).

⊙ Early surgical complications

One-third of complications arise within 1mo of operation, and 80% within 6mo. Most early complications are identified during the immediate post-operative hospital admission.

Vascular complications

Arterial occlusions (particularly hepatic artery thrombosis) are the most frequent of the post-operative vascular complications.

Arterial thrombosis

Arterial complications relate to the haemodynamic properties of transplant vessels, quality of vascular anastomoses, and the peri-operative hypercoagulable state. Symptoms vary according to timing: early thrombosis typically leads to graft ischaemia and necrosis (which may present with pain, jaundice, and elevated serum transaminases), whereas late thrombosis generally causes biliary complications (particularly intrahepatic bilomas and biliary stenoses) but with preserved graft function. Diagnosis is by Doppler US, contrast CT, or direct selective angiography.

Treatment depends on timing of thrombosis and its clinical consequences. Acute occlusions can be thrombolysed by an interventional radiologist, or removed surgically. Where these measures fail, urgent retransplantation may be required. For late occlusions, treatment is directed at preventing or managing biliary complications (see 'Biliary complications',

p. 345). Overall, 50–70% of patients diagnosed with arterial thrombosis require re-transplantation.

Portal vein thrombosis

The prevalence of portal vein thrombosis is 2–3%. Risk factors include pre-transplantation portal thrombosis, splenectomy, and prior surgery for portal hypertension. In the less common acute presentation, symptoms and signs are dominated by those of hepatic failure; however, portal vein thromboses more typically present late (with deranged LFT ± pain over the graft). Diagnosis is by Doppler US or contrast CT; direct angiography is rarely required. Management relies on anticoagulation, initially using heparin with subsequent conversion to warfarin. Bleeding risks from established GI varices may need to be addressed concurrently.

Occasionally, a similar clinical presentation results from stenosis of the venous anastomosis. This may be resolved by dilatation at angiography although, if this fails, surgical resection of the affected vessel segment, followed by repeat direct anastomosis or vein graft, may be necessary.

Biliary complications

Occur in 8–20% of patients. Common problems include bile leaks, fistulation, bilomas, stones/debris, and anastomotic strictures. Less frequent are hilar and intrahepatic strictures, papillary stenosis, sphincter of Oddi dysfunction, and mucocoeles. Bile leaks, bilomas, and strictures due to mismatched bile duct diameters tend to occur early. Suspect with abnormal LFT ± fever, anorexia, RUQ pain (may be absent following hepatic denervation), pruritus, or bilious ascites. Obtain Doppler US, and proceed to angiography if hepatic artery stenosed, MRCP with a view to ERCP if biliary dilatation (PTC in patients with Roux-en-Y anastomosis), or otherwise liver biopsy to exclude rejection/ischaemia.

Bile leaks and fistulae

Biliary leaks and fistulae may arise from the biliary anastomosis itself, damaged cystic or accessory bile ducts, the T-tube tract (suspect if abdominal pain post-withdrawal), or (rarely) incidental intrahepatic injuries (including the cut liver surface in live donor transplants). They predispose to future strictures. Most early post-operative leaks are anastomotic due to technical issues during surgery. Non-anastomotic leaks should prompt consideration of vascular compromise (particularly hepatic artery thrombosis), which should be investigated, as outlined in 'Arterial thrombosis under Vascular complications' (see p. 344).

If an indwelling T-tube is present (which is associated with bile leaks), this should be used to obtain a cholangiogram; confirmed leaks can then often be managed conservatively by leaving the T-tube open to divert bile flow. Otherwise, MRCP (or sometimes HIDA scan; sensitivity only 50%) should be performed, which, if positive, should proceed to ERCP with bile duct stenting. This is successful in >90%. Stents can be removed after 2–3mo. Nasobiliary tubes are sometimes employed in late bile leaks (often following T-tube removal), although be aware that biliary excreted drug levels fall.

Bilomas

Collections of bile within the abdominal cavity or hepatic parenchyma, resulting from bile leaks, often following ischaemic bile duct necrosis. They are identified on US or cross-sectional imaging. Small bilomas often respond to conservative management (± redirection of bile flow via T-tube or ERCP, with stenting if there is significant ongoing extravasation). Large bilomas should be drained percutaneously, with antibiotic cover if there is evidence of infection. Surgical intervention is reserved for patients in whom this approach fails, those with hepatic artery thrombosis or a duct-to-duct anastomotic defect too large to heal spontaneously, or overt peritonitis.

Haemorrhage

Post-operative haemorrhage occurs in up to 20%. It is typically diagnosed within 48h of transplantation, evidenced by increasing volumes of blood in abdominal drains, haemodynamic instability, and falling Hb levels. Haemorrhage subsides in most cases with expectant management, fluid resuscitation, and blood product support. Re-operation is required in 10–15%, but a source of haemorrhage is only found in ~50% of these.

① Rejection

Immunological rejection reactions are classified as hyper-acute (within 24h post-transplant), acute (1–2wk), or chronic (years).

Hyper-acute rejection

Caused by pre-existing antibodies and complement activation in transplants with donor-recipient mismatch. Massive hepatic necrosis necessitates urgent re-transplantation, although fortunately this is very rare.

Early and late acute rejection

Early acute rejection occurs in 30–70% of patients, usually within 5–30d post-transplant. When recognized, it does not prejudice graft or patient survival. Often clinically silent, although may present with general malaise and RUQ discomfort. Consider the diagnosis in transplant recipients whose serum transaminases are rising, particularly if accompanied by sub-therapeutic plasma levels of immunosuppressive drugs. Liver biopsy is mandatory to confirm the diagnosis.

Treatment involves escalation of immunosuppression, to which there is usually rapid response. This may include increasing doses of first-line drugs, switching to more potent agents (such as converting ciclosporin to tacrolimus), introducing additional agents (mycophenolate mofetil or anti-thymocyte globulin), or pulsed boluses of IV methylprednisolone.

Late acute rejection is defined as occurring after 180d (with some occurring up to 6y later) and arises in ~25% of patients. Of those, ¾ respond to pulsed IV steroids and increased immunosuppressants, as it is usually caused by insufficient levels.

Chronic rejection

Characterized by progressive bile duct loss, obliterative angiopathy, hepatic fibrosis, and cholestasis. Termed 'vanishing bile duct syndrome'. Occurs in 5% of patients, and more common in those with previous recurrent episodes of acute rejection, CMV infection, or hepatitis C. Diagnosis suggested by derangement of LFT (particularly bilirubin and ALP) several years after transplant. Chronic rejection is the major cause of graft failure at this time. Loss of synthetic function may not be evident until very late. Adjustment of immunosuppression delays progression, but eventual graft failure requiring re-transplantation is usual.

⊙ Chronic biliary complications

After the first post-operative year, the annual incidence of biliary complications falls to <4%.

Biliary strictures

Strictures account for 40% of post-transplant biliary complications, which occur in up to 15% patients with long-term follow-up. The majority arise within 12mo at (or just proximal to) the anastomosis. Their formation is insidious, and they are most often detected during investigation of deranged LFT in an asymptomatic patient (although cholangitis may be the presenting event). Absence of duct dilatation on sonography does not preclude the presence of stricturing in the transplanted liver. MRCP, cholangiography at ERCP, or percutaneous cholangiography following Roux-en-Y anastomosis are definitive.

Anastomotic strictures usually arise due to post-operative ischaemia with fibrotic tissue repair. They respond well to balloon dilatation and insertion of temporary stents. Strictures presenting early may require 2–3 attempts at dilatation but typically remain patent long-term (although recurrence can occur years after treatment). Those presenting late (after 6mo) often also respond transiently to dilatation, but patency is of shorter duration, requiring multiple repeated dilations with stent placement (e.g. 3-monthly for up to 2y, although recurrence thereafter is common). Surgical revision to Roux-en-Y occasionally necessary but unusual.

The natural history of non-anastomotic strictures (hilar, intrahepatic, or bile duct), which occur in up to 10% of patients, is less favourable. Risk factors include post-operative ischaemia, CMV, immunological mismatch causing vasculitis, and pre-transplantation diagnosis of PSC. Endoscopic or percutaneous balloon dilatation and stenting should be attempted, as 50% respond, but surgical revision is required in many cases. Diffuse disease of the intrahepatic ducts should prompt consideration of early re-transplantation; this is seen most frequently following non-heart beating donation where warm ischaemia prejudices the bile ducts selectively.

Biliary stone disease and cholangitis

Biliary obstruction can occur in the post-transplant patient as a result of strictures, stones, casts, or sludge. The clinical picture varies from elevation of bilirubin and ALP in the asymptomatic patient to septic shock secondary to bacterial cholangitis. Symptoms are often non-specific, and the RUQ pain typical of biliary disorders in non-transplant patients is usually absent due to hepatic denervation.

Obstruction is treated by endoscopic sphincterotomy ± stenting. Broad-spectrum antibiotics and IV fluid support are required in cholangitis; co-amoxiclav or cefuroxime are appropriate (ciprofloxacin in patients with severe penicillin allergy, although beware interaction with cytochrome P450). UDCA delays formation of new stones.

Sphincter of Oddi dysfunction

Occurs in 2–7% of patients with duct-to-duct anastomosis, probably secondary to denervation. Diagnosis usually based on clinical presentation and response to sphincterotomy. Confirmatory manometry is occasionally performed but rarely required. The diagnosis is supported by improvement in LFT if an indwelling T-tube is unclamped or if drainage of contrast is delayed at cholangiography or HIDA scan.

Mucocoele

Mucocoeles (collections of mucus from cells lining cystic duct remnants) are very rare. These expand over weeks to years, eventually compressing the adjacent bile duct. CT or US demonstrate a fluid collection in the porta hepatis, the differential diagnosis of which includes hepatic artery pseudoaneurysm, biloma, loculated ascites, abscess, liquefied haematoma, tumour, and adenopathy. Surgical excision/drainage is curative.

ⓘ Infections

Liver transplantation patients are predisposed to bacterial, viral, and fungal infections according to the duration since surgery and degree of immunosuppression. Immunosuppression often attenuates the typical symptoms and signs of infection, and antimicrobial therapies often interact with immunosuppressants. Infections may derive from:

- Donor liver.
- Transfused blood products.
- Exogenous organisms.
- Endogenous flora.
- Re-activation of latent infection.

Early post-operative infections

During the first post-operative month, nosocomial and endogenous bacterial infections predominate. These include:

- Superficial and deep wound infections.
- Intrahepatic abscesses (associated with ischaemia).
- Extrahepatic abscesses (super-infection of haematomas and bilomas).
- Peritonitis.
- Cholangitis (in the context of stenoses and choledocholithiasis).
- Nosocomial pneumonias (e.g. MRSA, *Pseudomonas*).
- *C. difficile*-associated diarrhoea.

Wound infections are usually staphylococcal; flucloxacillin is first-line therapy whilst cultures are pending (teicoplanin or vancomycin in MRSA-colonized patients). Intra-abdominal infections require cover for enterococci, Gram-negative organisms, and anaerobes; broad-spectrum cephalosporins + metronidazole are appropriate. Consider extending cover to *Candida* species if response is inadequate. Collections need to be drained percutaneously or surgically, and any biliary obstruction relieved.

Infections related to immunosuppression

Opportunistic infections related to iatrogenic immunosuppression arise from wk4 post-transplant until profound immunosuppression is no longer required (usually around the sixth month); they may also emerge when prophylaxis is stopped. Additionally, these infections can manifest if further immunosuppression is required to treat late acute rejection. Viral infections are most frequent, followed by fungi/yeast (*Pneumocystis jirovecii*, *Candida*, *Aspergillus*, and *Cryptococcus*) and bacteria (mycobacteria (18-fold relative risk post-transplant), *Nocardia*, and *Listeria*). After 6mo, levels of immunosuppression have usually reduced; therefore, standard community-acquired infections predominate, although with increased frequency.

In the absence of a clear septic focus, initial assessment of febrile immunocompromised patients should include: blood cultures (including fungal cultures), chest radiography, urine culture, and abdominal imaging (US or CT) for evidence of collection; and peripheral blood serology and PCR for CMV. When selecting antimicrobial therapies, be aware of cytochrome P450 interactions, as these will affect plasma levels of immunosuppressants (particularly ciclosporin and tacrolimus).

Cytomegalovirus

CMV is the most frequently isolated opportunistic pathogen. Infection may be primary (from a seropositive liver or blood donor into a seronegative recipient) or re-activation of endogenous latent infection. Patients present with fever, malaise, and peripheral blood lymphocytosis with atypia on blood film. CMV hepatitis manifests with elevated serum transaminases ± jaundice and pain over the graft; CMV pneumonitis with dyspnoea, cough, hypoxia, and bilateral infiltrates on chest radiography; and CMV colitis with diarrhoea (which may be bloody). CMV attenuates the immune response, increasing the risk of invasive bacterial and fungal infections. Diagnosis is principally through PCR quantification of CMV viraemia ± biopsy of the affected organ. Routine histology may show pathognomonic inclusion bodies, although these have limited sensitivity. *In situ* hybridization or immunohistochemistry improve virus detection.

CMV responds to ganciclovir 5mg/kg IV bd or valganciclovir 900mg PO bd. Duration is guided by clinical response and suppression of viraemia. Monitor U & E for nephrotoxicity, and FBC for myelosuppression. Cidofovir or foscarnet are alternatives. For patients at high risk of developing CMV disease (donor-positive/recipient-negative transplants, high blood transfusion requirements, immunological rejection with escalating immunosuppression, or use of anti-thymocyte antibodies), prophylaxis with valganciclovir 900mg PO od for up to 100d can be provided (and also has activity against HSV, VZV, and EBV).

Epstein–Barr virus

EBV is most frequently re-activated from latent infection. Clinical presentation is similar to CMV, with fever, malaise, atypical lymphocytosis, and elevated serum transaminases. Pneumonitis and colitis are much less common. Diagnosis is serological, and viral loads can be quantified by PCR. Treatment is with aciclovir 5mg/kg IV qds for severe disease or 800mg PO 5 times/d for mild-to-moderate infections. EBV is a risk factor for post-transplant lymphoproliferative disorders (see 'Secondary malignancy', 📖 p. 352).

Other viruses

Several other viruses may be acquired or re-activated, including adenoviruses, HSV, and VZV. Recurrence of hepatitis B and C are discussed in 'Disease recurrence and long-term prognosis' (see 📖 p. 354).

Pneumocystis jirovecii

Pneumocystis jirovecii pneumonia (PCP) presents insidiously with progressive exertional dyspnoea, fever, and non-productive cough. Patients are hypoxic and desaturate rapidly on exercise. Respiratory examination may be remarkably normal, given the degree of hypoxia. The classic CXR appearance is said to be diffuse bilateral infiltration, extending from both hila; however, it may be normal or infiltrates asymmetric. There is substantial overlap between the appearances of PCP and bacterial pneumonia. High-resolution CT demonstrates ground glass shadowing. The organism can be identified on microscopy of induced sputum or bronchoalveolar lavage samples; expectorated sputum has low sensitivity. Inform the laboratory that PCP is suspected.

Antibiotic therapy should be commenced with co-trimoxazole 120mg/kg PO or IV in 2–4 daily divided doses for 14d. Give adjunctive corticosteroids (prednisolone 50–80mg PO od for 5d, then taper over 2wk) to patients with pO_2 <9kPa on room air. Prophylaxis of PCP in high-risk patients should be provided (co-trimoxazole 960mg PO three times/wk) and virtually eliminates risk of infection.

Other fungi

Other fungi can cause localized or disseminated infection, and are identified on specific cultures. These include *Candida*, *Aspergillus*, and *Cryptococcus*. *Candida* is the predominant post-transplant fungal infection. Aspergillus accounts for ~20%, although it is found in 55% of brain abscesses. Treat with liposomal amphotericin (AmBisome®) 1mg/kg IV od (can increase up to 3–5mg/kg od if limited response). Caspofungin 70mg IV on d1, followed by 50mg IV od, is second-line. Duration is guided by clinical response. Fluconazole can be given as prophylaxis to those at risk.

! **Medical disorders**

Several medical disorders become more prevalent in liver transplant patients. Many are due to, or exacerbated by, immunosuppressants.

Hypertension

New occurrence in 15% post-transplant. Systolic BP may increase by 40–50mmHg within the first 6mo following transplantation but typically settles thereafter. This is principally due to endothelin-1-mediated systemic vasoconstriction, with minimal activation of the renin-aldosterone-angiotensin system. This is exacerbated by calcineurin inhibitors and corticosteroids.

Hypertension may improve with salt reduction and dose reduction of immunosuppressants as clinical state allows, but many patients require antihypertensive therapy. Vasodilatation using calcium channel blockers is the optimum initial treatment strategy; dihydropyridines (amlodipine 5–10mg od) are preferred to non-dihydropyridines (verapamil and diltiazem) due to less potential for cytochrome P450 interaction. β-blockers (atenolol 25–50mg od) and thiazide diuretics (bendroflumethiazide 2.5–5mg od) are second-line agents. ACE inhibitors are less effective but may have additional benefits in patients with co-morbid diabetes mellitus, renal failure, or heart failure.

Renal failure

In a representative study, renal failure developed in 15% and 25% patients 3y and 10y post-transplant, respectively. Renal impairment is closely related to use of calcineurin inhibitors, although other causes include hypertension, diabetes mellitus, and HCV-associated glomerulonephropathy. Use of serum creatinine alone underestimates the extent of renal dysfunction compared to GFR.

In mild renal impairment, dose de-escalation of calcineurin inhibitors may be sufficient to normalize GFR. Ensure that plasma drug levels do not exceed therapeutic range. It may be necessary to initiate a second immunosuppressive agent to maintain immunological response; non-nephrotoxic regimens, including sirolimus or mycophenolate mofetil, may be preferential, although rates of graft rejection are higher. Hypertension should be rigorously controlled, and use of other nephrotoxic drugs minimized. Patients should be screened regularly for albuminuria and deterioration in GFR. Refer to nephrology services early if renal dysfunction is moderate or severe, or does not normalize rapidly.

Disturbed carbohydrate and lipid metabolism

Diabetes mellitus develops in 13–25% patients. Consequently, rates of obesity and coronary heart disease are increased post-transplant. Glucose levels are initially elevated due to steroids but, subsequently, calcineurin inhibitors suppress insulin synthesis and secretion, and increase peripheral insulin resistance (ciclosporin less than tacrolimus). Management is identical to non-transplant patients.

Hypercholesterolaemia is common in patients with disturbed bile secretion and those on long-term corticosteroids, ciclosporin, or sirolimus.

Advise dietary changes first, followed by HMG-CoA reductase inhibitors (statins) if response inadequate.

Reduced bone mineral density

Osteopaenia and osteoporosis are very common in patients with advanced chronic liver disease, particularly those with cholestasis. Up to 40% of patients post-liver transplantation develop atraumatic fractures, particularly involving vertebrae and ribs. Provide calcium and vitamin D supplementation (check level), and initiate bisphosphonates (alendronic acid 70mg PO weekly, or by infusion 3-monthly or annually) in confirmed osteoporosis or osteopaenia with >2 associated fractures.

Neurological symptoms

A large proportion of patients on calcineurin inhibitors develop neuro-toxicity. Tremor is the most frequent side effect; others include headache, paraesthesia, and insomnia. These usually resolve with dose reduction ± standard medications for symptom control. An acute demyelinating leukencephalopathy can develop early post-transplant, presenting with disturbed consciousness, behavioural abnormalities, or coma. Whilst MRI may be helpful, diagnosis and management are largely empirical, based on high index of suspicion and early withdrawal of the calcineurin inhibitor and substitution with a calcineurin inhibitor-free regime until symptoms resolve. At this point, it is usually possible to re-introduce an alternative calcineurin inhibitor.

① Secondary malignancy

Malignancy arises de novo in 5–15% of patients after solid organ transplantation. Risk is proportional to duration and intensity of immunosuppression. Kaposi sarcomas occur earliest (but are least common), followed by lymphoproliferative disease/lymphoma. Squamous cell carcinomas usually manifest after 1y. Other malignancies are increased, e.g. GI and oropharyngeal. Patients should receive intermittent screening (e.g. skin exam, mammogram, Pap smear, PSA, colonoscopy).

- Kaposi sarcoma. HHV-8-associated neoplasm arising from endothelial cells. Typically presents with multifocal cutaneous and visceral lesions, which macroscopically appear as purple/red-brown papules or plaques. Reduction in immunosuppression, or switch to sirolimus, can induce regression. If unsuccessful, subsequent treatment often involves a combination of surgical excision, chemotherapy, and radiotherapy.
- Post-transplant lymphoproliferative disease (PTLD). EBV-driven proliferation of B lymphocytes, with a spectrum of presentations from polyclonal hyperplasias to aggressive non-Hodgkin's lymphomas. Longitudinal monitoring of EBV DNA load is highly sensitive for predicting emergence of PTLD and should prompt a search for developing tumours, although specificity is only ~50%. Withdrawal or reduction of immunosuppression in patients with pre-malignant disease may be effective, as are anti-viral therapies using interferon-α, IV immunoglobulin, or aciclovir. Response should be seen within

2–4wk. Elevated LDH, organ dysfunction, multiorgan involvement, and monoclonal disease predict failure of this approach. Localized disease has been successfully treated with surgery or radiotherapy, but disseminated malignancy requires chemotherapy ± B cell depletion with anti-CD20 monoclonal antibodies (rituximab).

- Squamous cell carcinoma (SCC). Can affect multiple organs in the post-transplant setting, with skin the most frequent. Peri-anal and vulval SCCs are also common. Oropharyngeal carcinomas are more prevalent in patients transplanted for alcoholic cirrhosis. Reduction in immunosuppressive therapy may delay progression of pre-malignant lesions. Treatment is principally surgical, although topical therapies are available for cutaneous SCCs. HPV immunization preventative.

Immunosuppressant medications

Most patients receive three immunosuppressants in the immediate post-transplant period, usually a calcineurin inhibitor (ciclosporin or tacrolimus), with either mycophenolate mofetil or, less commonly, azathioprine, together with a glucocorticoid such as prednisolone. Usually, only a calcineurin inhibitor is needed beyond 6mo.

- Ciclosporin. Calcineurin inhibitor that disrupts IL-2 signalling, reversibly blocking the lymphocyte cell cycle in the G_0/G_1 phases of cell division. Helper T cells are the primary targets. Dosing is individualized, as absorption and elimination vary, and based on plasma drug levels and renal function. Target levels have been derived by various centres, based principally on clinical experience. Generally, 2h post-dose levels are felt to reflect levels of immunosuppression better than trough values. Micro-emulsified formulations (e.g. Neoral®) provide more consistent blood levels. Side effects: acute nephrotoxicity (40–70%, usually reversible with dose reduction), chronic nephrotoxicity (often irreversible and may necessitate renal replacement therapy), hyperkalaemia, hypertension, venous thrombosis, tremor, headache, paraesthesia, gout, gingival hyperplasia.
- Tacrolimus (FK506). Macrolide antibiotic that also inhibits calcineurin; dosing based on plasma levels. Side effects: nephrotoxicity (similar to ciclosporin). Hypertension and hyperlipidaemia less common than with ciclosporin, but higher rates of diabetes mellitus and neurotoxicity. Graft and patient survival comparable to ciclosporin, but steroid requirements lower.
- Sirolimus. Structurally related to tacrolimus and disrupts IL-2 signalling but does not inhibit calcineurin. Dosing potentially more complex; serum levels require 3–5d to equilibrate and are often only measured by specialist laboratories. Used in place of calcineurin inhibitors if renal toxicity. Side effects: myelosuppression, hyperlipidaemia, peripheral oedema, delayed wound healing. Sirolimus does not appear to cause significant nephrotoxicity.
- Azathioprine. Thiopurine precursor of 6-mercaptopurine. Inhibits DNA synthesis, suppressing cell-mediated immunity and antibody production. Dosing and risk of toxicity guided by TPMT activity

(see Chapter 7). *Side effects*: myelosuppression, nausea and vomiting, pancreatitis, hepatotoxicity.

- Mycophenolate mofetil (MMF). Antibiotic that selectively inhibits purine synthesis, potently suppressing B and T lymphocyte proliferation. *Side effects*: neutropaenia (although causes less bone marrow suppression than azathioprine), GI symptoms.
- Corticosteroids. Pleiotropic immunosuppressive actions. Used long-term if immune-mediated disease caused transplant (e.g. PBC, PSC). Try to avoid in HCV infection. *Side effects*: hypertension, diabetes mellitus, dyslipidaemia, cataracts, weight gain, infection, depression/mania, osteoporosis, pancreatitis, proximal myopathy, avascular necrosis.

① Disease recurrence and long-term prognosis

- Pre-existing conditions other than congenital anomalies and metabolic diseases recur post-transplant.
- Hepatitis B. Graft re-infection may be limited/prevented using a combination of hepatitis B immunoglobulin (HBIg) at and following the transplant, and anti-viral therapy (lamivudine, tenofovir, adefovir, or entecavir).
- Hepatitis C. Re-infection of graft is universal and may cause accelerated cirrhosis and graft loss. Up to 45% develop cirrhosis within 10y. Of these, clinical decompensation then occurs in 40% within 1y and 60% within 3y, with overall survival rate <10% at 3y. This may occur more rapidly with more potent immunosuppressants such as tacrolimus and mycophenolate mofetil. Improved control may be achieved with a combination of pegylated interferon-α, ribavirin, and ciclosporin, but optimal treatment regimens for HCV have yet to be defined in the post-transplant setting. Interval liver biopsies allow rapid fibrosers to be identified early, which may guide initiation or adjustment of anti-viral therapy and immunosuppression, potentially leading to improved outcomes.
- Alcoholic liver disease. Up to 30% of patients return to drinking post-transplantation.
- Autoimmune hepatitis, PBC, and PSC recurrences post-transplantation are well described, although absolute risks difficult to estimate at present.

Overall mortality varies according to aetiology of the underlying liver disease. Causes of death >1y following transplantation are:

- End-stage liver failure (28%). Hepatitis C, need for re-transplantation, and post-transplantation diabetes mellitus/hypertension increase risk.
- Malignancy (22%).
- Cardiovascular disease (11%).
- Renal failure (6%).

Liver transplant patients

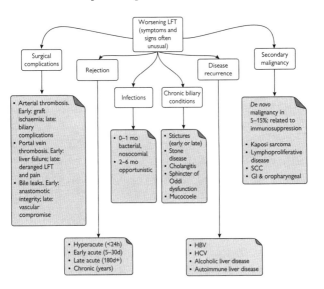

Worsening LFT (symptoms and signs often unusual)

Surgical complications

Rejection

Infections

Chronic biliary conditions

Disease recurrence

Secondary malignancy

- Arterial thrombosis. Early: graft ischaemia; late: biliary complications
- Portal vein thrombosis. Early: liver failure; late: deranged LFT and pain
- Bile leaks. Early: anastomotic integrity; late: vascular compromise

- 0–1 mo bacterial, nosocomial
- 2–6 mo opportunistic

- Stictures (early or late)
- Stone disease
- Cholangitis
- Sphincter of Oddi dysfunction
- Mucocoele

De novo malignancy in 5–15%; related to immunosuppression

- Kaposi sarcoma
- Lymphoproliferative disease
- SCC
- GI & oropharyngeal

- Hyperacute (<24h)
- Early acute (5–30d)
- Late acute (180d+)
- Chronic (years)

- HBV
- HCV
- Alcoholic liver disease
- Autoimmune liver disease

Appendix

Preparation for endoscopic procedures

Prior to performing endoscopy, patients should be made aware of possible complications. Diagnostic procedures (including biopsy) are low-risk, whereas those that involve cutting, cauterizing, dilating, or injecting tissues are deemed high-risk.

Management of antiplatelet and anticoagulant therapy

The risk of bleeding from the procedure needs to be balanced against the risks of stopping anti-thrombosis therapy. Conditions conferring higher risk of thrombosis are shown in Box A1.1.

> **Box A1.1 Conditions associated with high risk of thrombosis**
> - AF with:
>   - Valvular heart disease/mechanical valve.
>   - CCF or left ventricular ejection fraction <35%.
>   - Previous thromboembolic event.
>   - Hypertension, diabetes, or age >75y.
> - Mitral mechanical valve.
> - Mechanical aortic valve with previous thromboembolic event.
> - Coronary stenting within 1y (especially drug-eluting stents).
> - Acute coronary syndrome.
> - Non-stented percutaneous coronary intervention after MI.

Low-risk procedures

Antiplatelet drugs and anticoagulation can continue (although adjusted if supratherapeutic).

High-risk procedures

Antiplatelet drugs

If a high-risk procedure may be required (e.g. polypectomy, ERCP), stop NSAIDs and consider stopping antiplatelets (clopidogrel and dipyridamole) 7d beforehand, but continue aspirin. Be aware that coronary stent thrombosis carries ~50% mortality and, most frequently, occurs during the first year following placement if antiplatelet agents are stopped. The risk is higher with drug-eluting than bare metal stents. Delay elective procedures where possible. Discuss all patients at high risk of thrombosis with a cardiologist.

Anticoagulants

In patients at low risk of thrombosis, stop warfarin 5d, and dabigatran/rivaroxaban 1–2d (3–4d with GFR <50mL/min) beforehand. Ensure INR <1.4 on the morning of the procedure for those on warfarin, and a normal thrombin time in those on direct thrombin (e.g. dabigatran) or factor Xa (e.g. rivaroxaban) inhibitors. Therapies can be restarted the evening following the procedure.

In patients at high risk of thrombosis, consider 'bridge' therapy once INR <2, with either unfractionated heparin (stop 4h before procedure, and provisionally restart 4h after procedure and continue until INR >2) or LMWH (e.g. enoxaparin 1mg/kg SC bd; stop 8–24h before the procedure, and restart 4h afterwards). In general, anti-thrombotic therapy should be delayed for 5d after sphincterotomy, and up to 14d following polypectomy.

Prophylactic antibiotics

Prophylactic antibiotics are only recommended in patients with biliary sepsis, those undergoing percutaneous endoscopic gastrostomy/jejunostomy (PEG/PEJ), EUS-FNA of cystic lesions, treatment of varices, and patients with profound immunocompromise (e.g. severe neutropaenia) undergoing high-risk procedures (e.g. dilatation, laser therapy, sclerotherapy, or colonoscopy). Adhere to local policies when choosing antibiotic.

Sedation

Diagnostic upper GI endoscopy may be well tolerated with local anaesthetic throat spray (e.g. lidocaine 2%), but most procedures use conscious sedation (usually benzodiazepine ± opiate). Beware combining local anaesthesia with sedation, as risk of aspiration is increased.

- Use the lowest dose of sedation possible.
- An appropriate regimen is fentanyl 50–100µg and midazolam 1–5mg IV. In general, use the lowest possible dose.
- The following is required in any patient undergoing conscious sedation:
  - Supplemental oxygen (2–3L/min) via nasal cannulae.
  - Pulse oximetry.
  - IV access throughout procedure.
  - Cardiac monitoring.
- Sedation causes breathing problems in ~1/200 cases, although these are usually mild.
- If required, benzodiazepines can be reversed with flumazenil 250–500µg IV, and opiates with naloxone 400µg IM/IV.

Complications of endoscopy

This section provides a summary overview. Complications are also covered in relevant chapters throughout the book.

Gastroscopy

There is a very small risk of haemorrhage or perforation. Other rare complications include aspiration pneumonia and a slight risk to teeth or dental bridgework.

The risk of PEG can be quoted as 1/150 mortality, 1/30 serious morbidity, and 1/8 low-risk morbidity. All patients for PEG tubes should be reviewed by a gastroenterologist to determine the appropriateness of the request, ensure pre-procedural safety checks have been undertaken (abdominal examination, FBC, coagulation profile, and G & S), and ensure that informed consent has been obtained. In all cases, it is advisable to involve the relatives of the patient in these discussions.

Flexible sigmoidoscopy

There is a very small risk (1/15,000) of haemorrhage or perforation.

Colonoscopy

Overall, the risk of a perforation is ~1/800 and bleeding ~1/1,500. Surgery is usually required if this occurs. If polypectomy is performed, the risk of a perforation is ~1/600, but risk of bleeding is ~1/50–100, although this usually does not require blood transfusion.

ERCP

There is a 5% risk of pancreatitis. Haemorrhage, cholangitis, and perforation occur in ~1/500, but are up to 10-fold more common if sphincterotomy is performed. The procedure has a 1/500 mortality rate. Other complications are as for gastroscopy.

Capsule endoscopy

There is ~1/150 risk of capsule retention, which may result in surgery (although, in the majority, this turns out to be necessary due to underlying pathology). Therefore, 'unnecessary' surgery is only required in ~1/750 cases. This risk is largely abrogated by prior use of a patency capsule in any case where capsule retention is thought to be more likely (e.g. Crohn's disease).

☠ Management of major haemorrhage

Most hospitals have now established protocols in the event of a major haemorrhage. This is defined as blood loss >50% estimated blood volume (70mL/kg) in 3h, >100% within 24h, or >150mL/min.

Basic resuscitation

If suspected, initiate basic resuscitation:
- Airway. If airway is at risk, fast bleep anaesthetist. Consider use of adjuncts (e.g. nasopharyngeal tube). Give high-flow oxygen via face mask with a reservoir bag (unless contraindicated).
- Breathing. If ventilatory support required, put out a crash call and initiate bag-valve-mask ventilation.
- Circulation. Establish IV access (ideally, two large-bore cannulae in the antecubital fossae but, if this proves challenging, any access that can be achieved will do to initiate resuscitation). Start fluid resuscitation.

Who is contacted?

Call switchboard, and ask to activate the 'major haemorrhage protocol'. State where the patient is and which specialist team is required (i.e. medical or surgical). The following are automatically contacted:
- Haematology basic medical scientist, who should then call back to ask how quickly blood is required. Options are:
  - Immediate (≈2U of O-negative).
  - 10min from receipt of sample (≈group-compatible blood).
  - 30min from receipt of sample (≈fully cross-matched blood).
- ITU registrar.
- Haematology registrar.
- Porter.

What blood products will be available?

The following are automatically authorized on activation of a major haemorrhage protocol:
- 6U of packed red cells.
- 2 packs of FFP.
- 1 pool of platelets.

What tests need to be sent?

- Cross-match.
- FBC.
- Coagulation screen.
- Fibrinogen (if low, indicates need for cryoprecipitate).

These may need to be re-checked, until the patient is stable. Aim for platelets >50 × 10^9/L, INR <1.5, and fibrinogen >1g/L.

Estimating blood losses

	Class I	Class II	Class III	Class IV
Blood loss				
Percentage (%)	<15	15–30	30–40	>40
Volume (mL)	<750	750–1,500	1,500–2000	>2000
Vital signs				
HR (bpm)	<100	100–120	120–140	>140
BP	Normal	Normal	↓	↓
Pulse pressure	Normal/↑	↓	↓	↓
RR (min⁻¹)	14–20	20–30	30–40	>40
Urine output (mL/h)	>30	20–30	5–15	<5
Mental state	Anxious	Anxious	Confused	Confused/ unconscious
Fluid replacement	Crystalloid	Crystalloid	Crystalloid + blood	Crystalloid + blood

Adapted from Advanced Trauma and Life Support Guidelines, 2004 (see ⓡ http://www.resus. org.uk/pages/guide.htm).

Complications of blood transfusion

Assess for the following if transfuse ≥4U:

- Depletion of clotting factors and platelets. If ongoing bleeding:
  - If platelet count <50 × 10^9/L, give 1–2 pools of platelets.
  - If INR >1.4, give 10–15mL/kg FFP + 10mg vitamin K IV.
  - If fibrinogen <1g/L, give 4–8U cryoprecipitate.
- Hypothermia. If core temperature <36°C, use blood warmers and warmed fluids.
- Acidosis. Ensure adequate correction of hypovolaemia.
- Hyperkalaemia:
  - Perform ECG to look for tall tented T waves, small P waves, and broadening of the QRS complex. Give 10mL of 10% calcium gluconate if present.
  - Correct with 10U soluble insulin and 100mL of 20% glucose.
- Hypocalcaemia. Give 10mL of 10% calcium gluconate for every 4U transfused.
- DIC. Can be caused by massive blood transfusion. Call haematologist for advice.

Useful UK contacts

Liver transplant units

- Addenbrooke's Hospital (Cambridge)   01223 245 151
- Edinburgh Royal Infirmary (Edinburgh)   0131 536 1000
- Freeman Hospital (Newcastle-upon-Tyne)   0191 233 6161
- King's College Hospital (London)   0203 299 9000
- Queen Elizabeth Hospital (Birmingham)   0121 472 1311
- Royal Free Hospital (London)   0207 794 0500
- St. James's University Hospital (Leeds)   0113 243 3144

Toxicology

- National Poisons Information Service   0844 892 0111

Tropical diseases

- Hospital for Tropical Diseases (London)   0203 456 7891
- Liverpool   0151 706 2000
- Glasgow   0141 211 1000

Patient support groups

- British Liver Trust: see ✍ www.britishlivertrust.org.uk
- Cancer Research UK: see ✍ www.cancerresearchuk.org
- Coeliac UK: see ✍ www.coeliac.org.uk
- Crohn's and Colitis UK: see ✍ www.nacc.org.uk
- PBC Foundation: see ✍ www.pbcfoundation.org.uk
- UK Transplant: see ✍ www.uktransplant.org.uk

Normal laboratory ranges

Haematology

- Hb   Male: 13–18g/dL; female: 11.5–16g/dL
- MCV   78–87fL
- Haematocrit   0.36–0.46
- WCC $4–11 \times 10^9$/L
- Neutrophils $2–7.5 \times 10^9$/L
- Lymphocytes $1.5–4 \times 10^9$/L
- Eosinophils $0.04–0.4 \times 10^9$/L
- Platelets $150–400 \times 10^9$/L
- ESR   1–12mm/h
- IgG   5.3–16.5g/L
- IgA   0.8–4.0g/L
- IgM   0.5–2.0g/L

Biochemistry

- Urea   2–7.5mmol/L
- Creatinine   50–120μmol/L
- Sodium   135–145mmol/L
- Potassium   3.5–5mmol/L
- Calcium   2.15–2.6mmol/L
- Phosphate   0.8–1.48mmol/L
- Magnesium   0.7–1.0mmol/L
- Glucose   3.6–7mmol/L
- Bicarbonate   22–28mmol/L
- CRP   0–10mg/L
- Amylase   20–80U/L
- Cholesterol   3.3–5.5mmol/L
- Triglycerides   0.8–2.0mmol/L
- Total protein   60–80g/L
- LDH   70–250IU/L

Liver function tests

- Bilirubin   3–17μmol/L
- ALT   5–50IU/L
- AST   5–45IU/L
- ALP   40–165IU/L
- γGT   10–60IU/L
- Albumin   35–50g/L
- PTT/APTT   Laboratory-specific
- INR   0.8–1.2
- α-FP   1–10ng/mL
- Ammonia   10–80μg/dL

Haematinics

- Ferritin   11–307ng/mL
- Serum iron   10–32μmol/L
- Transferrin saturation   Male: 15–50%; female: 12–45%
- Total iron-binding capacity   45–72μmol/L
- Red cell folate   100–600μg/L
- Vitamin B12   150–700ng/L

Index